The End of World Population Growth in the 21st Century

The International Institute for Applied Systems Analysis

is an interdisciplinary, nongovernmental research institution founded in 1972 by leading scientific organizations in 12 countries. Situated near Vienna, in the center of Europe, IIASA has been producing valuable scientific research on economic, technological, and environmental issues for nearly three decades.

IIASA was one of the first international institutes to systematically study global issues of environment, technology, and development. IIASA's Governing Council states that the Institute's goal is: *to conduct international and interdisciplinary scientific studies to provide timely and relevant information and options, addressing critical issues of global environmental, economic, and social change, for the benefit of the public, the scientific community, and national and international institutions.* Research is organized around three central themes:

- Energy and Technology;
- Environment and Natural Resources;
- Population and Society.

The Institute now has National Member Organizations in the following countries:

Austria
The Austrian Academy of Sciences

China
National Natural Science
Foundation of China

Czech Republic
The Academy of Sciences of the
Czech Republic

Egypt
Academy of Scientific Research and
Technology (ASRT)

Estonia
Estonian Association for
Systems Analysis

Finland
The Finnish Committee for IIASA

Germany
The Association for the Advancement
of IIASA

Hungary
The Hungarian Committee for Applied
Systems Analysis

Japan
The Japan Committee for IIASA

Netherlands
The Netherlands Organization for
Scientific Research (NWO)

Norway
The Research Council of Norway

Poland
The Polish Academy of Sciences

Russian Federation
The Russian Academy of Sciences

Sweden
The Swedish Research Council for
Environment, Agricultural Sciences
and Spatial Planning (FORMAS)

Ukraine
The Ukrainian Academy of Sciences

United States of America
The National Academy of
Sciences

Population and Sustainable Development Series

The End of World Population Growth in the 21st Century

New Challenges for Human Capital Formation and Sustainable Development

Edited by

Wolfgang Lutz, Warren C. Sanderson, and Sergei Scherbov

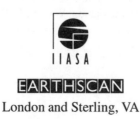

IIASA

EARTHSCAN
London and Sterling, VA

First published by Earthscan in the UK and USA in 2004

Copyright © International Institute for Applied Systems Analysis, 2004

ISBN: 1-84407-099-9 paperback
      1-84407-089-1 hardback

Printed and bound in the UK by Creative Print and Design Wales
Cover design by Yvonne Booth

For a full list of publications please contact:

Earthscan
8–12 Camden High Street
London, NW1 0JH, UK
Tel: +44 (0)20 7387 8558
Fax: +44 (0)20 7387 8998
Email: earthinfo@earthscan.co.uk
Web: **www.earthscan.co.uk**

22883 Quicksilver Drive, Sterling, VA 20166-2012, USA

Earthscan publishes in association with WWF-UK and the International Institute for
Environment and Development

A catalogue record for this book is available from the British Library

Library of Congress Cataloging-in-Publication Data

The end of world population growth in the 21st century: new challenges for human
capital formation and sustainable development / edited by Wolfgang Lutz, Warren C.
Sanderson, and Sergei Scherbov.
    p. cm.
  Includes bibliographical references and index.
  ISBN 1-84407-099-9 (pbk.) – ISBN 1-84407-089-1 (hardback)
    1. Population forecasting. 2. Twenty-first century–Forecasts. 3. Demographic
transition. I. Lutz, Wolfgang. II. Sanderson, Warren, C. III. Scherbov, Sergei.

HB849.53.E53 2004
304.6'2'0112–dc22

2003025468

Contents

List of Acronyms

ADLI	agricultural development led industrialization
AIDS	acquired immune deficiency syndrome; the last and most severe stage of the clinical spectrum of HIV-related diseases
ANDI	Africa Nutrition Database Initiative
ASF	Atmospheric Stabilization Framework
CBR	crude birth rate
CDR	crude death rate
CFCs	chlorofluorocarbons
CSA	Central Statistical Authority, Addis Ababa, Ethiopia
DHS	Demographic and Health Survey
ENSO	El Niño–Southern Oscillation
EU	European Union
FAO	Food and Agriculture Organization of the United Nations
FAOSTAT	FAO Statistical Databases
FFS	Fertility and Family Surveys
FSU Europe	European part of the former Soviet Union
GCMs	general circulation models
GDP	gross domestic product
GED	Global Education Database
GHG	greenhouse gas
GNP	gross national product
GWP	global warming potential
HCFCs	hydrochlorofluorocarbons
HDI	Human Development Index
HFCs	hydrofluorocarbons
HIV	human immunodeficiency virus; a retrovirus that damages the human immune system, thus permitting opportunistic infections to cause eventually fatal diseases. The causal agent for AIDS
ICPD	International Conference on Population and Development held in Cairo in 1994

IIASA	International Institute for Applied Systems Analysis, Laxenburg, Austria
ILO	International Labour Organization
I=PAT	Describes the environmental impact (I) of human activities as the product of three factors: population size (P), affluence (A), and technology (T)
IPCC	Intergovernmental Panel on Climate Change
ISCED	international standard classification of education
IUSSP	International Union for the Scientific Study of Population
LDCs	less developed countries
LDRs	less developed regions
LLE	literate life expectancy
MDCs	more developed countries
MDRs	more developed regions
NAS	(US) National Academy of Sciences
NGO	nongovernmental organization
NRC	(US) National Research Council
OECD	Organisation for Economic Co-operation and Development
PDE	population–development–environment
PEDA	population–environment–development–agriculture
PFCs	perfluorocarbons
RIDR	relative interdecile range
SDD	Sustainable Development Division of UNECA
SRES	Special Report on Emissions Scenarios
TFR	total fertility rate
UN	United Nations
UNAIDS	Joint United Nations Programme on HIV/AIDS
UNDP	United Nations Development Programme
UNECA	United Nations Economic Commission for Africa
UNESCO	United Nations Educational, Scientific and Cultural Organization
UNU	United Nations University
WFP	World Food Programme

Chapter 1

Introduction

Wolfgang Lutz and Warren C. Sanderson

While the 20th century was the century of population growth—with the world's population increasing from 1.6 to 6.1 billion—the 21st century is likely to see the end of world population growth and become the century of population aging. At the moment, we are at the crossroads of these two different demographic regimes, with some countries still experiencing high rates of population growth and others already facing rapid population aging. Demographic changes will make the 21st century like no other. Forecasting these changes, understanding their consequences, and formulating appropriate policies will, indeed, be challenging. This book is a step toward meeting those challenges.

Rapid population growth in the 20th century, and especially the acceleration in the growth rate after World War II, gave rise to notions such as the "population explosion" and associated fears of hunger, socio-economic collapse, and ecological catastrophe. More recently, the prospect of the substantial aging of populations has led to fears that public pension plans will fail and that those countries most affected (mainly in Europe, along with Japan) will enter an era of economic, social, political, and cultural stagnation.

This book deals with the anticipated population trends of the 21st century in a comprehensive manner. It highlights the population dimension that matters most in the context of sustainable development, namely, human capital, which is usually approximated here by level of education. It also attempts to combine methodological innovations (in probabilistic forecasting, multistate projections, and dynamic

1

modeling) with a focus on the most relevant population-related challenges of the century ahead.

New forecasts of world and regional populations are presented here and are combined with an outlook for future human capital in different parts of the world. The picture is complemented by a series of more specific chapters that deal with the key elements of population change in the context of sustainable development, which include studies on the

- interactions between population growth, education, and food security in Ethiopia;
- interactions between HIV prevalence and education in Botswana;
- interactions between urbanization and education in China's population outlook; and
- the impact of population trends on greenhouse-gas emissions and climate change.

All of these studies were produced in and around the Population Project of the International Institute for Applied Systems Analysis (IIASA) over the past few years. They were driven by the common agenda of deepening our understanding of the role of population in sustainable development in a model-based and quantitative manner and applying what we learn to forecasting.

The different chapters of this volume are fully consistent with one another, both in terms of serving this goal and in terms of the specific assumptions made in the forecasts presented in the individual chapters. They also provide the basis for a new approach to thinking about population trends. The new concept of population balance, which is discussed in the concluding chapter (Chapter 10), provides a common framework within which to address the challenges associated with both rapid population growth and rapid population aging. These two demographic regimes, at whose intersection we now stand, seem to be very different from one another, but our new analysis shows them to be two sides of the same coin. We do not have two separate phenomena to study—population growth and population aging—but rather a single one, namely, age-structure imbalance that results from specific forms of demographic transition.

The acceleration and subsequent deceleration of population growth, which are a consequence of the universal and ongoing process of demographic transition (which we discuss below), have not occurred simultaneously in all parts of the world. Europe and Japan have been experiencing fertility levels well below the replacement level (an average of around 2.1 births per woman) for two to three decades, while in most of Africa and some parts of Asia more than half the population is under 20 years of age and family size is still above four children per woman.

Hence, today we see a demographically divided world in which those countries that are further developed not only have reached very low fertility and high life expectancy, but also have high human capital (education) and high levels of material well-being. The latest entrants into the process of demographic transition not only have lower life expectancy and higher fertility, but also are much more affected by poverty, malnutrition, and lack of education. Although we expect these countries to complete their transitions during the 21st century, low human capital, weak institutions, political instability, and high economic and environmental vulnerability pose significant limits to their prospects for social and economic development in the near term.

The expectation that almost all the countries in the world will complete their demographic transitions by the end of this century is central to the arguments made in this book. Before discussing why we believe this, it is worthwhile to consider different public perceptions about the demographic future. We do this in a rather simple manner by highlighting two of the most prominent, and also most extreme, positions in the public discourse.

1.1 Contrasting Perceptions of the Demographic Future: From "Population Explosion" to "Gray Dawn"

Population and especially the related issues of changing family forms, abortion, and migration are topics on which many people (scientists and nonscientists alike) have strong views. This may be because, unlike many other objects of scientific analysis, these topics directly touch upon the lives of almost everybody. Everyone has a family of origin of one form or another that is of the highest emotional importance. A large number of people either have or are considering having children. Similarly, most people are involved in the labor market and are concerned personally about the security of their pensions. However, even aggregate-level population considerations beyond personal experience and based on abstract reasoning about conditions in the rather distant future tend to excite people. Obviously, questions concerning changes in the size and structure of our own species, our nation, or our ethnic group interest us in a rather existential way. Even many people who do not subscribe to collective goals and who are interested only in the possible implications of population trends for their own welfare believe that, at least in the medium to long run, population trends do matter, be it in terms of population growth or population aging. Since we stand today at the crossroads of two demographic regimes, it is not surprising that people hold deeply felt, but divergent, views about our demographic future.

Since his 1968 book *The Population Bomb*, which was followed in 1990 by *The Population Explosion*, Paul Ehrlich has been one of the most vocal proponents of the group of scientists who warn of the disastrous consequences of rapid population growth and the resultant overpopulation. From his biological and ecological background, he has no doubts that "overpopulation is a major factor in problems as diverse as African famines, global warming, acid rain, the threat of nuclear war, the garbage crisis, and the danger of epidemics" (Ehrlich and Ehrlich 1990, p. 238). However, there still is some optimism, as "people can learn to treat growth as the cancer-like disease it is and move toward a sustainable society" (Ehrlich and Ehrlich 1990, p. 23). For them, "there is no question that the population explosion will end soon. What remains in doubt is whether the end will come humanely because birth rates have been lowered, or tragically through rises in death rates" (Ehrlich and Ehrlich 1990, p. 238). "Action to end the population explosion *humanely* and start a gradual population *decline* must become a top item on the human agenda" (Ehrlich and Ehrlich 1990, p. 23).

The latest population forecasts presented in this book show that it is likely that world population growth will come to an end during the 21st century and that this "will come humanely because birth rates have been lowered" (Ehrlich and Ehrlich 1990, p. 238). Still, the world's population is expected to grow by at least two billion before leveling off and possibly beginning to decrease. The end of world population growth is now on the horizon because the past decades have seen significant fertility declines around the world, and these declines are unlikely to stop at the replacement level of around 2.1 children per woman. Armenia, Bahamas, Barbados, Costa Rica, Cuba, Kazakhstan, Mauritius, Seychelles, Sri Lanka, Thailand, Trinadad and Tobago, Tunisia, and Ukraine are among a considerably larger group of developing countries that now have below-replacement fertility (Population Reference Bureau 2003). Indeed, fertility in countries that together account for 45 percent of the total world population is already below the replacement level. Unfortunately, in some parts of the world—mostly in Africa—increasing death rates due to the acquired immune deficiency syndrome (AIDS) pandemic have contributed to this new outlook of lower future population growth. But this HIV/AIDS tragedy is not immediately related to overpopulation; actually, the countries hit worst are among the least overpopulated.

The population aging that results from low fertility combined with a general increase in life expectancy is not an issue in Ehrlich's analysis. This is in sharp contrast to another highly political book concerned with population trends. *Gray Dawn* by Peter Peterson starts out by saying, "The challenge of global aging, like a massive iceberg, looms ahead ... . Lurking beneath the waves, and not yet widely understood, are the wrenching economic and social costs that will accompany this demographic transformation—costs that threaten to bankrupt even the greatest of powers ... " (Peterson 1999, pp. 3–4). Referring to Ehrlich, Peterson—a well-known investment banker and former US Secretary of Commerce—describes the change in concern: "Thirty years ago, the future was crowded with babies. Today, it's crowded with elders" (Peterson 1999, p. 27). He claims that the social transformation associated with the expected massive aging is comparable to some of the great economic and social revolutions of the past. Population aging will constitute an "unprecedented economic burden" (Peterson 1999, p. 31) and make existing pension and health programs "unsustainable" (Peterson 1999, p. 66). Peterson also discusses the necessary policy responses, which range from later retirement to more and better education and raising more children. Although such policies can all be parts of a response, they cannot lead to a reversal of the aging trend in the foreseeable future, as is demonstrated clearly in the projections given below. Landis MacKellar, in a review of *Gray Dawn*, says that "aging is not a problem so much as it is a predicament. Problems have solutions, predicaments do not" (MacKellar 2000, p. 365).

When reading through these books, one wonders whether the authors are writing about the same world. They express serious population-related concerns, but the differences could hardly be greater. A critical reader might be tempted to conclude that, since both views cannot be right at the same time, both are gross exaggerations and, in reality, population may not matter much in either way. Unfortunately, the view that population growth and aging may cancel each other and thus there is no reason for concern is a simple-minded short circuit. Both aspects refer to genuine population-related concerns that operate at different levels, tend to affect different societies in different intensities at different times, and in some cases even simultaneously burden a country. China may be the most prominent example. Some consider it already "overpopulated," but around 200 million more people are expected through population momentum (see below), while at the same time the one-child family is already causing serious problems in terms of the support of the rapidly increasing number of elderly. Indeed, during the first part of the 21st century, a large number of countries will experience population growth and aging simultaneously.

The demographic divide between young and still-growing populations, on the one hand, and rapidly aging and even shrinking populations, on the other, means that we are living in a seemingly paradoxical situation, which tends to confuse commentators who do not know whether they should be in favor of lower or higher fertility. Such seemingly contradictory developments and concerns cannot be explained adequately by one or the other of the existing conventional analytical frameworks used to study population. What is required is a new, broader, multidimensional population paradigm. In Chapter 10 of this book, we offer such a paradigm, which we call "population balance." Unlike older concepts such as "population stabilization" that narrowly focus on population size, population balance simultaneously takes population size, age structure, and the educational composition of the population into account.

1.2   The Continuing Demographic Transition

How can we understand such a demographically diverse world, and how can we make meaningful assumptions for the future? How can we find the right policies to respond to trends that pose different challenges in different parts of the world? Since the answers to these questions always refer to the secular process of demographic transition, which was the reason for the "population explosion" in the 20th century and is the basis for our expectation of an end to the growth in world population in the 21st century, we start this volume with a short description of the nature of this demographic transition process.

The *demographic transition* began in today's more developed countries (MDCs) in the late 18th and 19th centuries and spread to today's less developed countries (LDCs) in the last half of the 20th century (Notestein 1945; Davis 1954, 1991; Coale 1973). The conventional theory of demographic transition predicts that as living standards rise and health conditions improve, mortality rates decline and then, somewhat later, fertility rates decline. Demographic transition theory has evolved as a generalization of the typical sequence of events in what are now MDCs, in which mortality rates declined comparatively gradually from the late 1700s and more rapidly in the late 1800s, and in which, after a varying lag of up to 100 years, fertility rates declined as well. Different societies experienced the transition in different ways, and today various regions of the world are following distinctive paths (Tabah 1989). Nonetheless, the broad result was, and is, a gradual transition from a smaller, slowly growing population with high mortality and high fertility rates to a larger, slowly growing or even slowly shrinking population with low mortality and low fertility rates. During the transition itself, population growth accelerates because the decline in death rates precedes the decline in birth rates.

A number of theories of the causal structure of the demographic transition have appeared in the literature. An excellent review of these is given in Kirk (1996). Kirk examined economic theories of the transition, the anthropological theories of Caldwell, cultural and ideational theories, historical views, the role of the government, and the role of diffusion. He concluded, "No unique cause exists. Perhaps all aspects of modernization may be described as related to the demographic transition, which in itself is an essential part of modernization" (Kirk 1996, p. 380).

In the same article, Kirk (1996, pp. 381–383) provides eight summary propositions about the state of the demographic transition today:

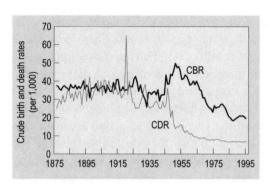

Figure 1.1. Crude birth rate (CBR) and crude death rate (CDR) in Mauritius since 1875. *Source:* Mauritius Central Statistical Office.

- "given a modicum of domestic and international peace, mortality has fallen in every country and has been part of socioeconomic progress";
- "the fertility transition has reached every major region";
- "once a country has started firmly on the path of fertility decline, it has been successful in reducing it to low levels";
- "fertility decline in the less developed countries (excluding China) did not really slow up during the 1980s";
- "the timing of decline in countries with non-European traditions conformed to the forecasts by the original authors of transition theory";
- "in Europe fertility has declined to well below-replacement level, and in a few areas the population has actually declined";
- "except for a few outliers, like Iceland, Ireland and Albania, fertility has been below replacement in *all* European countries"; and
- "the transition is now beginning at increasingly lower levels of development."

Figure 1.1 illustrates the demographic transition in Mauritius, a developing country that has good records for birth and death rates that go back more than a century. Until around World War II, the birth and death rates show a pattern of strong annual fluctuations, caused mostly by diseases and changing weather conditions, typical of "pre-transition" societies. Whenever birth rates are consistently above death rates, the population grows, as was the case in Mauritius during the late 19th century. After World War II, death rates in Mauritius declined precipitously because of malaria eradication and the introduction of European medical technology. Birth rates, however, remained high or even increased, partly through the better health status of women (a typical phenomenon in the early phase of demographic transition). By 1950, this had resulted in a population growth rate of more than 3 percent per year, one of the highest at that time. Later, birth rates declined, with the bulk of the transition occurring during the late 1960s and early 1970s, when the total fertility rate (TFR) declined from above six to below three children per woman within only seven years, one of the world's most rapid national fertility declines. This happened on a strictly voluntary basis, the result of a high female educational status together with successful family planning programs (Lutz 1994). As a result of the very young age structure of the Mauritian population, current birth rates are still higher than death rates and the population is growing by about 1 percent per year despite fertility below replacement level. Such growth induced by age structure is called population momentum.

Empirically observed trends in all parts of the world overwhelmingly confirm the relevance as well as the predictive power of the concept of demographic transition for LDCs (Tabah 1989; Cleland 1996; Westoff 1996; United Nations 2001). With the exception of pockets in which religious or cultural beliefs are strongly pro-natalist, fertility decline is well advanced in all regions except sub-Saharan Africa, and even in that region many signs of a fertility transition can be observed. In Southeast Asia and many countries in Latin America, fertility rates are on par with those seen in MDCs only several decades ago, and in an increasing number of developing countries and in territories such as the Commonwealth of Puerto Rico, fertility is at subreplacement levels.

An important difference between the demographic transition process in today's MDCs and LDCs has been the speed of mortality decline. Mortality decline in Europe, North America, and Japan came about over the course of two centuries as a result of reduced variability in the food supply, better housing, improved sanitation, and, finally, progress in preventive and curative medicine. Mortality decline in LDCs, by contrast, occurred very quickly after World War II as a result of the application of Western medical and public health technology to infectious, parasitic, and diarrheal diseases. Life expectancy in Europe rose gradually from about 35 years in 1800 to about 50 in 1900, 66.5 at the end of World War II, and 74.4 in 1995. In LDCs, it shot up from 40.9 years at the end of World War II to 63 in 2000. The increase that took MDCs about 150 years to achieve came to pass in LDCs in less than 50 years. As a result of the speed of this mortality decline, together with higher pre-transition fertility, typically through nearly universal marriage at a young age, populations in LDCs are growing three times faster today than did the populations of today's MDCs at the comparable stage of their own demographic transition.

The consistency of the demographic transition framework with the regularities in observed patterns of fertility and mortality change is the basis for our expectation that fertility will decline in countries or even subregions of a country that have already seen a mortality decline but still show high levels of childbearing. Despite this important predictive power, the demographic transition model is imprecise in three important aspects that result in significant uncertainties about the future population trends. First, it does not tell us exactly the time lag with which the fertility decline follows the mortality decline. Second, it does not specify how steep the decline will be once it has started. There is considerable diversity in the historical record on both counts. The third important uncertainty is about the level of fertility at the end of the demographic transition, whether it will be near the replacement level of around two surviving children per woman, or whether it will stay below that level for extended periods.

While the well-founded, general notion of demographic transition is the basis for our expectation that world population growth will come to an end during the second half of the 21st century, the uncertainty about the speed of fertility decline translates into uncertainty about the evolution of world population size. Depending on whether we expect long-term, post-transition fertility to be around replacement level or below it, we will see stabilization of population size or a global population decline after a peak. As discussed in the following chapter, we consider the second to be more likely.

There are, of course, further demographic uncertainties associated with future mortality and migration trends that influence the population outlook. For example, the question of whether we are already close to the limit of the human life span in the lowest-mortality countries, or whether at some point we will be able to have average life expectancies well over 100 years, is still the subject of scientific debate. Another newly emerged uncertainty is how the AIDS pandemic will evolve in different parts of the world.

1.3 Antecedents

This book combines scientific analyses using the latest tools and methods of population forecasting with a comprehensive conceptual framework that includes the natural environment, human capital, and human well-being. In a way, it is an ambitious attempt to define, empirically describe, and quantitatively project the role of population factors in a way that links them more closely to the broader framework of sustainable development.

Substantively and methodologically, this volume builds on five other books published in recent years, four of which were IIASA books. It is a direct follow-up to *The Future Population of the World: What Can We Assume Today?* (Lutz 1996), which presented and justified the previous IIASA world population projections. The 1996 edition consisted of substantive background chapters by leading population scholars that summarized what is known about the past trends and determinants of fertility, mortality, and migration in different parts of the world, and what can be assumed meaningfully for the future, on the basis of scientific arguments. It presented the first probabilistic population projections for the world and its 13 major regions. Most of the analyses presented in that volume—even most of the specific projection assumptions defined, discussed, and justified there—are still valid and form the basis of the projections presented in this book. The main substantive difference between the 1996 projections and those presented here lies in the starting conditions, which now reflect the year 2000 rather than 1995. Only in a few instances did we find reasons for significant changes in the assumptions—most notably concerning the more serious impact of AIDS in Africa and the lower assumed future fertility for China. In this book, reference is often made to the extensive discussions published in Lutz (1996), and the full argumentation and justification of specific assumptions are not repeated.

Methodologically, the population projections given in this book are more advanced than the earlier ones in several important aspects. The way to these improvements was paved by a *Population and Development Review* special supplement entitled *Frontiers of Population Forecasting* (Lutz *et al.* 1999). The contributions in this supplement centered on three major new issues in population projections:

- How to deal with uncertainty.
- How to include explicitly sources of population heterogeneity other than age and sex.
- How to deal with environmental constraints and feedbacks.

Based on the discussions and recommendations in that volume, advances on these fronts have been incorporated into the new projections presented here. The probabilistic forecasts discussed in Chapters 2 and 3 are based on a more sophisticated methodology. The deterministic multistate forecasts in Chapter 4 present, among other things, the first ever global-level projection of the population by educational attainment. The forecasts in Chapters 5 through 8 explicitly consider sources of population heterogeneity, such as level of education, rural or urban place of residence, and HIV status.

A recent report by the Panel on Population Projections of the US National Academy of Sciences (NAS) entitled *Beyond Six Billion: Forecasting the World's Population* (National Research Council 2000) provides a highly useful summary of the state of the art and different arguments in favor of alternative assumptions, as well as a discussion of what the most likely trends are from today's perspective. The forecasts in this book are consistent with *Beyond Six Billion* in four important ways:

- The report states that "fertility in countries that have not completed transition should eventually reach levels similar to those now observed in low fertility countries" (National Research Council 2000, p. 106). This is consistent with the views of the authors in Lutz (1996). The forecasts herein utilize this assumption.
- The report states that forecasts should not assume that the evolution of mortality rates will be constrained in the future by a hypothetical limit to human life expectancy. We do not make such an assumption. Our mortality assumptions are consistent with the views expressed in Chapter 5 of *Beyond Six Billion*.
- The report talks about the importance of replacing the "probabilistically inconsistent" variants approach to expressing the uncertainty of forecasts with a procedure that is probabilistically consistent. This is one of the chief contributions of the new forecasts.
- The report suggests that the probabilistic forecasts make use of information about the range of errors in past population projections, exactly as is done here.

The NAS Panel did not produce its own projections. The projections presented here are the first to follow the NAS recommendations in all four of the aspects mentioned.

Two other recent IIASA books paved the way for comprehensively relating the anticipated future population trends to key aspects of the natural environment and sustainable development in a broader sense. *Population and Climate Change* (O'Neill *et al.* 2001) gives a systematic assessment of how population trends drive greenhouse-gas emissions and how, in turn, population health and migration may be affected by environmental change. It also translates the results of the 1996 IIASA projections into different possible emissions paths. A summary of the most important lessons learned from this analysis is included in Chapter 9. Most recently, another *Population and Development Review* special supplement, entitled *Population and Environment: Methods of Analysis* (Lutz *et al.* 2002a), discussed in detail new methods for studying the complex population–environment interactions. These methods are applied in the analyses presented in the chapters of this volume.

Finally, this volume has been inspired greatly by the work of the Global Science Panel on Population and Environment, an international group of distinguished experts that produced an assessment of our knowledge about the complex population–development–environment (PDE) interactions as background for the Johannesburg World Summit on Sustainable Development. This Global Science Panel was organized by IIASA together with the International Union for the Scientific Study of Population (IUSSP) and the United Nations University (UNU). It also published a policy statement entitled "Population in Sustainable Development" (Lutz and Shah 2002; Lutz *et al.* 2002b). Since the Panel was coordinated by IIASA at the same time as this book was finalized, there were important cross-fertilizations. The work of the Global Science Panel and the content of its concluding statement are discussed in the final chapter.

1.4   Structure of the Volume

Following this introduction, Chapters 2 and 3 present the results of the latest probabilistic world population projections made by IIASA for 13 world regions. Since the methods and assumptions that underlie these projections are discussed extensively in the above-mentioned books, these chapters focus only on the presentation and discussion of the most salient assumptions and results. More detailed supplementary information is posted on the IIASA Web site (www.iiasa.ac.at).

Chapter 2 focuses on future population size and is entitled "The End of World Population Growth." This was also the title of a recent contribution in *Nature* (Lutz *et al.* 2001) that first presented these new forecasts and received extensive media coverage around the globe. Chapter 2 starts with a discussion of why we need new world population forecasts and introduces the probabilistic framework to deal with uncertainty. It goes on to summarize the results of the thousands of simulations of alternative future population paths. This is first done for the aggregate world population and then for individual world regions. Special attention is given to the probability that the population size will reach a peak during the 21st century and to the changing regional population shares. The chapter concludes with a comparison of these new projections with other published world population forecasts.

Chapter 3, "Applications of Probabilistic Population Forecasting," presents three distinct aspects of these new forecasts. The first section discusses the changing age distribution under the heading "Massive Population Aging." It describes the uncertainty distributions for individual age groups as well as derived measures such as the old-age dependency ratios in different parts of the world. The second section deals with the concept of conditional probabilistic population forecasting. Since policy makers are not only interested in full uncertainty distributions, but also want to know what happens if, for example, fertility follows a specific low path, the 1996 IIASA volume (Lutz 1996) included traditional if-then scenarios, in addition to the probabilistic forecasts. The approach to conditional forecasting presented here can be used to answer such questions in a consistent probabilistic framework. The third section introduces an entirely new concept, probabilistic future jump-off date forecasting. It addresses the question, To what degree are population forecasts modified through the passage of time as new empirical information becomes available? Users know that past projections have been modified every few years, and they want to know what changes they can expect in the future. We show how a distribution of probabilistic paths can allow us to predict the forecast that we would make at future times, conditional on our observations between now and then.

Chapter 4 goes beyond the strictly demographic variables of age and sex. It describes the first global-level projections of the population by level of education, a summary of which was published recently in *Population and Development Review* (Lutz and Goujon 2001) under the title "The World's Changing Human Capital Stock." The regional fertility, mortality, and migration assumptions of these educational projections are consistent with those in the probabilistic population projections described in Chapters 2 and 3. Alternative scenarios of future trends in school enrollment show that the educational composition of the adult population changes only very slowly. This results from the great demographic momentum of educational changes; it takes a long time for more-educated children to grow up and slowly replace less-educated adults. The resultant regional distribution of the future labor force by educational attainment shows, for example, that over the coming decades, China is likely to have a much better-educated labor force than India. It also shows that, within a few decades, China is likely to have more working-age people with some secondary or tertiary education than Europe and North America together. Such projected changes in human capital may have significant consequences for international competitiveness. Forecasts of the educational composition may also provide an important analytical handle with which to assess societies' future capacities to adapt to inevitable environmental changes and to other sustainable development challenges.

Chapter 5 introduces a useful social development indicator called literate life expectancy (LLE). It is calculated by combining age-specific proportions of people who are literate with a life table. This results in a summary indicator that gives the average number of years that a man or woman can expect to be alive and be able to read and write. This indicator also captures the social development side of the United Nations Development Programme (UNDP) Human Development Index (HDI), because it includes two of its three components, leaving out the material well-being (income). LLE is introduced here for two reasons. First, it is a practical way to combine demographic information and information on human capital in a single, easily interpretable variable. Second, LLE is one of the few (if not the only) social indicators that not only can be used to describe past and current differentials, but that also can be projected readily into the future. Such projections based on alternative scenarios are presented in Chapter 5.

Chapter 6 further broadens the analysis by adding consideration of rural or urban place of residence and food-security status to the demographic dimensions of age, sex, and education already discussed. This broader population definition is integrated into a model that includes food production, food distribution, and land degradation. Its approach to dealing with food production and food distribution allows the number of food-insecure people to be easily computed. The model expands upon a similar one, which was developed in collaboration with the United Nations Economic Commission for Africa (UNECA), and is called PEDA (population–environment–development–agriculture). PEDA is one of the few modeling frameworks that explicitly links population change and the incidence of poverty and food insecurity. The expanded model is illustrated here using the example of Ethiopia, one of the world's least food-secure countries.

Chapter 7 remains in Africa and moves to a consideration of HIV/AIDS in Botswana, the country most severely hit by this pandemic. In the context of this volume, Chapter 7 serves a dual purpose. It discusses a procedure to estimate the demographic impacts of AIDS that incorporates a new way to capture explicitly the changing pattern of HIV infection by level of education. This analysis also provides a background for our assumptions on future HIV/AIDS in the mortality assumptions of the global population projections discussed above. In addition, it presents the results of models (developed in the context of IIASA's series of in-depth case studies on the interactions of population, development, and the environment) that have been used to assess the consequences of AIDS for sustainable development.

Chapter 8 moves from Africa to Asia, presenting projections that include the dimensions of education and rural or urban place of residence for the world's most populous country, China. This chapter also serves a dual purpose. It considers in detail the specific fertility assumptions made for China in Chapters 2 and 3 and concludes that a continuation of below-replacement fertility there is likely. At the same time, it illustrates the additional insights that can be gained by combining educational projections with rural–urban projections. This chapter provides a case study of one of the world's most rapid and quantitatively most significant urbanization processes.

Chapter 9 brings us back to the global level. The projected global population trends for the 21st century are discussed in terms of their interactions with what is perceived today as the primary environmental challenge of the 21st century, global climate change. The chapter looks not only at population size, as is usually done in this context, but also considers age structure and the impact of changes in the number of households. It highlights some of the findings of O'Neill *et al.* (2001) dealing with the multidimensional global- and regional-level interactions between population and climate change. This analysis demonstrates that alternative population paths over the 21st century would substantially influence greenhouse-gas emissions in the long run and at the same time affect the ability of societies to adapt to inevitable climate change impacts. It addresses the role of population in a key global sustainable development challenge, and hence adds another important piece toward the development of a broader framework to describe these interdependencies.

The concluding chapter pulls together the analyses presented and discusses them using the new concept of population balance. It integrates the different pieces presented in this book (future trends in population size, age distribution, educational composition, urbanization, and various forms of their interactions) with the natural environment, including food security, water, and global climate change. This integration is at the heart of the concept of population balance, which we propose as a replacement for the traditional, one-dimensional goal of population stabilization. In contrast with the breadth of the idea of population balance, population stabilization deals only with the quantity of people and ignores their age structure, education, and productivity. This chapter not only discusses this new concept in qualitative terms, but also develops a highly simplified quantitative model that captures the salient dynamics and that can be used for simulations to demonstrate the effects on intergenerational equity of different trends in population and education, and their interactions with the environment.

This last chapter also discusses past and current international policy rationales in the field of population, including the recent work of the Global Science Panel on Population and Environment. Against this policy background, the different pieces of analysis presented in this book prove to have significant political relevance. We show that population research, when linked with research on human empowerment and productivity and on environmental change, can make a serious and relevant contribution to preparing the scientific basis for efforts toward sustainable development in this decisive 21st century.

References

Cleland J (1996). A regional review of fertility trends in developing countries: 1960 to 1995. In *The Future Population of the World: What Can We Assume Today?* Revised Edition, ed. Lutz W, pp. 47–72. London, UK: Earthscan.

Coale AJ (1973). The demographic transition. In *Proceedings of the International Population Conference*, Vol. 1, 53–73. Liege, Belgium: International Union for the Scientific Study of Population.

Davis K (1954). The world demographic transition. *Annals of the American Academy of Political and Social Science* **237**:1–11.

Davis K (1991). Population and resources: Fact and interpretation. In *Resources, Environment and Population: Present Knowledge*, eds. Davis K & Bernstam MS, pp. 1–21. Oxford, UK: Oxford University Press.

Ehrlich P (1968). *The Population Bomb*. New York, NY, USA: Ballantine.

Ehrlich PR & Ehrlich AH (1990). *The Population Explosion*. New York, NY, USA: Simon and Schuster.

Kirk D (1996). Demographic transition theory. *Population Studies* **50**:361–387.

Lutz W (1994). *Population–Development–Environment: Understanding Their Interactions in Mauritius*. Berlin, Germany: Springer-Verlag.

Lutz W (1996). *The Future Population of the World. What Can We Assume Today?*, Revised Edition. London, UK: Earthscan.

Lutz W & Goujon A (2001). The world's changing human capital stock: Multi-state population projections by educational attainment. *Population and Development Review* **27**:323–339.

Lutz W & Shah M (2002). Population should be on the Johannesburg agenda. *Nature* **418**:17.

Lutz W, Vaupel JW & Ahlburg DA (1999). *Frontiers of Population Forecasting*. Supplement to *Population and Development Review*, 1998, **24**. New York, NY, USA: The Population Council.

Lutz W, Sanderson W & Scherbov S (2001). The end of world population growth. *Nature* **412**:543–545.

Lutz W, Prskawetz A & Sanderson WC (2002a). *Population and Environment. Methods of Analysis*. Supplement to *Population and Development Review*, 2002, **28**. New York, NY, USA: The Population Council.

Lutz W, Shah M, Bilsborrow RE, Bongaarts J, Dasgupta P, Entwisle B, Fischer G, Garcia B, Hogan DJ, Jernelöv A., Jiang Z, Kates RW, Lall S, MacKellar FL, Makinwa-Adebusoye PK, McMichael AJ, Mishra V, Myers N, Nakicenovic N, Nilsson S, O'Neill BC, Peng X, Presser HB, Sadik N, Sanderson WC, Sen G, Torrey B, van de Kaa D, van Ginkel HJA, Yeoh B & Zurayk H (2002b). The Global Science Panel on Population in Sustainable Development. *Population and Development Review* **28**:367–369.

MacKellar FL (2000). The predicament of population aging: A review essay. *Population and Development Review* **26**:365–397.

National Research Council (2000). *Beyond Six Billion: Forecasting the World's Population*, eds. Bongaarts J and Bulatao RA, Panel on Population Projections. Committee on Population, Commission on Behavioral and Social Sciences and Education. Washington, DC, USA: National Academy Press.

Notestein FW (1945). Population—The long view. In *Food for the World*, ed. Schultz TW, pp. 36–57. Chicago, IL, USA: University of Chicago Press.

O'Neill BC, MacKellar FL & Lutz W (2001). *Population and Climate Change*. Cambridge, UK: Cambridge University Press

Peterson PG (1999). *Gray Dawn. How the Coming Age Wave Will Transform America—and the World*. New York, NY, USA: Times Books.

Population Reference Bureau (2003). *2003 World Population Data Sheet of the Population Reference Bureau: Demographic Data and Estimates for Countries and Regions of the World*. Washington, DC, USA: Population Reference Bureau.

Tabah L (1989). From one demographic transition to another. *Population Bulletin of the United Nations* **28**:1–24.

United Nations (2001). *World Population Prospects. The 2000 Revision*. New York, NY, USA: United Nations.

Westoff CF (1996). Reproductive preferences and future fertility in developing countries. In *The Future Population of the World: What Can We Assume Today?*, Revised Edition, ed. Lutz W, pp. 73–87. London, UK: Earthscan.

Chapter 2

The End of World Population Growth

Wolfgang Lutz, Warren C. Sanderson, and Sergei Scherbov

Over the past two decades, roughly two billion people were added to the world's population. No other period in human history has seen such an increase in numbers, and the coming decades will continue to see significant world population growth. Population size will most likely increase by at least another two billion to over eight billion people. However, during the second half of the 21st century, the world is likely to experience no further population growth and possibly even see the beginning of a decline. Sometime before 2100, the great centuries-long expansion of the world's population will have come to an end. This chapter presents, explains, and draws out a few of the implications of this striking new outlook.

In this chapter we present the main findings of the new International Institute for Applied Systems Analysis (IIASA) population projections for the world and 13 major regions (a list of the countries belonging to each region is given in Appendix 2.1). In Section 2.1, we discuss the need for population forecasts that incorporate uncertainty. In Section 2.2, we introduce our approach to making such forecasts, which we call "expert argument-based probabilistic forecasting." This is followed by a short summary of the arguments that led to the specific assumptions made concerning future fertility, mortality, and migration paths in different parts of the world. The projection results and the likely timing of the end of world population growth are discussed in Section 2.4. We obtain our results for the world by making interrelated forecasts for 13 major regions and present these regional forecasts and their uncertainties in Section 2.5. We then discuss the implications of these findings for the changing shares that different world regions will have in the world population. Finally, in Section 2.7 we compare the results of our population projections with those of other groups.

During the past 300 years, the population of the world has increased around 10-fold, but this amazing transition to a much larger population is likely to come to an end during the 21st century. In the final section of this chapter, we return to the larger picture and comment on the importance of understanding our likely demographic future.

2.1   Why Do We Need New Forecasts?

Why did we make new forecasts? After all, the United Nations (UN), the US Census Bureau, and other agencies have been making similar forecasts every few years for quite some time. There are three main reasons:

- We make better estimates of the uncertainty of population forecasts.
- Our forecasts are based on the most recent scientific evidence on all three components of population change—fertility, mortality, and migration.
- The new results challenge out-of-date thinking about world population prospects.

2.1.1   Uncertainty of population forecasts

Over two decades ago, Nathan Keyfitz, one of the great demographers of the 20th century, wrote:

> Demographers can no more be held responsible for inaccuracy in fore-
> casting 20 years ahead than geologists, meteorologists, or economists
> when they fail to announce earthquakes, cold winters, or depressions
> 20 years ahead. What we can be held responsible for is warning one
> another and our public what the error of our estimates is likely to be.
> (Keyfitz 1981, p. 579)

Keyfitz was undoubtedly right. Nevertheless, many agencies still make forecasts with no indication of their uncertainty. Others, like the UN and many national statistical agencies, use a procedure that is problematic in several respects. The United Nations Population Division uses "variants" to address the uncertainty issue. The "medium variant" is their best guess as to what will happen. The "high variant" uses the same assumptions as the "medium variant," except that the average number of births per woman is around one-half a child higher. The "low variant" uses the same assumptions as the "medium variant," except that the average number of births per woman is around one-half a child lower. These variants are said to cover a "plausible range" of future population trends.

Unfortunately, this approach is imprecise, incomplete, and statistically deficient. It is imprecise in the sense that it does not tell the user what "plausible" means. Do the high–low ranges of results include 99 percent or only 50 percent of possible future outcomes? The approach is incomplete because it ignores uncertainties in mortality and in migration. It is statistically deficient because when high or low variants for regions or for the world are computed, all the high or low variants for each country are simply added up. But the likelihood of *all* the countries in the world, for example, following their high-variant paths simultaneously is much lower than the likelihood of an individual country following its high-variant path. For this reason, a panel of the US National Academy of Sciences (NAS) called this approach "inherently inconsistent from a probabilistic point of view" (National Research Council 2000, p. 192).

The population projections presented here avoid the problems of the "variants approach," because they are explicit in stating probabilities, they fully incorporate uncertainties in mortality and migration as well as in fertility, and they scale up from regions to the world in a statistically consistent manner. They are also an improvement over other global projections made by the World Bank and the US Census Bureau, because those give no indication of the uncertainties of their forecasts at all.

2.1.2 Assumptions on fertility, mortality, and migration

Aside from the question of how population forecasts deal with the issue of uncertainty, another main difference between forecasts lies in the choice of specific assumptions as to the most likely future paths of fertility, mortality, and migration in different parts of the world. There are clearly different views among population experts about what, for instance, is the most likely future path of life expectancy in any particular country. Are we already close to a possible maximum of human life expectancy, or might life expectancy increase to well over 100 years? A population forecaster, when choosing his or her assumptions, needs to study and evaluate these alternative views carefully to make an informed choice. This process is undoubtedly carried out in one way or another in all forecasting agencies, but it is almost never documented for the users. The users can only trust that the forecasters made the best possible choice and really considered all relevant arguments carefully. However, even as trusting users of the projections, we would like to be able to look up the evidence and scientific arguments upon which the specific assumptions were made. Unfortunately, most forecasting groups do not provide such systematic substantive justifications of the assumptions made.

The population projections presented here are based directly on assumptions that have been discussed extensively and defined on the basis of empirical evidence and the comparative evaluation of competing arguments. The full account of this complex process is published and open to anyone wishing to have a closer look. The IIASA book *The Future Population of the World: What Can We Assume Today?* (Lutz 1996a) systematically discusses recent trends and arguments for assuming certain future trends separately for the three determinants of population change (namely, fertility, mortality, and migration), and also separately for developed and developing countries. The more recent assessment published by the National Research Council (2000) complements the earlier book in many respects. Together, these two volumes provide a comprehensive state-of-the-art assessment of what we can assume today and, most importantly, for what reasons. In this volume, we can give only a short summary of the literature and highlight some of the main arguments behind certain assumptions (see Section 2.2).

2.1.3   Challenging out-of-date views

There is still another reason for making new forecasts. The worldview shared by many people is based on old forecasts that are now out of date. Many textbooks used in high schools and colleges around the world still tell future decision makers that the world population will likely increase to 12 billion or more. Even worse, many people still tend to believe that world population growth will be stopped only through higher death rates resulting from food shortages and environmental catastrophes. In contrast to these views, we demonstrate in this book that world population growth will likely come to an end during the 21st century through the benign process of declining fertility rather than the disastrous process of increasing death rates caused by our overshooting the global carrying capacity. This does not mean that there will be no environmental problems and no local food shortages. There certainly are real dangers, especially in the parts of the world that still have widespread poverty together with high population growth, and addressing these problems needs to be given priority. They will be easier to solve, however, using a more realistic perspective on future world population growth.

2.2   Our Approach to Population Forecasting

The approach we used to produce this set of new world population forecasts is called expert argument-based probabilistic forecasting. It was developed over the past decade at IIASA.

The word "probabilistic" indicates that we try to quantify the uncertainties involved in the population outlook presented. Importantly, our use of the term refers to what is called subjective or judgmental probability. This is different from what some people may associate with the term "probability" in the context of, for example, throwing a perfect die. Simply put, there are no perfect ways to predict the probabilities of future demographic changes. Instead, our task is to collect the best available information from which to make an informed judgment. The statistician Richard Jeffrey defines subjective probabilities in the following way: "If you say the probability of rain is 70% you are reporting that, all things considered, you would bet on rain at odds of 7:3, thinking of longer or shorter odds as giving an unmerited advantage to one side or the other. A more familiar mode of judgment is flat, 'dogmatic' assertion or denial, as in 'It will rain' or 'It will not rain.' In place of this 'dogmatism,' the probabilistic mode of judgment offers a richer palate for depicting your state of mind" (Jeffrey 2002, p. ii).

The scientists involved in the development of this expert argument-based probabilistic approach included specialists in population forecasting as well as leading demographers from different parts of the world and an experimental psychologist with expertise in cognitive science. The main question in this context was, What are the best assumptions we can make today about possible and likely future paths of fertility, mortality, and migration in different parts of the world and their associated uncertainties? If we have accurate information about the current size and sex and age distribution of a population, as well as reliable estimates of the current levels of fertility, mortality, and migration, assumptions on the future distributions of the paths for these three factors are the only further prerequisite for producing forecasts. In this sense, population forecasts are less complicated than, for instance, economic forecasts or climate forecasts, which must make assumptions on many more parameters.

There are essentially two different approaches to providing such assumptions for the future. One is based on mathematical extrapolation and the other, on expert views. Mathematical extrapolation also requires the input of experts in the choice of the mathematical model, the decision of how to test the model against alternatives, the choice of the empirical database with which to establish the model parameters, and the evaluation of the results. This approach has the advantage of being reproducible, once the rules have been set. The drawback is that it is completely blind in the sense that it is uninformed about knowledge that one may have about the driving forces of the process, about structural change, or about possible limits and interactions with other exogenous processes. The demographic transition described in the previous chapter is a good example of a structural change that we know about and that informs all serious projections of the world population. We know that it would be foolish to assume that a country that has not yet begun its fertility decline and where average fertility is more than six children per woman will stay at that level for the coming decades simply because it has been around that level for the past few decades.

Experts who have carefully studied demographic processes for many years know the relevant literature well, and they know about competing hypotheses on the driving forces. There seems to be a generally accepted guideline that it takes at least 10 years until one becomes an expert in a specific field (Lutz *et al.* 2000). No mathematical rule could possibly include the same kind of information that an experienced expert has accumulated over his or her career. The only problem with experts is that they are human. Like all human beings, they have their personal biases, they may be overly impressed by the most recent trends, or they may underestimate the uncertainty involved in their judgment. One strategy to try to avoid some of these problems with expert opinion is to ask larger groups of experts, as is often done in Delphi studies. Doing so can avoid individual biases, but it does not help against biases that collectively affect many experts. Unfortunately, many studies have shown that such collective biases exist. Hence, majority opinion or even voting among experts is no guarantee of obtaining the best assumptions.

What should forecasters do when faced with this difficult choice between two deficient approaches to predicting the future? In the field of population forecasting, practically all the forecasting agencies have clearly chosen the expert-based approach. Presumably, the driving forces of the three demographic factors are considered to be so complex that agencies tend to believe that possible structural changes and limits to population trends can better be perceived intuitively rather than formally and that no mathematical model could replace this sort of expert knowledge. Only when it comes to assessing the uncertainty ranges (variance) around a trend assumed by experts do some authors prefer to refer to mathematical rules rather than expert judgment (Keilman 1999; Lee 1999). Since, however, it is the same model of the future and the same intuition about the process that generates the demographic trend (e.g., future fertility rates) and its variance, it is not clear to us why it is sensible to derive the median and the associated distribution around it from entirely different sources. As opposed to previous forecasts based on expert opinions, our new approach of expert argument-based assumptions takes an important step forward in the direction of making expert-based assumptions more objective. It also builds in additional checks against any underestimation of uncertainty by experts as it includes the empirical errors of past population projections (*ex post facto* error analysis) in assessing the uncertainty distributions assumed for the future.

The *ex post facto* analysis of past errors enters our study in two ways: the substantive assumptions made on fertility and mortality changes are informed by the analysis of previous errors in those components (Keilman 1999; National Research Council 2000), and our results at the regional level have been compared, wherever possible, with the results of an *ex post facto* error analysis of global UN projections documented in the National Research Council (NRC) report.

Our approach distinguishes between two kinds of experts, resource experts and meta-experts. While the former provide the substantive knowledge and arguments for assuming certain future trends, the latter coordinate the process of argument evaluation and translation into operational projections. The resource experts are scientists with in-depth knowledge in specific areas relevant to population forecasting. The group of resource experts should be as broad as possible, and one should try hard to include leading experts on all three demographic factors as well as on different parts of the world. It is also important to try to include key proponents of alternative views about the likely future trends, with special efforts made to capture dissenting views outside the mainstream of the field. Including such people reduces the risk that some important factors ignored by the mainstream will be missed. These resource experts are invited to specify their views about likely future trends and uncertainties and, most importantly, to specify explicitly the reasons and arguments they see as supporting their views. This explicit reasoning is the basis for the process of scientific discourse and the comparative evaluation of arguments that is at the heart of our approach and distinguishes it from purely subjective expert opinion, on the one hand, and mechanistic projection rules, on the other.

This process of specification of alternative assumptions and the underlying chains of argumentation can be achieved in different ways. Over the past few years, IIASA's Population Project has experimented with two of these. The more traditional way, used to produce the world population projections presented in this chapter, is based on the writing of scientific articles that review the empirical evidence and describe specific arguments in a scholarly manner. Where arguments or data were weak, we always preferred to err on the side of a higher variance because this lowers the probability that population growth will end during the 21st century. An alternative way, which was applied recently to produce forecasts for individual countries in Southeast Asia, consists of a combination of questionnaires and interviews. In the questionnaires, resource experts were asked to describe their views about future demographic developments numerically and briefly sketch the key arguments upon which their views were based. In subsequent extensive in-depth interviews, those experts were asked deeper questions about their arguments, including the degree to which they were convinced or doubtful about them. In this specific case, the resource experts were a large group of national population experts from the region (Lutz and Scherbov 2003).

2.3 Summary of Arguments and Specific Assumptions

The world population projections presented here are based on the fertility, mortality, and migration assumptions described in *Tables 2.1* and *2.2* for the 13 world regions, as defined in Appendix 2.1. *Tables 2.1* and *2.2*, respectively, give the assumptions for the average number of births per woman (the total fertility rate, TFR) and for life expectancies at birth for men and women ($e0$). The figures give the mean of the assumed distribution; those in parentheses specify the 80 percent uncertainty interval based on an assumed normal distribution. In other words, it is assumed that four out of five possible future fertility and mortality levels at the stated time lie within the intervals given in parentheses. The remaining fifth lie in the tails outside this range and may be significantly lower or higher than the stated values.

Below, we give a concise description of the individual assumptions and a summary of the arguments that led to the choice of these assumptions. For further analysis, see Lutz (1996a) and National Research Council (2000), as well as other sources as cited.

2.3.1 Future fertility in today's high fertility countries

In the year 2000, the world region with the highest fertility was sub-Saharan Africa with about 5.3 children per woman. This was followed by the Middle East with 4.0, North Africa with 3.3, South Asia and Central Asia with 3.1 each, Latin America with 2.6, and Pacific Asia with 2.5. All these fertility levels are significantly lower than they were in 1995, which was the base year for the 1996 IIASA projections. Just to mention a few examples, only five years earlier, fertility in sub-Saharan Africa was estimated at 6.2, in the Middle East at 5.5, and in North Africa at 4.4. This is another strong confirmation of the predictive power of the theory of demographic transition discussed in Chapter 1, which suggests that once countries enter the secular fertility decline, fertility continues to fall until levels at or below replacement are reached. This theory is also the primary basis for the assumption that fertility in these world regions will continue to fall in the years to come.

As far as region-specific future fertility trends are concerned, the keys lie in assumptions regarding the timing of the onset of the fertility transition, the pace of fertility decline, and the level of fertility after the completion of the transition. Empirical analyses presented by the National Research Council (2000, p. 54) show that by the mid-1990s almost all countries in Latin America, Asia, the Middle East, and North Africa had started their fertility declines. Only sub-Saharan Africa generally lagged behind; but even there some countries have shown a very rapid change. While in 1980 less than 10 percent of the countries there had started the fertility decline (Casterline 2001), this proportion increased to more than 60 percent by

Table 2.1. Assumptions about the total fertility rate.

TFR[a]	North Africa	Sub-Saharan Africa	North America	Latin America	Central Asia	Middle East	South Asia	China region	Pacific Asia	Pacific OECD[b]	Western Europe	Eastern Europe	FSU Europe[c]
2000	3.3	5.3	1.9	2.6	3.1	4.0	3.1	1.9	2.5	1.5	1.6	1.4	1.3
2025–2029	2.1	3.0	1.9	2.1	2.1	2.1	2.1	1.8	2.1	1.7	1.7	1.7	1.7
	(1.5–2.7)	(2.0–4.0)	(1.4–2.4)	(1.5–2.7)	(1.5–2.7)	(1.5–2.7)	(1.5–2.7)	(1.3–2.3)	(1.5–2.7)	(1.2–2.2)	(1.2–2.2)	(1.2–2.2)	(1.2–2.2)
2080–2084	1.9	1.8	2.0	2.0	1.8	1.8	1.5	1.7	1.6	1.6	1.7	1.7	1.9
	(1.4–2.4)	(1.3–2.3)	(1.5–2.5)	(1.5–2.5)	(1.3–2.3)	(1.3–2.3)	(1.0–2.0)	(1.2–2.2)	(1.1–2.1)	(1.1–2.1)	(1.2–2.2)	(1.2–2.2)	(1.4–2.4)

[a]Total fertility rate.

[b]Organisation for Economic Co-operation and Development members in the Pacific region.

[c]European part of the former Soviet Union.

Note: The figures give the mean of the assumed distribution; those in parentheses give the 80 percent uncertainty interval based on an assumed normal distribution.

Table 2.2. Assumptions about life expectancy at birth, e0, for men and women.

Period	North Africa	Sub-Saharan Africa	North America	Latin America	Central Asia	Middle East	South Asia	China region	Pacific Asia	Pacific OECD[a]	Western Europe	Eastern Europe	FSU Europe[b]
Males													
2000	63.9	45.6	74.1	66.5	64.1	67.4	62.1	68.0	65.0	77.1	73.7	68.4	62.4
2010–2014	66.8 (64.2–69.4)	43.0 (40.1–45.9)	76.6 (74.0–79.2)	69.0 (66.4–71.6)	66.6 (64.0–69.2)	70.3 (67.7–72.9)	64.0 (61.4–66.6)	69.9 (67.3–72.5)	67.5 (64.9–70.1)	79.6 (77.0–82.2)	76.2 (73.6–78.8)	70.9 (68.3–73.5)	64.9 (62.3–67.5)
2030–2034	71.4 (64.8–78.0)	51.0 (48.0–54.0)	80.6 (74.0–87.2)	73.0 (66.4–79.6)	70.6 (64.0–77.2)	74.9 (68.3–81.5)	67.0 (60.4–73.6)	72.9 (66.3–79.5)	71.5 (64.9–78.1)	83.6 (77.0–90.2)	80.2 (73.6–86.8)	74.9 (68.3–81.5)	68.9 (62.3–75.5)
2100–2104	85.4 (65.4–105.4)	65.0 (45.0–85.0)	94.6 (74.6–114.6)	87.0 (67.0–107.0)	84.6 (64.6–104.6)	88.9 (68.9–108.9)	81.0 (61.0–101.0)	86.9 (66.9–106.9)	85.5 (65.5–105.5)	97.6 (77.6–117.6)	94.2 (74.2–114.2)	88.9 (68.9–108.9)	82.9 (62.9–102.9)
Females													
2000	67.0	48.3	80.7	73.0	71.6	69.8	63.0	72.2	69.3	83.1	79.9	76.3	73.7
2010–2014	69.8 (67.2–72.4)	45.0 (42.1–47.9)	83.2 (80.6–85.8)	75.5 (72.9–78.1)	74.1 (71.5–76.7)	72.6 (70.0–75.2)	65.5 (62.9–68.1)	74.7 (72.1–77.3)	71.8 (69.2–74.4)	85.6 (83.0–88.2)	82.4 (79.8–85.0)	78.8 (76.2–81.4)	76.2 (73.6–78.8)
2030–2034	74.4 (67.8–81.0)	55.0 (52.0–58.0)	87.2 (80.6–93.9)	79.5 (72.9–86.1)	78.1 (71.5–84.7)	77.2 (70.6–83.8)	69.5 (62.9–76.1)	78.7 (72.1–85.3)	75.8 (69.2–82.4)	89.6 (83.0–96.2)	86.4 (79.8–93.0)	82.8 (76.2–89.4)	80.2 (73.6–86.8)
2100–2104	88.4 (68.4–108.4)	69.0 (49.0–89.0)	101.2 (81.2–121.2)	93.5 (73.5–113.5)	92.1 (72.1–112.1)	91.2 (71.2–111.2)	83.5 (63.5–103.5)	92.7 (72.7–112.7)	89.8 (69.8–109.8)	103.6 (83.6–123.6)	100.4 (80.4–120.4)	96.8 (76.8–116.8)	94.2 (74.2–114.2)

[a] Organisation for Economic Co-operation and Development members in the Pacific region.
[b] European part of the former Soviet Union.
Note: The figures give the mean of the assumed distribution; those in parentheses give the 80 percent uncertainty interval based on an assumed normal distribution. Because of the life tables used, life expectancies in our computations had to be truncated at 120.

the mid-1990s. As the fertility transition has started in almost all countries of the world, very little uncertainty remains about its onset date. Therefore, most of the fertility uncertainty lies in the speed of the fertility decline and the assumed level of post-transitional fertility.

Our assumptions with respect to the speed of fertility decline are quite similar to those of the United Nations (2003a). The main differences are in the levels of post-transition fertility. The means of the regional fertility levels have been defined for the periods 2025–2029 and 2080–2084, with interpolations in between. The TFRs assumed for 2025–2029 are similar to those chosen by the UN, but for 2080–2084 and beyond they are assumed to be constant and to range between 1.5 and 2.0, with lower levels for regions with higher population density in 2030. This assumed dependence of the level of fertility on population density is extensively discussed in Lutz and Ren (2002). The variances in the TFRs are assumed to depend on the level of fertility. If the TFR is above 3.0, we assume that there is an 80 percent chance that fertility will be within one child of the mean. When it is below 2.0, the same probability is attached to the range that lies within one-half a child on either side of the mean. Between the two TFR levels, the variance is interpolated.

The level of post-transition fertility (i.e., the level at which individual countries and regions are assumed to stop their decline) has recently been hotly debated. In their 2000 assessment, the United Nations Population Division still assumed that all countries above replacement fertility would ultimately converge at the level of 2.1 (United Nations 2001). This traditional assumption had already been challenged by the 1996 IIASA projections (Lutz 1996a), in which it was assumed that the fertility decline would not magically stop at 2.1, but would continue below replacement fertility. This corresponds to the empirical evidence, which shows that almost all countries that approached replacement fertility in their declines also went below 2.1. As a consequence, in their 2002 assessment (United Nations 2003a), the United Nations Population Division changed their methodology and assumed that all countries converge to a TFR of 1.85. In our forecasts we do not insist on a universal convergence in fertility levels, but specify that average TFRs in all regions will end up within a range of fertility of between 1.5 and 2.0. Where, within this range, a region falls is determined by its population density (as assessed in 2030), a rationale based on the finding that, other things being equal, a higher population density is associated with lower fertility (see Lutz and Ren 2002). The assumption of a range of post-transition fertility levels rather than a single target value is consistent with the conclusions of the NAS panel, which states, after a thorough review of the literature on the subject, that "fertility in countries that have not completed the transition should eventually reach levels similar to those now observed in low fertility countries" (National Research Council 2000, p. 106).

2.3.2 Future fertility in today's low fertility countries

As to future fertility levels in the regions that are already below replacement level, no consistent theory is available as a guiding principle. In one sense, forecasting is easier than for today's high fertility regions because, as a result of the irreversibility of the demographic transition, the possible range of future fertility levels is assumed to be rather narrow. For modern, largely urban societies in which the economic activity of women is increasing, it is unlikely that fertility will be significantly above replacement level in the future; it is equally unlikely that fertility will remain permanently below half the replacement level without creating a societal response. In another sense, the task is more difficult than in high fertility countries, because even the direction of future changes is uncertain. In many industrialized countries it is completely unclear whether fertility will increase or decrease over the coming years.

The arguments reviewed in Lutz (1996b) in favor of assuming further fertility declines and others supporting the assumption of moderate fertility increases over the coming years are still valid. One argument in favor of a recovery of fertility is that of homeostatic responses (see Vishnevsky 1991). The mechanisms through which such responses could operate range from pro-natalist government policies to value changes, but few researchers currently support this view. In recent years there has been a heated debate concerning another reason for an increase, the so-called "tempo effect" on fertility. This refers to the fact that during periods in which the mean age of childbearing increases, the period fertility rates are lower than they would be without this effect (as measured by the "quantum" of fertility or "tempo-adjusted" fertility). Bongaarts (2002) estimated that this effect depressed the TFR in 10 European Union (EU) countries by around 0.3 per woman during the 1990s. Because increases in the mean age at childbearing must eventually come to an end, a rise in TFRs in the EU and elsewhere where changes in the timing of births have been significant is certainly possible. However, because of "tempo-quantum interactions" (Kohler and Philipov 2001), that is, the fact that some of the postponed births may not happen at a later point, it is not clear how significant this effect could be (Frejka and Calot 2001).

Many arguments also point toward lower fertility. These range from the weakening of the family because of declining marriage rates, to increasing divorce rates, to the increasing career orientation of women, to an increasing reluctance to make long-term commitments. Having children is undoubtedly a long-term commitment. These factors, together with the increasing amounts of money, time, and effort that people believe should be devoted to children, are likely to result in few couples having more than one or two children and an increasing prevalence of childlessness. Also, the proportion of unplanned pregnancies is still high in most industrialized countries, and future improvements in contraceptive technologies may result in further fertility declines.

There is no clear consensus about the likely direction of change of fertility in today's low fertility countries. The "tempo effect" however, is still likely to be operative. After a critical evaluation of all these different arguments, it was assumed that in Eastern Europe, Western Europe, the Pacific OECD,[1] and FSU Europe[2] fertility would be at around a level of 1.7 in 2025–2029. The assumed 80 percent interval around this mean is 1.2–2.2. The mean of 1.7 in 2025–2029 is above its level in 2000 in all four regions. The consistently somewhat higher fertility in the United States means a similar distribution around a mean of 1.9 has been specified for North America.

2.3.3   Fertility in China

While most of the assumptions of the projections presented in this volume are quite similar to those made in the 1996 IIASA projections, one quantitatively significant change in fertility assumptions has been made for China and warrants further discussion. China, because of its enormous population weight, provides a particularly good example of how new information about the most recent demographic developments can have a major impact.

Over the past few decades, China has experienced a precipitous fertility decline of a speed that is hard to find even among much smaller populations. In the late 1960s, China still had a fertility rate of around 6 children per woman. This declined steeply to around 4 children per woman by the mid-1970s. It first fell below 3.0 in the late 1970s and came close to 2.0 in the early 1980s. A detailed analysis of these trends, which also considers changes in marriage rates and birth-order-specific fertility, was given in Feeney (1996) in a study that served as the main basis for the assumptions in the 1996 IIASA projections. The late 1980s saw a reversal of this trend, with some increases in fertility. From this analysis, Feeney concluded that for the coming decades a plausible fertility range would be from 1.5 to 3.0 children per woman. Assuming a symmetric distribution, this implied 2.25 as the most likely trend. Substantively, the expectation behind this assumption was that economic reforms and a gradual liberalization of the society would result in a loosening of the strict one-child family policy, which in turn could result in an end to the fertility decline and even in some increase.

Today we know that this has not happened. All recently received pieces of information point toward a continuation of the fertility decline. In the late 1990s, the government of China announced that the fertility level was 1.85. The fertility level derived from the 2000 census has not yet been announced officially, but several

---

[1]Organisation for Economic Co-operation and Development members in the Pacific region.

[2]European part of the former Soviet Union.

other pieces of information seem to imply that fertility may lie below 1.85 (Zhai *et al.* 2000). Fertility intentions as collected in surveys also seem to be falling (CPIRC 1998). There is evidence from Shanghai that many couples who are now officially allowed to have two children because they are both single children themselves, do not want to use this option, possibly because they may have already internalized the one-child norm (CPIRC 2001). Furthermore, the strong educational and urban/rural fertility differentials in China, combined with the high expected urbanization and increases in educational attainment (discussed in Chapters 5 and 8 of this book), point to rather low future fertility. The assumptions on future fertility in China made for the projections presented here take into account the recent empirical trends and the new substantive arguments related to future education and urbanization. The choice of the specific numerical assumptions (an average TFR of 1.8 and an 80 percent range of between 1.3 and 2.3 in 2025–2029) was defined in 2000 on the basis of intensive personal communication with Professor Jiang Zhenghua, one of China's most senior population experts and deputy chairman of the People's Congress of China.

These new fertility assumptions for China, which are almost half a child lower on average than the previous ones, result in a markedly lower expected future population growth rate for the China region. This is a good example of how assumptions made based the best information available at the time need to be revised as new information is gathered.

2.3.4   Future mortality in today's higher mortality countries

The outlook for future mortality trends has become much more uncertain over recent years. While in the past it seemed safe to assume a continued improvement in life expectancy throughout the developing world until the level of the industrialized countries was reached, such an expectation is no longer valid. This is mostly because of acquired immune deficiency syndrome (AIDS), but also because of other infectious diseases and because of structural problems in the health sectors of some countries.

After World War II, virtually all countries in the developing world saw phenomenal declines in child and adult mortality, mostly because of a reduction of the infectious disease burden. The improvements were most impressive in Asia, where life expectancy at birth increased from 41 years in the early 1950s to almost 70 years today. Between 1950–1955 and 1980–1985, life expectancy in China increased by 26 years, which is an annual increase of almost one year (Bucht 1996). Africa also did fairly well in terms of life expectancy gains (increasing from 38 years in 1950–1955 to 50 years in 1980–1985) until the late 1980s, when the improvements leveled off. Although this leveling off was not the result of AIDS alone, the HIV pandemic certainly has changed the outlook dramatically for many African countries. AIDS in Africa is discussed specifically below.

Detailed analyses of past mortality trends in developing countries can give very useful indications as to exactly what happened and through which mechanisms mortality rates changed. However, the unprecedented uncertainties with respect to the possible impacts of new infectious diseases in a globalizing world, the worsening environmental conditions in certain regions (which foster old infectious diseases, such as malaria, or cause new chronic conditions through air pollution), and the increases in conditions that appear more often in affluent countries, such as obesity and diabetes, mean we cannot rule out the possibility of bleaker health prospects in the coming decades. Yet there may be significant positive impacts of new medical interventions that could quickly improve life expectancies at a low cost for large segments of the population. At the moment, we know very little about both the possible new threats and the possible new blessings. All we know is that this considerable uncertainty needs to be taken into account in our projections. For this reason, as a general rule we assumed that life expectancy on average increases by two years per decade (this follows the assumptions discussed extensively in Lutz 1996a) and that the 80 percent uncertainty interval lies between no gains in life expectancy on the lower side and a very optimistic gain of four years per decade on the upper side. The specific assumptions, which appear in *Table 2.2*, generally follow this rule, although some region-specific assumptions for sub-Saharan Africa and, to a lesser extent, for South Asia and the China region are associated with the uncertainty about the future spread of HIV/AIDS.

This approach of assuming very broad uncertainty intervals about future changes in life expectancy is radically different from the conventional approach, used by the UN, of only considering one mortality variant in combination with several fertility variants.

2.3.5 Future AIDS mortality in Africa

Notably, the 2001 projections are more pessimistic than the 1996 projections in terms of the impact of AIDS in sub-Saharan Africa. The HIV pandemic has spread more rapidly to greater segments of the population than had been assumed some years ago. This also implies a bleaker outlook for the coming years, since a cure, a vaccine, or an affordable treatment for high proportions of the infected seems unlikely.

Unfortunately, all population projections produced during the mid-1990s underestimated the extent of the disease. For the period 1995–2000 for sub-Saharan Africa, the UN 1996 assessment assumed an average life expectancy of 52 years; for 2010–2015 it was 59 years (United Nations 1998). Only four years later, in the 2000 assessment, these figures were reduced to 48 and 53 years, respectively. For individual countries the changes in outlook are even more dramatic. For Botswana the life expectancy assumption for 2010–2015 changed from more than 60 years in the 1996 assessment to 49 years in the 2000 assessment and to only 32 years in the most recent 2002 assessment (United Nations 2003a). In other words, over the course of only six years, the life expectancy assumptions for Botswana in the next decade were cut by almost half. For South Africa, a much more populous country than Botswana, the corresponding assumptions were reduced by as much as 29 years of life expectancy.

The 1996 IIASA population projections made significantly more pessimistic assumptions than the 1996 UN assessment. For 2010–2014, IIASA assumed a median life expectancy for both sexes combined of 54 years in sub-Saharan Africa, as opposed to the 59 years assumed by the UN. Even this turned out to be too optimistic. Unlike the UN, IIASA also defined an uncertainty range, and it turns out that the unexpectedly tragic actual development still lies within the 95 percent range as defined in 1996. The 2001 IIASA forecasts presented here assume a median life expectancy for both sexes combined in 2010–2014 of 44 years; after that, there is initially a slow and later a more rapid recovery to 53 years in 2030–2034. The uncertainty ranges assumed around this trend are even wider than those for the other world regions. While over the coming decade the median life expectancy for both sexes combined is assumed to decline by three years, the 80 percent uncertainty range is from a decline of six years to constancy. In the subsequent decade, we assume an uncertainty interval of six years of life expectancy with the generally increasing trend described above. An extensive substantive discussion of the modeling of the dynamics of future AIDS mortality is given in Chapter 7 of this book. We re-emphasize that both the empirical information about the current HIV prevalence and the possible future developments with respect to behavioral changes and possible medication are extremely uncertain.

2.3.6   Future mortality in today's low mortality countries

Until recently, most forecasting agencies assumed that life expectancy would level off fairly soon and then remain constant. As time went on and mortality improved beyond the previously assumed limits, those limits were shifted further and further upward, but the idea of a limit was not abandoned (Oeppen and Vaupel 2002). In their 1978 assessment, the UN assumed that 73.5 years would be the upper limit of life expectancy for men and 80.0 for women (United Nations 1981). However, less than 10 years later, in the mid-1980s, Japanese men and women surpassed these limits. Sam Preston (2001) called this unexpected increase in longevity the biggest demographic surprise of recent decades.

Whether there exists a fixed biological limit to the human life span is unclear at the moment. The more traditional view is that aging is considered to be an intrinsic process to all cells of the human body. Under this view, recent and possible future mortality improvements are interpreted as a rectangularization of the survival curve through the elimination of premature deaths and a concentration shortly before the maximum age. Based on this idea, a life table can be calculated with a maximum life span of 115 years and an average age for natural death of around 90 years (Duchêne and Wunsch 1991). This view clearly implies lower rates of improvement in the future. Such lower rates may also be induced by worsening living conditions, unhealthy behavior, or worsening environmental pollution (see Day 1991). Olshansky *et al.* (1990) argue that an increase in life expectancy beyond 85 years is unlikely.

The alternative view considers aging as a multidimensional process of interaction in which partial loss of function in one organ can be synergistically compensated by the functioning of others, so only total loss of a necessary organ system results in death (Manton 1991). If conditions are favorable—through improved living conditions or possible direct intervention in the process of cell replication and aging—this could result in much higher average life expectancies in the future. Manton *et al.* (1991) present an impressive list of evidence from small special populations followed for short periods of time that show average life expectancies of well above 90 years. Further evidence for the position that we are not close to an upper limit on human life expectancy is provided by studies of changes in very old-age mortality over time (Vaupel *et al.* 1998). Using reliable Swedish data since 1900, Vaupel and Lundström (1996) show that mortality rates at ages 85, 90, and 95 have declined at an accelerating rate, which over the past decades averaged 1 to 2 percent for women and 0.5 percent for men. Oeppen and Vaupel (2002) recently showed that the world's highest national-level life expectancies have increased almost linearly from year to year and show no sign of leveling off.

As a result of this great uncertainty about the development of old-age mortality over the course of the 21st century, the 80 percent uncertainty intervals assumed for today's low mortality countries are as wide as those assumed for the developing countries. The median path of two years' improvement per decade, as supported by Mesle (1993), still seems a plausible assumption and is roughly consistent with the findings in Oeppen and Vaupel (2002). The 80 percent interval around that path for each year is the median value plus or minus two years. By making these assumptions, we are clearly rejecting the position that there is a limit to human life expectancy that will soon be constraining further gains, but we do allow for the possibility of slower improvements in the future than were experienced in the past.

When discussing the typically very low or "conservative" assumptions about future gains in life expectancy with forecasting agencies, the argument is often heard that it is best to be "on the safe side." This may well be true for individual expectations of longevity. When it comes to aging and the future viability of pension systems, however, such low assumptions turn out to be very unsafe. In any case, in the projections presented here, we prefer to err toward assuming too much uncertainty rather than too little.

2.3.7   Future international migration

Recent immigration trends in Western Europe clearly demonstrate the volatility of migratory streams. During the early 1970s, West Germany had an annual net migration gain of more than 300,000; five years later, this had declined to only around 6,000, and even further to 3,000 during the early 1980s. During 1985–1990, however, the annual net gain increased sharply to 378,000, 100 times that of the previous period. Few other countries show fluctuations as extreme as those of Germany, but even the traditional immigration countries—the United States, Canada, and Australia—show remarkable ups and downs. Annual net migration to Australia declined from 112,000 in the early 1970s to 54,000 in the late 1970s. During the 1980s it increased again to over 100,000. For the United States and Canada, data show an increase from around 280,000 per year during the early 1960s to around 800,000 in the mid-1990s.

Labor migration from Asia has also been quite variable over the past few decades. For instance, during the late 1980s, more than 430,000 workers left the Philippines annually, with around 280,000 of them going to the Middle East. The Republic of Korea lost an average of 170,000 workers per year during the early 1980s; India lost 240,000 and Pakistan lost 130,000 annually during the same period. The largest proportion of these workers went to the oil-rich countries in the Middle East. During the late 1980s, these migratory streams showed significant declines.

The volatility of these flows and the great role that short-term political changes play in both the receiving and sending countries mean it is more difficult to forecast future migratory streams than future trends in fertility and mortality. Furthermore, net migration always results from the combination of two partly independent migration streams, people entering the country and people leaving it.

The potential for further increases in interregional migration seems to be great because of better communication between the regions, cheap mass transport facilities, and the persistent gap between the North (which is not only richer, but is also rapidly aging and most likely in need of young labor) and the South (which has many young people with rising skill levels, but low income opportunities in their home countries). In addition to these economic factors, expected environmental changes in many parts of the world may cause further significant pressure to migrate to other regions where conditions are perceived to be better. This issue and the associated notion of "environmental refugees" are discussed at length in Chapter 5.

Still, the actual extent of future South–North migration streams not only depends on "pull" and "push" factors, but also on the migrant acceptance policies in the receiving countries. Four regions of in-migration have been specified, North America, Western Europe, the Pacific OECD, and the Middle East. If the European Community, for instance, decided to enforce a policy of closed outside borders, this could result in a situation of almost no net migration. Hence, for all four receiving regions the low value (the lower end of the 80 percent uncertainty range) chosen for net migration was zero. This does not mean that the borders would be closed to migrants entirely; it only assumes that, on average, the number of in-migrants would approximately equal the number of out-migrants. For the high end of the uncertainty range, annual net migration gains of two million in North America, one million in Western Europe, 350,000 in the Pacific OECD (Japan, Australia, and New Zealand combined), and 50,000 in the Middle East have been assumed. Given a symmetric distribution, the median assumption lies at half these levels. The distribution of migrants from the assumed sending regions to the receiving regions and migration patterns among the developing regions are based mostly on recently observed migratory streams as given in Zlotnik (1996) and are made consistent in each year with the random flows into the receiving areas. Model migration schedules by Rogers and Castro (1981) were used to determine the age patterns of migrants. The full international migration matrix is given in Appendix 2.2.

2.3.8   Generating 2,000 different simulations

The population projections were carried out using the cohort-component method for single years of age and single years in time. This method calculates the population by age and sex as it changes from one year to the next, subject to a set of assumed age-specific fertility, mortality, and net migration rates. Such projections are carried out jointly for all 13 world regions. The forecasts presented here give neither one such cohort-component projection (as is done for a best-guess projection) nor a small number of alternative scenarios or variants, but rather the distribution of the results of 2,000 different cohort-component projections. For these stochastic simulations, the fertility, mortality, and migration paths that underlie the individual projection runs were derived randomly from the uncertainty distributions, described above, for each of the world regions. The mathematical details of how these alternative paths were generated are summarized in Appendix 2.3.

In the 1996 IIASA projections, the assumed individual paths of fertility, mortality, and migration in the 13 regions were piecewise linear. Since observed vital rates are not piecewise linear and show annual fluctuations, we developed a new approach for these forecasts that incorporates these fluctuations. The characterization of year-to-year variability was chosen after considerable sensitivity analysis and comparison with observations (see Appendix 2.3).

When simultaneously projecting the populations of different regions, correlations between the differences from the assumed averages in those regions need to be considered. For example, if fertility in Europe turns out to be below the average level assumed for it at a particular date, does this also mean that fertility in China is also likely to be below its assumed average at that time? Or is future fertility in China completely independent of fertility in Europe? The truth is probably somewhere in between perfect correlation and complete independence. We assumed an interregional correlation of 0.7 for fertility and 0.9 for mortality deviations, with no correlation between fertility and mortality deviations from their assumed trends and perfect correlation between male and female life expectancy. These choices also followed extensive sensitivity analyses, which are also documented in Appendix 2.3. The main rationale behind these choices is that, under modern post-demographic transition conditions, correlations between deviations from assumed fertility and mortality trends are unlikely to be large. On the other hand, we assume that globalization of communication is likely to bring correlated fluctuations of rates among world regions. We assume that interregional correlations of mortality will be higher than fertility correlations, because of the faster communication of medical technology and the faster spread of new health hazards. In Appendix 2.3, we show that our main conclusion, that there is around an 85 percent chance that a peak in world population size will occur in the 21st century, is quite robust to plausible changes in those correlations.

Using the fertility, life expectancy, and migration distributions discussed above, and the initial age and sex distributions, we made 2,000 population forecasts for the world at the level of 13 major regions for each year of the 21st century.[3] We have selected nine of these 2,000 and plotted them in *Figure 2.1*. The uncertainty with regard to future population size is clearly evident. We could follow Path 6, in which the world's population falls dramatically after 2070, or Path 7, in which it rises rapidly over the same period. Indeed, each of the time paths in the graph, along with the 1,991 that we did not plot, is equally likely.

Time paths, such as those in *Figure 2.1*, are the raw material of this chapter and the next. Our forecasts are not single numbers some time in the future, but a set of 2,000 paths over 100 years. One way to present our results, therefore, would be to list 2,000 numbers at each date, but if we were to do this, our findings would be unintelligible. The complete set of all 2,000 paths is accessible from the IIASA Web site (www.iiasa.ac.at) for anyone who wishes to analyze the data independently.

To discuss 2,000 numbers as a group without listing them all, we use the concepts of the median and the deciles of the distribution that they generate. Usually

---

[3]In general, the more forecast time paths used, the better. We made 2,000 forecasts because of limitations of computer software and time.

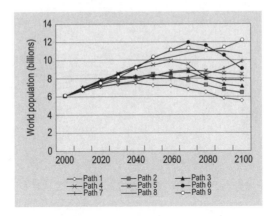

Figure 2.1. Nine (of 2,000) paths of world population from 2000 to 2100. *Source*: Authors' calculations.

when we need to characterize the entire set of forecasts with a single number, we use the median of the distribution. The median is the center of the distribution in a particular year, in the sense that the population size that we expect to experience in that year has a 50 percent chance of being above the median and a 50 percent chance of being below it.[4] If we had to collapse our predicted distribution into one best guess, it would be the median.

When we describe the uncertainty of our forecast distributions, we usually use the inner 80 percent interval. The ninth decile forms the upper bound of this interval, and the first decile forms the lower bound. Often, we produce an uncertainty measure by dividing the difference between the ninth and first deciles by the median. This measure of uncertainty has the advantage that it does not change when we change the unit of measurement (say, from thousands of people to millions of people).

The inner 80 percent interval is not a familiar concept from standard statistical analysis, in which 95 percent prediction intervals are more commonly used. We prefer to use the 80 percent interval here because the forecast distributions are themselves uncertain, but they are most uncertain at the extremities. The 80 percent intervals are far more robust to the technicalities in the forecasting methodology than are the 95 percent intervals. An additional advantage of using the 80 percent intervals is that doing so serves as a reminder that we are not using standard statistical analysis here, but are augmenting the analysis with expert opinion.

The results of taking the 2,000 simulated world population paths and creating deciles from their distributions is shown in *Figure 2.2*. The paths of deciles are smooth, but they are not just smoothed examples of the paths in *Figure 2.1*. They

---

[4]The median is not necessarily the most likely population size.

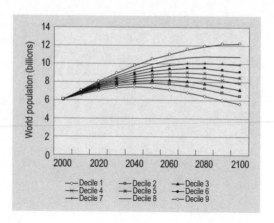

Figure 2.2. Deciles of 2,000 world population paths, 2000 to 2100. *Source*: Authors' calculations.

are derived from the distributions of population size outcomes. Real population paths look like those in *Figure 2.1*, not like those in *Figure 2.2*. Nevertheless, characteristics of ensembles of population paths, such as the median, are useful for descriptive purposes, as long as we keep in mind exactly what they mean and what they do not mean.

2.4 The Future Population of the World and Its Uncertainty

The full scale of recent world population growth and the significance of the uncertainty involved in our outlook only become visible when we examine them over a longer time horizon. *Figure 2.3* shows the population of the world from the years 1000 to 2100. For the period 1000 to 2000, we use figures from different sources.[5] From 2010[6] to 2100, we show the deciles of our forecast distributions. As uncertain as our forecasts are, the likely end of the world's population growth toward the end of the 21st century is impossible to overlook.

Figure 2.4 provides another perspective on the end of world population growth. It shows the proportion of our 2,000 simulated world population paths that have a peak value prior to the date indicated on the *x*-axis. Around 22 percent of these paths have a peak prior to 2050, 56 percent prior to 2075, and 86 percent before

---

[5]For earlier data, we use *Historical Estimates of World Population*, downloaded from www.census.gov/ipc/www/worldhis.html on 16 November 2002. For data from 1950 through 2000, the source of the figures is United Nations (2001).

[6]For simplicity, we plot population sizes at 10-year intervals.

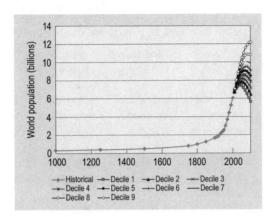

Figure 2.3. World population from the year 1000 to 2100: Historical data from 1000 to 2000; forecasts from 2010 to 2100. *Sources*: Estimates from 1000 to 2000, *Historical Estimates of World Population*, downloaded from www.census.gov/ipc/www/worldhis.html on 16 November 2002, and United Nations (2001). Forecasts from authors' calculations.

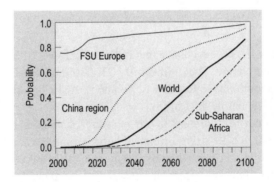

Figure 2.4. Proportion of simulated world population paths peaking prior to indicated year (out of 2,000 simulated population paths for the world and for each region). *Source*: Authors' calculations.

2100. According to our forecasts, we cannot say with confidence when the world's population growth will come to an end, but we can say that there is a high probability that the end will, indeed, occur sometime during the 21st century.

Table 2.3 shows deciles of the world population at 10-year intervals from 2000 to 2100 and our measure of population uncertainty. In 2000, the world population was 6.06 billion people. In the median forecast, the world's population grows to 8.98 billion by 2070 and then declines to 8.41 billion by the end of the 21st century. The uncertainty of this forecast increases with time. In 2010, the median forecast is

Table 2.3. First, third, fifth (median), seventh, and ninth deciles of the forecast distribution of world population size at 10-year intervals from 2000 to 2100.

Year	1st decile (10% of cases below this number)	3rd decile (30% of cases below this number)	Median (50% of cases below this number)	7th decile (70% of cases below this number)	9th decile (90% of cases below this number)	RIDR[a]
2000	6.055	6.055	6.055	6.055	6.055	–
2010	6.612	6.743	6.828	6.915	7.038	0.062
2020	7.034	7.337	7.539	7.731	8.006	0.129
2030	7.317	7.765	8.086	8.425	8.898	0.196
2040	7.442	8.037	8.525	9.034	9.740	0.270
2050	7.347	8.157	8.797	9.492	10.447	0.352
2060	7.140	8.162	8.936	9.794	10.958	0.427
2070	6.834	8.038	8.975	9.981	11.496	0.519
2080	6.446	7.782	8.890	10.020	11.835	0.606
2090	5.998	7.478	8.682	9.964	12.105	0.703
2100	5.573	7.124	8.414	9.845	12.123	0.778

[a]The relative interdecile range (RIDR) is the difference between the ninth decile of the distribution and the first decile divided by the median.
Source: Authors' calculations.

6.83 billion, with a 10 percent chance that it will be below 6.61 billion and an equal chance that it will be above 7.04 billion. By 2100, the uncertainty is much larger. There is a 10 percent chance that it will be above 12.12 billion and a 10 percent chance that it will be below 5.57 billion.

The final column in *Table 2.3* is our measure of uncertainty, the relative interdecile range (RIDR). It is the difference between the ninth decile and the first decile, the interdecile range, divided by the median. When the measure is 0.5, for example, this means that the difference between the ninth decile and the first decile is half the median. When the measure is 1.0, for example, the interdecile range is exactly as large as the median value. In *Table 2.3*, the uncertainty of our population forecasts increases with time. It is interesting that the graph of the RIDR (not shown here) looks very much like an upward-sloping straight line. In 2050, the RIDR is 0.35 and in 2100 it is 0.78.

Table 2.4 shows forecast average annual world population growth rates for 2000–2050 and for 2050–2100 by presenting the first, third, fifth (median), seventh, and ninth deciles of their distributions. In the median forecast, world population grows at an average annual rate of 0.75 percent during 2000–2050. The growth rates vary from 0.39 percent for the first decile to 1.10 percent for the ninth. Between 2050 and 2100, all the deciles below the median show the world population slowly decreasing. In the median forecast, the world's population shrinks at an

Table 2.4. First, third, fifth (median), seventh, and ninth deciles of the forecast average annual rates of world population growth, 2000 to 2050 and 2050 to 2100.

Period	1st decile	3rd decile	Median	7th decile	9th decile
2000–2050	0.39	0.60	0.75	0.90	1.10
2050–2100	−0.55	−0.27	−0.09	0.07	0.30

Source: Authors' calculations.

average annual rate of 0.09 percent. Even at the ninth decile, the world's population only grows at 0.30 percent per year. During the final decade of the 21st century, the rate of population growth even in the ninth decile falls to around 0.01 percent (one one-hundredth of one percent).

Dividing the century into halves masks that, in the median forecast, world population grows until 2070 and then begins to shrink. Over the 2050–2070 period, our median grows at an annual rate of 0.1 percent per year. Over 2070–2100, it shrinks at 0.2 percent per year. Both the growth and the shrinkage are slow after 2050.

It is easy to gain the wrong impression from what we have shown here. The typical population path looks nothing like the median or any other of the deciles. Population forecasts typically wander around in the sense that they could be at the eighth decile in one year and at the median in another. When we say that world population growth is likely to come to an end during the 21st century, we are not referring to the median or any particular decile. We mean that when we look over the set of 2,000 century-long population futures, in around 85 percent of the cases population growth comes to an end before 2100. Other interesting pieces of information about the world's population can be gleaned as well. For example, there is around a 60 percent chance that the world's population will not exceed 10 billion in 2100, and around a 15 percent chance that it will be smaller in 2100 than it was in 2000.

2.5 The Population of World Regions and Their Uncertainties

Table 2.5 contains information about the dates of population peaks for our 13 regions and for the world. In around 76 percent of our simulated population paths, the peak 21st century population of European countries that were part of the former Soviet Union (FSU Europe) had already been reached in 2000. In other words, there is around a 76 percent chance that, between 2001 and 2100, the population of FSU Europe will never be larger than it was in 2000. In Eastern Europe, around 24 percent of the paths peaked in 2000. Shrinking population sizes are not something that we foresee in the distant future. It is likely that during most of the 21st century, the population size of FSU Europe will not be as high as it was in 2000, and there

Table 2.5. Proportion of 2,000 population paths that peak prior to the indicated date, selected years 2000 to 2100.

Region	2000	2025	2050	2060	2070	2075	2080	2085	2090	2095	2100
World	0.000	0.015	0.223	0.354	0.486	0.557	0.630	0.678	0.733	0.790	0.860
North Africa	0.000	0.005	0.094	0.184	0.292	0.363	0.439	0.500	0.569	0.653	0.753
Sub-Saharan Africa	0.000	0.010	0.061	0.130	0.253	0.337	0.421	0.497	0.569	0.643	0.734
North America	0.000	0.010	0.144	0.225	0.315	0.367	0.425	0.479	0.543	0.616	0.703
Latin America	0.000	0.008	0.104	0.180	0.270	0.324	0.385	0.435	0.492	0.569	0.666
Central Asia	0.000	0.002	0.093	0.194	0.302	0.379	0.460	0.529	0.583	0.665	0.754
Middle East	0.000	0.000	0.043	0.121	0.229	0.313	0.398	0.470	0.529	0.614	0.715
South Asia	0.000	0.009	0.260	0.431	0.598	0.681	0.747	0.787	0.835	0.877	0.924
China region	0.000	0.241	0.644	0.726	0.788	0.814	0.834	0.856	0.879	0.908	0.937
Pacific Asia	0.000	0.020	0.254	0.391	0.518	0.592	0.653	0.699	0.748	0.811	0.869
Pacific OECD[a]	0.000	0.391	0.657	0.727	0.807	0.839	0.872	0.898	0.923	0.938	0.959
Western Europe	0.000	0.271	0.583	0.675	0.752	0.782	0.816	0.843	0.870	0.904	0.939
Eastern Europe	0.235	0.768	0.869	0.890	0.913	0.928	0.936	0.943	0.950	0.960	0.972
FSU Europe[b]	0.755	0.876	0.909	0.918	0.929	0.935	0.942	0.947	0.951	0.961	0.973

[a]Organisation for Economic Co-operation and Development members in the Pacific region.
[b]European part of the former Soviet Union.
Source: Authors' calculations.

is a significant chance that this will also be the case in Eastern Europe. In some parts of the world, population is already shrinking.

There is an almost 40 percent chance that the population will peak sometime prior to 2025 in the Pacific OECD region, and an almost one-quarter chance that this will happen in the China region. The comparable figure for South Asia for that year is 0.9 percent. The population of the China region is dominated by China, whose policy of limiting the numbers of children that couples can have has put it among those regions with a high probability of a relatively early population decline. North America is an outlier among the more developed regions. By 2025, the probability of its having reached its population peak is only 1 percent.

By 2050, the chances of having reached a peak increase substantially. They are highest in Europe, the Pacific OECD, and the China region. Substantial migration means the proportion of our 2,000 paths that reach a peak before 2050 remains low in North America, at around the same levels as in Latin America and Central Asia, and well below the levels of Pacific Asia and South Asia.

By 2100, our regions are divided into two distinct groups, those in which the chance of a peak is above 80 percent and those in which it is below. The first group includes South Asia, the China region, Pacific Asia, the Pacific OECD, Western Europe, Eastern Europe, and FSU Europe. The second group is composed of North Africa, sub-Saharan Africa, North America, Latin America, Central Asia, and the Middle East. Fertility differences are the main reason for this division. Fertility starts high in North Africa, sub-Saharan Africa, Central Asia, and the Middle East, and decreases gradually. We assume that the level of long-term fertility, within the 1.5–2.0 range, is inversely related to population density. This produces relatively high long-term fertility rates in Africa and the Americas.

Figure 2.4 shows the peaking probabilities for the world and for three regions: FSU Europe, in which population decrease is likely to be under way already; sub-Saharan Africa, in which the probability of peaking is the lowest for most of the century; and the China region, which is in between these two. As these span the types of population size futures that we expect to see, we focus on them in the discussion below.

Table 2.6 shows the first decile, median, and ninth decile of our population forecasts and the RIDR for the world and for the 13 regions for 2000, 2050, and 2100. Of those regions, six have higher median forecast populations in 2100 than in 2050: North Africa, sub-Saharan Africa, North America, Latin America, Central Asia, and the Middle East. Seven regions are forecast to have lower populations in 2100 than in 2050: South Asia, the China region, Pacific Asia, the Pacific OECD, Western Europe, Eastern Europe, and FSU Europe.

This separation of the world into areas that we expect to have an increasing population between 2050 and 2100 and those that we expect to have a decreasing

Table 2.6. First, fifth (median), and ninth deciles of population sizes (in millions) of the world and 13 regions, and RIDR, for various years.

Region	Year	1st decile	Median	9th decile	RIDR[a]
World	2000	6,055	6,055	6,055	–
	2050	7,347	8,797	10,443	0.352
	2100	5,577	8,414	12,123	0.778
North Africa	2000	173	173	173	–
	2050	249	311	398	0.479
	2100	215	333	484	0.808
Sub-Saharan Africa	2000	611	611	611	–
	2050	1,010	1,319	1,701	0.524
	2100	878	1,500	2,450	1.048
North America	2000	314	314	314	–
	2050	358	422	498	0.332
	2100	313	454	631	0.700
Latin America	2000	515	515	515	–
	2050	679	840	1,005	0.388
	2100	585	934	1,383	0.854
Central Asia	2000	56	56	56	–
	2050	80	100	121	0.410
	2100	66	106	159	0.877
Middle East	2000	172	172	172	–
	2050	301	368	445	0.391
	2100	259	413	597	0.818
South Asia	2000	1,367	1,367	1,367	–
	2050	1,795	2,249	2,776	0.436
	2100	1,186	1,958	3,035	0.944
China region	2000	1,408	1,408	1,408	–
	2050	1,305	1,580	1,849	0.344
	2100	765	1,250	1,870	0.884
Pacific Asia	2000	476	476	476	–
	2050	575	702	842	0.380
	2100	410	654	949	0.824
Pacific OECD[b]	2000	150	150	150	–
	2050	125	148	174	0.331
	2100	79	123	173	0.764
Western Europe	2000	456	456	456	–
	2050	399	470	549	0.319
	2100	257	392	568	0.793
Eastern Europe	2000	121	121	121	–
	2050	86	104	124	0.365
	2100	44	74	115	0.959
FSU Europe[c]	2000	236	236	236	–
	2050	154	187	225	0.380
	2100	85	141	218	0.943

[a]The relative interdecile range (RIDR) is the difference between the ninth decile of the distribution and the first decile divided by the median.

[b]Organisation for Economic Co-operation and Development members in the Pacific region.

[c]European part of the former Soviet Union.

Source: Authors' calculations.

population is not the usual North–South divide. The Americas and Africa are together in one group; Europe and most of Asia are together in the other.

Even with the HIV/AIDS pandemic, sub-Saharan Africa is expected to have the world's fastest population growth. Its population in 2100 is expected to be around 2.5 times higher than that in 2000. Indeed, sub-Saharan Africa is expected to be the world's second most populous region, exceeded only by South Asia. In 2100, the China region is in third place. The population of the Middle East is expected to grow almost as fast as that of sub-Saharan Africa. By 2100, the population of the Middle East is expected to be greater than that of Western Europe, including Turkey.

Eastern Europe and FSU Europe are almost tied for having the fastest rates of population shrinkage over the 21st century. Both regions are expected to have around 40 percent fewer people in 2100 than in 2000.

Regional population uncertainties arise because of uncertainties in fertility, mortality, and migration and their interactions with the age structure of the region. The uncertainty about future population size is greatest in sub-Saharan Africa, both in 2050 and 2100. This is primarily because of the HIV/AIDS pandemic in the region; but even if HIV/AIDS were eliminated, there would be significant uncertainties about life expectancy improvements. The population sizes in Eastern Europe and FSU Europe are also quite uncertain over the longer run. The uncertainty here arises mainly on the mortality side. Life expectancies are currently relatively low in those regions. Over the 21st century, we anticipate that they will rise comparatively rapidly, but we are uncertain about the timing of the catch-up.

Areas that have high population uncertainty in 2050 are those that currently have high fertility: North Africa, sub-Saharan Africa, Central Asia, and South Asia. Fertility is falling in these regions, but the speed of the decline is quite uncertain today. The three richest areas of the world—North America, Western Europe, and the Pacific OECD—are the regions with the smallest population uncertainties. Long-term fertility decline is not expected in these regions, so the speed of fertility decline does not contribute to the uncertainty. Also, there are no special reasons for uncertainties in mortality, unlike in other regions.

Now let us consider the populations of FSU Europe, the China region, and sub-Saharan Africa in more detail. *Table 2.7* provides the forecast distribution of the population of FSU Europe. According to the median forecast, the population will decline from 236 million people in 2000 to 141 million in 2100, a decrease of around 40 percent. In all the columns of *Table 2.7*, except that for the ninth decile, population shrinkage occurs in all decades of the century. Even in the ninth decile, we see only a small amount of population growth between 2000 and 2010, and then again at the end of the 21st century.

Table 2.7. Distribution of population (in millions) and RIDR for FSU Europe[a] at 10-year intervals from 2000 to 2100.

Year	1st decile	3rd decile	Median	7th decile	9th decile	RIDR[b]
2000	236	236	236	236	236	–
2010	226	229	231	234	237	0.048
2020	211	219	223	228	236	0.112
2030	194	206	213	222	233	0.183
2040	175	190	202	214	231	0.277
2050	154	173	187	203	225	0.380
2060	135	157	175	195	221	0.491
2070	118	142	164	186	217	0.604
2080	103	130	154	182	216	0.734
2090	93	123	147	176	218	0.850
2100	85	116	141	173	218	0.943

[a]European part of the former Soviet Union.
[b]The relative interdecile range (RIDR) is the difference between the ninth decile of the distribution and the first decile divided by the median.
Source: Authors' calculations.

Table 2.8. Distribution of average annual population growth rates (in percent) from 2000 to 2050 and 2050 to 2100 in FSU Europe.[a]

Period	1st decile	3rd decile	Median	7th decile	9th decile
2000–2050	–0.85	–0.62	–0.46	–0.30	–0.10
2050–2100	–1.18	–0.80	–0.56	–0.32	–0.06

[a]European part of the former Soviet Union.
Source: Authors' calculations.

Table 2.8 shows the average annual population growth rates over 50-year periods. All the figures in this table are negative, which indicates a high likelihood of long-term population shrinkage. In the median forecast, the population of FSU Europe falls roughly at a rate of 0.5 percent per year throughout the century. We are quite uncertain about what the rate of decline will be, but we are quite confident that the population will, indeed, shrink.

FSU Europe already has a fertility rate far below replacement level and is expected to have low fertility (although not as low as it currently is) for the remainder of the century. Life expectancy in this region is also relatively low, particularly for males. We expect life expectancy to remain depressed for a while longer and then to begin to catch up to levels in the rest of Europe. We also forecast that the region will continue to experience out-migration. In addition, the region already has a relatively old age distribution. These four factors taken together explain why the expectation of a declining population is so strong.

Table 2.9. Distribution of population (in billions) and RIDR for the China region at 10-year intervals from 2000 to 2100.

Year	1st decile	3rd decile	Median	7th decile	9th decile	RIDR[a]
2000	1.408	1.408	1.408	1.408	1.408	–
2010	1.468	1.491	1.507	1.521	1.544	0.050
2020	1.496	1.550	1.586	1.622	1.669	0.109
2030	1.474	1.561	1.618	1.673	1.754	0.173
2040	1.404	1.529	1.614	1.700	1.822	0.259
2050	1.305	1.466	1.580	1.692	1.850	0.345
2060	1.177	1.365	1.517	1.656	1.871	0.457
2070	1.058	1.283	1.443	1.625	1.886	0.574
2080	0.945	1.200	1.388	1.573	1.885	0.677
2090	0.850	1.101	1.314	1.534	1.868	0.775
2100	0.764	1.022	1.250	1.493	1.871	0.886

[a]The relative interdecile range (RIDR) is the difference between the ninth decile of the distribution and the first decile divided by the median.
Source: Authors' calculations.

Table 2.10. Distribution of average annual population growth rates (in percent) from 2000 to 2050 and 2050 to 2100 in the China region.

Period	1st decile	3rd decile	Median	7th decile	9th decile
2000–2050	–0.15	0.08	0.23	0.37	0.55
2050–2100	–1.07	–0.72	–0.47	–0.25	0.02

Source: Authors' calculations.

The China region often comes up in these discussions, because currently it is the region with the most people. In *Tables 2.9* and *2.10*, we look at our forecast of the population of that region in more detail.

The population in the China region was 1.41 billion in 2000. In the median forecast, the population rises to 1.62 billion in 2030 and then declines to 1.25 billion in 2100. The growth rate of the population averages 0.23 percent per year between 2000 and 2050. From 2050 to 2100, the population shrinks at an average rate of 0.47 percent a year. The population of the China region will almost certainly shrink between 2050 and 2100. Even using the ninth decile as a yardstick, its population grows at a rate of only 0.02 percent per year. Chapter 8 of this book gives a more detailed discussion of China and also presents forecasts of its rural and urban population by level of education.

We began our discussion of the three regions in *Figure 2.4* with FSU Europe, the region in which we expect relatively rapid population shrinkage. We moved on to the China region, for which we forecast population growth early in the 21st century, followed by population shrinkage. We now turn to sub-Saharan Africa (*Tables 2.11* and *2.12*), the region of the world in which we expect the highest

Table 2.11. Distribution of population (in billions) and RIDR in sub-Saharan Africa at 10-year intervals from 2000 to 2100.

Year	1st decile	3rd decile	Median	7th decile	9th decile	RIDR[a]
2000	0.611	0.611	0.611	0.611	0.611	–
2010	0.727	0.748	0.760	0.775	0.796	0.091
2020	0.815	0.869	0.903	0.938	0.993	0.197
2030	0.888	0.985	1.047	1.114	1.212	0.309
2040	0.956	1.094	1.186	1.297	1.458	0.423
2050	1.009	1.183	1.319	1.468	1.701	0.525
2060	1.039	1.248	1.421	1.619	1.922	0.621
2070	1.032	1.289	1.499	1.738	2.113	0.721
2080	1.006	1.291	1.541	1.820	2.268	0.819
2090	0.937	1.256	1.533	1.855	2.379	0.941
2100	0.877	1.215	1.500	1.859	2.451	1.049

[a]The relative interdecile range (RIDR) is the difference between the ninth decile of the distribution and the first decile divided by the median.
Source: Authors' calculations.

Table 2.12. Distribution of average annual population growth rates (in percent) from 2000 to 2050 and 2050 to 2100 in sub-Saharan Africa.

Period	1st decile	3rd decile	Median	7th decile	9th decile
2000–2050	1.01	1.33	1.55	1.77	2.07
2050–2100	–0.28	0.05	0.26	0.47	0.73

Source: Authors' calculations.

rate of population growth, even after we have taken into account the HIV/AIDS pandemic there.

During the first half of the 21st century, when the HIV/AIDS pandemic is likely to have its greatest effect, we expect the population of sub-Saharan Africa to grow at somewhere between 1 and 2 percent per year (see *Table 2.12*). In the median forecast in *Table 2.11*, the population is expected to more than double, but the chance that it will more than triple, around 30 percent, is not trivial. Between 2000 and 2020, the median forecast foresees an increase in the sub-Saharan African population of around 50 percent. Even with rapid population growth early in the 21st century, we see population decline in the median forecast for the last two decades.

It is interesting to compare the development of population uncertainty in the three regions (see *Tables 2.7, 2.9*, and *2.11*). In 2010, uncertainty is low in both FSU Europe and the China region, but because of uncertainties with regard to both fertility and mortality, it is much higher in sub-Saharan Africa. Uncertainty initially increases more rapidly in sub-Saharan Africa as well, so around mid-century the difference in uncertainty measures between sub-Saharan Africa and the other two regions reaches its maximum. It is easy to see why this is the case. If an effective vaccine against HIV is developed quickly, there could be almost no AIDS deaths by that time. However, the HIV virus could mutate and become even more deadly. This uncertainty is reflected in our forecasts.

The uncertainty rises more slowly over time in the China region than it does in FSU Europe. At the time of writing, FSU Europe has an unusual combination of very low fertility and relatively low life expectancy (particularly for males). We expect that its demographic situation will evolve to look more like that of Western Europe, but the timing of this evolution is unclear, causing the greater current uncertainty about FSU Europe's future population.

2.6 Regional Population Shares

From a number of perspectives, regional shares of the world population, in addition to regional population sizes, are of interest. *Table 2.13* shows the distribution of shares of the world's population and the uncertainty attached to those distributions. In addition, it considers two extreme cases, one in which the world's population is below its current level of 6 billion in 2100 (labeled "low" in the table), and another in which the world's population is above 12 billion in 2100 (labeled "high").

The regions that are expected to increase their proportions of the world population significantly are North Africa, sub-Saharan Africa, Central Asia, and the Middle East. North America, Latin America, South Asia, and Pacific Asia are expected to have roughly the same proportion of the world's population in 2100 as they have today. The China region, the Pacific OECD, Western Europe, Eastern Europe, and FSU Europe are forecast to have noticeably smaller shares.

This listing may seem somewhat surprising. The China region currently is home to around 23 percent of all the people in the world. By 2100, the median forecast shows it as having only around 15 percent. Even in the ninth decile of the distribution of shares in 2100, it has only 18 percent. The future decrease in the share of the world's population in the China region is quite certain.

The situation in South Asia is also interesting. Using the median projection, its share rises from around 23 percent of the world's population in 2000 to around 26 percent in 2050 and then declines back to around 23 percent in 2100. Given the uncertainties involved, we can only safely say that the share of South Asia in the future population of the world is unlikely to be very different from what it is today.

Another interesting feature of *Table 2.13* is that the uncertainty in population shares is much lower in all regions than the uncertainty in population sizes. One reason for this is the increasing globalization of social and medical trends. Technically, this is expressed through interregional correlations in fertility and mortality.

Table 2.13. Distribution of regional population shares, RIDR,[a] and the regional shares conditional on whether world population is below 6 billion people in 2100 (low) or above 12 billion in 2100 (high), for 2000, 2050, and 2100.

Region	Year	1st dec.	3rd dec.	Med.[b]	7th dec.	9th dec.	RIDR	Low	High
North Africa	2000	0.029	0.029	0.029	0.029	0.029	–	–	–
	2050	0.031	0.033	0.035	0.037	0.040	0.239	0.036	0.035
	2100	0.031	0.036	0.039	0.044	0.050	0.493	0.043	0.036
Sub-Saharan Africa	2000	0.101	0.101	0.101	0.101	0.101	–	–	–
	2050	0.130	0.142	0.150	0.159	0.172	0.283	0.141	0.161
	2100	0.137	0.163	0.180	0.199	0.228	0.502	0.167	0.199
North America	2000	0.052	0.052	0.052	0.052	0.052	–	–	–
	2050	0.043	0.046	0.048	0.051	0.054	0.245	0.051	0.046
	2100	0.043	0.049	0.054	0.059	0.068	0.479	0.062	0.047
Latin America	2000	0.085	0.085	0.085	0.085	0.085	–	–	–
	2050	0.085	0.091	0.095	0.099	0.105	0.212	0.095	0.095
	2100	0.088	0.102	0.111	0.121	0.138	0.451	0.113	0.107
Central Asia	2000	0.009	0.009	0.009	0.009	0.009	–	–	–
	2050	0.010	0.011	0.011	0.012	0.013	0.254	0.011	0.011
	2100	0.010	0.011	0.013	0.014	0.016	0.500	0.013	0.012
Middle East	2000	0.028	0.028	0.028	0.028	0.028	–	–	–
	2050	0.037	0.040	0.042	0.044	0.047	0.235	0.042	0.041
	2100	0.038	0.044	0.049	0.053	0.062	0.475	0.050	0.046
South Asia	2000	0.226	0.226	0.226	0.226	0.226	–	–	–
	2050	0.232	0.246	0.255	0.265	0.279	0.184	0.252	0.261
	2100	0.190	0.216	0.234	0.252	0.279	0.381	0.225	0.246
China region	2000	0.232	0.232	0.232	0.232	0.232	–	–	–
	2050	0.163	0.172	0.178	0.185	0.195	0.178	0.184	0.173
	2100	0.117	0.135	0.148	0.160	0.183	0.442	0.147	0.146
Pacific Asia	2000	0.079	0.079	0.079	0.079	0.079	–	–	–
	2050	0.072	0.076	0.080	0.083	0.088	0.200	0.081	0.079
	2100	0.061	0.071	0.078	0.084	0.096	0.447	0.080	0.075
Pacific OECD[c]	2000	0.025	0.025	0.025	0.025	0.025	–	–	–
	2050	0.015	0.016	0.017	0.018	0.019	0.226	0.018	0.016
	2100	0.011	0.013	0.014	0.016	0.018	0.467	0.015	0.013
Western Europe	2000	0.075	0.075	0.075	0.075	0.075	–	–	–
	2050	0.048	0.051	0.053	0.056	0.060	0.217	0.056	0.050
	2100	0.037	0.043	0.047	0.051	0.059	0.454	0.050	0.043
Eastern Europe	2000	0.020	0.020	0.020	0.020	0.020	–	–	–
	2050	0.010	0.011	0.012	0.012	0.013	0.229	0.012	0.011
	2100	0.007	0.008	0.009	0.010	0.011	0.539	0.009	0.009
FSU Europe[d]	2000	0.039	0.039	0.039	0.039	0.039	–	–	–
	2050	0.019	0.020	0.021	0.022	0.024	0.219	0.022	0.021
	2100	0.013	0.015	0.017	0.019	0.021	0.503	0.017	0.017

[a] The relative interdecile range (RIDR) is the difference between the ninth decile of the distribution and the first decile divided by the median.
[b] The median of the forecast distribution of population sizes.
[c] Organisation for Economic Co-operation and Development members in the Pacific region.
[d] European part of the former Soviet Union.
Source: Authors' calculations.

As patterns of female labor market employment and smaller family size preferences spread around the world, so does the corresponding fertility behavior. Neither diseases nor cures remain in any region for long without spreading to all the others. The lower uncertainty in population shares than in population sizes is simply a manifestation of an increasingly interconnected world.

It is especially interesting to look at the distribution of population shares across regions in two special cases:

- Where world population size is less than 6 billion in 2100.
- Where world population size is above 12 billion in 2100.

We call these "low" and "high" populations, respectively, but it is important to state clearly that these populations are low and high relative to the distribution of population sizes in 2100 and not to the ability of the Earth to support that population in the long run or to any other criterion.

Perhaps the most striking findings from considering high and low world populations in 2100 is that population shares in these extreme cases are not themselves extreme. Almost without exception, the median shares in the extreme cases fall within the third and seventh deciles of the overall distribution. In other words, extreme world population sizes are not particularly associated with extreme values of regional population shares.

FSU Europe is an interesting example. For this region we expect the population to fall throughout the 21st century. If the population of the world turns out to be less than 6 billion in 2100, then FSU Europe will contain an average of 1.7 percent of that relatively small population. If, instead, the population of the world is over 12 billion in 2100, the region will also have 1.7 percent of that much larger population.

South Asia is another intriguing example. For cases in which the world population is low in 2100, South Asia will contain 22.5 percent of that population in 2100. For a high world population in 2100, South Asia's share will be 24.6 percent, less than the seventh decile of its share distribution in 2100.

Like South Asia, sub-Saharan Africa would have a larger share of a high world population in 2100 than it would have of a low one. In North Africa, the situation is reversed. Its share of a high world population would be smaller than its share of a low world population.

Generally, paths that lead to the extremes of the distribution of population sizes do not lead to the extremes in the regional distributions of population. This is another manifestation of the fact that our forecasts build on the notion of a highly interconnected world.

2.7   Comparison with Other World Population Forecasts

In this section, we compare our forecasts with those of the United Nations (2003a), the World Bank (2002), and the US Census Bureau (2003) over the 2000–2050 period. We cannot extend the comparison further because all three of the other forecasts end in 2050. A postscript has been added to the end of this section addressing the newly released UN long-range projections.

Table 2.14 shows population sizes for the world and for the 13 regions for 2000, 2025, and 2050. The size of the world's population in 2000 is not a number known with certainty. Population sizes in 2000 differ slightly across the agencies for reasons such as different estimating techniques and slight differences in geographic coverage. The differences across the four forecasts in regional and world population sizes are small enough to ignore, but are included here for completeness.

In 2025, our median forecast for the world's population is 7.827 billion, almost exactly the same as the 7.836 billion predicted by the US Census Bureau. The UN and the World Bank bracket those two middle forecasts. The UN is the highest at 7.851 billion, and the World Bank is the lowest at 7.701 billion. In the 2000–2025 period, our median world population grows at an average rate of 1.03 percent per year. The US Census Bureau forecast grows at an average rate of 1.02 percent per year, while the comparable figures for the World Bank and the UN are 0.98 and 1.03 percent per year, respectively. The differences between these average growth rates are quite small.

By 2050, there is slightly more variation. Our median forecast for the world's population is 8.797 billion, which is quite close to the World Bank's figure of 8.806 billion. The UN and the US Census Bureau numbers are slightly higher at 8.919 billion and 9.084 billion, respectively. Over the interval from 2025 to 2050, our median world population estimate grows at an average rate of 0.47 percent per year. We are closest to the UN rate of 0.51 percent per year. The World Bank and the US Census Bureau have somewhat higher figures at 0.53 and 0.59 percent per year, respectively. The difference between our 25-year average growth rate and that of the UN is four one-hundredths of 1 percent. The IIASA and World Bank growth rates differ by six one-hundredths of 1 percent. The greatest difference, that between the IIASA forecasts and those of the US Census Bureau, is only 12 one-hundredths of 1 percent. For all practical purposes, the differences in these growth rates are small.

Clearly, up to 2050 our forecasts of world population growth agree quite closely with those made by the UN, the World Bank, and the US Census Bureau. There is much more difference in the regional populations, particularly sub-Saharan Africa. Our median forecast in 2050 and that of the World Bank are almost exactly the same: we predict 1.319 billion people, while the World Bank forecasts 1.324 billion. In contrast, the UN forecasts 1.497 billion and the US Census Bureau, 1.454

Table 2.14. Comparison of forecast population size (in millions) in 2025 and 2050, our forecasts (IIASA) and those of the United Nations (UN), the World Bank (WB), and the US Census Bureau (USCB).

Region	2000				2025				2050			
	IIASA	UN	WB	USCB	IIASA (median)	UN (medium)	WB	USCB	IIASA (median)	UN (medium)	WB	USCB
North Africa	173	174	169	182	257	254	243	272	311	306	295	339
Sub-Saharan Africa	611	622	628	622	976	1,038	990	978	1,319	1,497	1,324	1,454
North America	314	320	316	318	379	399	377	392	422	452	394	466
Latin America	515	516	513	519	709	683	689	682	840	764	808	772
Central Asia	56	56	56	57	81	70	73	81	100	76	85	105
Middle East	172	173	168	170	285	285	268	283	368	391	343	401
South Asia	1,367	1,363	1,355	1,347	1,940	1,936	1,871	1,892	2,249	2,282	2,245	2,298
China region	1,408	1,404	1,390	1,413	1,608	1,617	1,629	1,645	1,580	1,593	1,694	1,635
Pacific Asia	476	479	477	490	625	615	620	644	702	670	707	722
Pacific OECD[a]	150	150	150	150	155	151	146	148	148	140	132	129
Western Europe	456	459	455	457	478	487	467	483	470	480	448	465
Eastern Europe	121	121	121	121	117	115	118	118	104	101	110	105
FSU Europe[b]	236	233	234	234	218	202	209	219	187	166	190	195
World	6,055	6,070	6,033	6,079	7,827	7,851	7,701	7,836	8,797	8,919	8,806	9,084

[a]Organisation for Economic Co-operation and Development members in the Pacific region.
[b]European part of the former Soviet Union.

Note: Rounding and slight difference in the coverage of small countries result in small differences between agencies by region and in small differences in totals.

Sources: Lutz *et al.* (2001); United Nations (2003a); US Census Bureau (2003); World Bank (2002).

billion. The average rate of world population growth from 2000 to 2050, excluding sub-Saharan Africa, is 0.64, 0.62, 0.65, and 0.67 percent per year, respectively, for IIASA (median), the UN (medium), the World Bank, and the US Census Bureau. These growth rates are practically identical. Differences in forecasts of the population of sub-Saharan Africa are the main contributor to differences in world population forecasts across the four agencies.

No region has greater population uncertainty than sub-Saharan Africa. This is not only because of its high HIV/AIDS prevalence, but also because of the uncertain prospects of economic development in that region. Our views on future demographic prospects for sub-Saharan Africa are similar to those incorporated into the World Bank forecasts. Sub-Saharan Africa provides a clear reason why probabilistic forecasts are needed. Opinions differ as to what will happen there. Forecasts need to recognize and incorporate these kinds of uncertainties.

Another difference in regional forecasts arises in the case of Central Asia, consisting only of Kazakhstan, Kyrgyzstan, Tajikistan, Turkmenistan, and Uzbekistan. In 2000, this was the region with the smallest population, and so disagreements about it have a much more limited effect on world population size. Our median forecast in 2050 for the region's population is 100 million. We agree closely with the US Census Bureau, which forecasts 105 million at that time. We disagree significantly with the UN and the World Bank, which forecast 76 and 85 million, respectively. The UN and the World Bank foresee much worse mortality conditions there in the future than the US Census Bureau and we do.

Sub-Saharan Africa and Central Asia aside, there is a great deal of agreement between the four forecasts at the regional level. It is worth noting that, for all regions, the forecasts of the other three agencies, except those of the UN for Central Asia and for FSU Europe (in 2025), fall within our 80 percent uncertainty intervals in both 2025 and 2050.[7] IIASA's forecasts differ from those of the UN in both FSU Europe and Central Asia for the same reason: we foresee more rapidly improving mortality conditions in those parts of the world than does the UN.

The UN is the only one of the three other agencies that produces some indication of the uncertainty of their forecasts. The UN provides three variants. Its medium variant is its best guess and is similar to our median. The high and low variants are quite different from our 80 percent uncertainty ranges. First, our ranges incorporate uncertainty with respect to fertility, mortality, and migration, whereas the UN high and low variants only incorporate variation in fertility. Second, our intervals are probabilistically consistent across regions and for the world. The UN variants are not, because they obtain regional and world high and low variants simply by summing the corresponding high or low variants for all the countries

---

[7]In 2025, the UN and the World Bank forecasts fall outside our 80 percent uncertainty range only in the case of Central Asia.

involved. In other words, in determining the high variant for a region, the UN assumes that every country in the region is simultaneously on its high variant path. This kind of perfect correlation is extremely unlikely to occur in reality.

Tables 2.15 and *2.16* show our forecasts for 2025 and 2050, respectively, with the bounds of our 80 percent uncertainty intervals and the UN forecasts with their associated high and low variants. These tables have four additional columns. For the UN, we present the differences between the high and low variants; for our forecasts, we present the differences between the ninth and the first deciles. The two other columns show the ratios of those differences to the medium variant, in the case of the UN, and to the median forecast in our case. As these ratios are independent of the size of the regional populations, they are directly comparable across regions. In the case of the IIASA forecasts, this column is the RIDR statistic discussed above. Both the IIASA and UN ratios are measures of uncertainty.

Let us begin by looking at the comparison for 2025 (*Table 2.15*). The differences between the UN high and low variants are almost always considerably smaller than the differences between our first and ninth deciles. The only exception is the China region, for which the difference between the UN high and low variants is slightly larger than the difference between our first and ninth deciles. This indicates that the differences between the UN high and low variants generally account for far less than the 80 percent range between our highest and lowest deciles. If the differences and the uncertainty measures showed a uniform pattern across the regions, we could simply conclude that the range between the UN's high and low variants had a lower probability content and be done with the comparison. However, the pattern is so varied region by region that nothing consistent appears.

In 2025 in sub-Saharan Africa, the difference between our first and ninth deciles is 244 million people. The difference between the UN's high and low variants is only 130 million people. Our uncertainty measure, 25 percent, is the highest for any of the regions. The UN uncertainty measure for this is only 13 percent and is exceeded by 7 of the 12 other regions. Given the high HIV prevalence in sub-Saharan Africa, its significant effect on population growth, and the uncertainty as to whether the epidemic will improve or worsen, it seems plausible to us that sub-Saharan Africa should have the highest population uncertainty. The UN variants approach does not capture this uncertainty because it considers only variability in fertility, not in mortality or migration.

There are other cases for which taking the uncertainty in mortality into account matters. Consider the case of the Pacific OECD, a region whose population is dominated by that of Japan. Our uncertainty measure for the Pacific OECD in 2025 is 14 percent. The UN uncertainty measure is 4 percent. The Pacific OECD region has the world's oldest population. Mortality variability, which is especially important in this case, is reflected in our measure, but not that of the UN.

Table 2.15. Comparison of our 80 percent prediction intervals with those covered by the UN high and low variants, for the world and 13 regions, 2025 (population in millions).

Region	UN low	UN medium	UN high	UN high – low	UN uncertainty	IIASA 1st decile	IIASA median	IIASA 9th decile	IIASA 9th decile – 1st decile	IIASA uncertainty (RIDR)
North Africa	235	254	273	38	0.15	228	257	285	57	0.22
Sub-Saharan Africa	973	1,038	1,103	130	0.13	856	976	1,100	244	0.25
North America	380	399	417	37	0.09	351	379	410	59	0.16
Latin America	631	683	730	99	0.15	643	709	775	132	0.19
Central Asia	65	70	76	11	0.16	73	81	90	17	0.21
Middle East	265	285	305	39	0.14	252	285	318	66	0.23
South Asia	1,795	1,936	2,079	284	0.15	1,735	1,940	2,154	419	0.22
China region	1,499	1,617	1,736	237	0.15	1,494	1,608	1,714	220	0.14
Pacific Asia	569	615	660	92	0.15	569	625	682	113	0.18
Pacific OECD[a]	148	151	154	7	0.04	144	155	165	21	0.14
Western Europe	467	487	506	40	0.08	445	478	508	63	0.13
Eastern Europe	112	115	118	6	0.05	109	117	125	16	0.14
FSU Europe[b]	196	202	207	11	0.06	203	218	234	31	0.14
World	7,334	7,851	8,365	1,031	0.13	7,219	7,827	8,459	1,240	0.16

[a]Organisation for Economic Co-operation and Development members in the Pacific region.
[b]European part of the former Soviet Union.
Note: For the UN forecasts, uncertainty is defined as high variant minus low variant divided by medium variant.
For the IIASA forecasts, uncertainty is defined as 9th decile minus 1st decile divided by median. It is the RIDR.
Sources: United Nations (2003a); authors' calculations.

Table 2.16. Comparison of our 80 percent prediction intervals with those covered by the UN high and low variants, for the world and 13 regions, 2050 (population in millions).

Region	UN low	UN medium	UN high	UN high – low	UN uncertainty	IIASA 1st decile	IIASA median	IIASA 9th decile	IIASA 9th decile – 1st decile	IIASA uncertainty (RIDR)
North Africa	251	306	368	118	0.38	249	311	378	129	0.41
Sub-Saharan Africa	1,265	1,497	1,753	489	0.33	1,010	1,319	1,701	691	0.52
North America	394	452	517	123	0.27	358	422	498	140	0.33
Latin America	620	764	919	299	0.39	679	840	1,005	326	0.39
Central Asia	61	76	93	32	0.42	80	100	121	41	0.41
Middle East	327	391	461	134	0.34	301	368	445	144	0.39
South Asia	1,867	2,282	2,761	893	0.39	1,795	2,249	2,776	981	0.44
China region	1,291	1,593	1,947	656	0.41	1,305	1,580	1,849	544	0.34
Pacific Asia	545	670	814	268	0.40	575	702	842	267	0.38
Pacific OECD[a]	128	140	153	25	0.18	125	148	174	49	0.33
Western Europe	420	480	547	127	0.26	399	470	549	150	0.32
Eastern Europe	91	101	113	23	0.22	86	104	124	38	0.37
FSU Europe[b]	148	166	186	38	0.23	154	187	225	71	0.38
World	7,409	8,919	10,633	3,225	0.36	7,347	8,797	10,443	3,096	0.35

[a] Organisation for Economic Co-operation and Development members in the Pacific region.
[b] European part of the former Soviet Union.

Note: For the UN forecasts, uncertainty is defined as high variant minus low variant divided by medium variant.
For the IIASA forecasts, uncertainty is defined as 9th decile minus 1st decile divided by median. It is the RIDR.
Sources: Lutz *et al.* (2001); United Nations (2003a); authors' calculations.

The same sorts of differences appear in 2050 (*Table 2.16*). For example, according to the UN, sub-Saharan Africa still does not have a particularly uncertain population size. In the IIASA forecasts, sub-Saharan Africa clearly has the most uncertain population, with an uncertainty measure of 52 percent. The region with the second most uncertain population in our forecasts is South Asia, for which the uncertainty measure is 44 percent. In contrast, in the UN's forecasts sub-Saharan Africa has a population uncertainty in the middle of the range, with only 5 of the 13 regions having less uncertainty.

In addition to a region-by-region analysis, it is also important to look at the broad comparison between uncertainty in 2025 and in 2050. In 2025, the difference in world population size between the UN high variant and its low variant is 1.031 billion. In the same year, the difference between the first and ninth deciles of our distribution of population outcomes is 1.240 billion. The UN difference is 17 percent smaller than ours. In 2050, the situation is reversed. The UN has a difference of 3.225 billion between its high and low variants, while we have a difference of 3.096 billion. The UN difference in 2050 is 4 percent higher than ours. The UN difference is initially smaller than ours because the UN does not include uncertainties in mortality and migration in its high and low variants. Their difference grows more rapidly than ours because UN fertility differentials are permanently high or low. This persistent variability expands uncertainty rapidly compared with our forecasting methodology, which does not assume that fertility will always be above or below its trend value. Using the IIASA forecasts as a basis, it appears that the probability of the world population's being within the UN high and low variants changes over time.

Postscript: The latest UN long-range projections

About a month before the final editing of this book was scheduled to be completed and almost a year and a half after the publication of Lutz *et al.* (2001), the UN published a draft of its latest long-run population forecasts on the Internet (UN 2003b). The new UN long-run forecasts closely corroborate our earlier findings. This can be seen clearly from *Figure 2.5*. The three lines in the center of the figure show, from top to bottom, the UN (2003b) medium variant world population forecast, the Lutz *et al.* (2001) mean world population forecast, and the Lutz *et al.* (2001) median world population forecast. In 2050, the UN medium forecast is 8.919 billion. Our median is 8.797 and our mean is 8.862. The UN forecast is 1.38 percent higher than our median and 0.64 percent higher than our mean. In 2075, the UN medium forecast (9.221 billion) is 3.02 percent higher than our median (8.951 billion) and 1.66 percent higher than our mean (9.070 billion). By the end of the century the differences grow a bit larger. In 2100, the UN medium forecast is 9.064 billion, 7.73 percent higher than our median and 4.55 percent

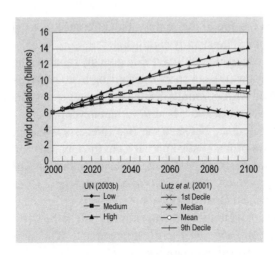

Figure 2.5. Comparison of world population forecasts for the 21st century from Lutz *et al.* (2001) and United Nations (2003b). Sources: Lutz *et al.* (2001), United Nations (2003b).

higher than our mean. It is remarkable that the two forecasts differ only by, at most, 7.73 percent after 100 years.

The bottom two lines show the UN low variant forecast and the first decile of our forecast population distribution. They are almost identical. In 2100, the two forecasts differ by only 1.54 percent. The top two lines show the UN high variant and the ninth decile of our forecast population distribution. After mid-century, the two forecasts diverge significantly. In 2100, the UN forecast is 15.64 percent higher than our ninth decile. The difference between the UN high variant and our ninth decile is the largest difference between the two sets of forecasts, and we will discuss its origin in more detail below.

From our perspective, the most important similarity between the UN forecasts and ours is that they both foresee a peak in world population size in the 21st century, followed by a decline. The UN presents its population forecasts in five-year intervals, so for comparability we use the same intervals for our forecasts. According to the UN (2003b) medium variant forecast, the world's population will peak in 2075 at 9.221 billion and will fall to 9.064 billion by 2100. According of ours, the median of our forecast population distribution will peak in 2070 at 8.973 billion and then decrease to 8.414 billion in 2100. In 2070, the UN medium variant forecast is only 2.60 percent higher than ours. According to the UN medium variant, there will be a 1.60 percent decrease in the world's population over the 25-year period from 2075 to 2100. Using our median forecast, we foresee a 6.23 percent decrease over the 30-year period from 2070 to 2100. Given the massive uncertainty about population sizes at the end of the century, the difference in the sizes of the declines would certainly not be statistically significant.

The UN low variant and our first decile give the same perspective on the end of world population growth. Both show it occurring in 2040. Again, a comparison of the UN high variant with our ninth decile shows the greatest difference. Our ninth decile peaks in 2095, while the UN high variant never peaks.

The greatest difference between the two forecasts is the clarity that is gained through the use of a probabilistic approach. In the UN forecasts, the end of world population growth during the 21st century occurs in the low and medium variants, but not in the high variant. How is this to be interpreted? Does it mean that there is a two-thirds chance that world population growth will come to an end during the 21st century? World population growth ends in 2040 in the UN low variant, in 2075 in the medium variant, and never in the high variant. What does this mean for the timing of the end of world population growth?

Probabilistic forecasts provide clear answers to these questions. Our calculations show that there is an 86 percent chance that world population growth will come to an end during this century. They also tell us the chance that it will come to an end during any given period. In particular, they assumed that 80 percent of the cases lie between a matrix with all zeros say that there is only a 14 percent chance that the end of world population growth will occur in the decade from 2070 to 2080. Our results shows that if we were to bet that the end of world population growth would come in the decade indicated by the UN medium variant, we would likely be on the losing side of the wager. Our probabilistic forecasts teach us that the end of world population growth is almost as likely to occur in each decade from 2040–2050 to 2090–2100.

Now that the UN has also projected a peak and then a decline in the world population during the 21st century, recognition of its likelihood is moving from being on the frontiers of scientific research to being widely accepted and acknowledged.

2.8 Conclusions

This text was first drafted just after the 15th anniversary of the first World Population Day, the day on which the human population reached five billion. As in recent years, World Population Day passed largely unnoticed. It is easy to understand why the day no longer excites much public interest. It was invented to draw our attention to problems associated with rapid population growth. The usual way to commemorate it was with reports that highlighted such troubles.

The problems were so serious and the solutions apparently so remote that people just stopped listening and caring. But in our rapidly changing world it is time to re-evaluate our thinking. For example, women who live on the island of Puerto Rico no longer bear enough children over their lifetimes to replace themselves. Their fertility is now lower than that of the average American woman living outside Puerto Rico.

Women in a long list of places, including, for example, Thailand, South Korea, Barbados, the British Virgin Islands, and several states in south India, now have fertility levels below those needed to reproduce their populations in the long run. The average Bangladeshi woman today knows about as many contraceptive methods as the average American woman. Spain and Italy used to be relatively high fertility countries. Today, fertility levels there are so low that, on average, 100 women of reproductive age will produce only 65 daughters to follow them as potential mothers in the next generation.

These examples help explain why we are expecting a period of near zero population growth, or even population decline, toward the end of the 21st century. The idea that the world will experience unbounded exponential population growth must now be discarded decisively. This does not mean, however, that the future will be free of population-related problems. There are still some major pockets of very rapid population growth, particularly in Africa, the Middle East, and in the north of the Indian subcontinent. Over the coming decades, these regions are still likely to experience many of the well-known social, economic, and environmental problems of rapid population growth. Yet the low fertility countries will be faced with the new challenge of rapid population aging, as is discussed extensively in Chapter 3.

Despite the slowing pace of world population growth and the prospect of its end, there is every reason to continue with current programs of reproductive health and family planning provision. Today, too many people still have children they do not want because they lack access to modern contraceptive methods or education about how to use them correctly. Too many children die needlessly from easily preventable causes. Too many mothers still die in childbirth.

As is discussed in more detail in the subsequent chapters of this book, and particularly in the concluding chapter, education, especially universal basic education for young women, is a key priority in this field. It will not only contribute directly to the amelioration of these health and population problems, but it also will enhance productivity in a wide variety of activities. As is shown throughout much of the rest of this book, the recognition that an explosive world population growth is not our future will allow a more realistic focus on investments in human capital, better health, and poverty eradication.

Doomsday prophesies about global collapse through a continuing population explosion are not only wrong, but they also divert our attention from the essential next steps. We must stop our fixation on the numbers of human beings, move from quantity to quality concerns, and think about how best to invest in the well-being of people.

The recognition of the likely end of world population growth can help us put the myriad challenges of sustainable development into a more realistic context. Hopefully, this will make understanding those challenges and surmounting them easier.

Appendix 2.1:
Definition of World Regions

Thirteen World Regions

I. North Africa

Algeria	Morocco
Egypt	Sudan
Libya	Tunisia

II. Sub-Saharan Africa

Angola	Madagascar
Benin	Malawi
Botswana	Mali
British Indian Ocean Territory	Mauritania
Burkina Faso	Mauritius
Burundi	Mozambique
Cameroon	Namibia
Cape Verde	Niger
Central African Republic	Nigeria
Chad	Réunion
Comoros	Rwanda
Congo	St. Helena
Côte d'Ivoire	Sao Tomé and Príncipe
Djibouti	Senegal
Equatorial Guinea	Seychelles
Eritrea	Sierra Leone
Ethiopia	Somalia
Gabon	South Africa
Gambia	Swaziland
Ghana	Tanzania
Guinea	Togo
Guinea-Bissau	Uganda
Kenya	Zaire
Lesotho	Zambia
Liberia	Zimbabwe

III. China region

Cambodia	Mongolia
China	North Korea
Hong Kong	Taiwan
Laos	Viet Nam

Thirteen World Regions (continued)

IV. Pacific Asia

American Samoa	Papua New Guinea
Brunei Darussalem	Philippines
East Timor	Singapore
Fiji	Solomon Islands
French Polynesia	South Korea
Indonesia	Thailand
Kiribati (Gilbert Islands)	Tonga
Malaysia	Vanuatu
Myanmar	Western Samoa
New Caledonia	

V. Pacific OECD

Australia	New Zealand
Japan	

VI. Central Asia

Kazakhstan	Turkmenistan
Kyrgyzstan	Uzbekistan
Tajikistan	

VII. Middle East

Bahrain	Oman
Iran	Qatar
Iraq	Saudi Arabia
Israel	Syria
Jordan	United Arab Emirates
Kuwait	Yemen
Lebanon	

VIII. South Asia

Afghanistan	Maldives
Bangladesh	Nepal
Bhutan	Pakistan
India	Sri Lanka

IX. Eastern Europe

Albania	Macedonia
Bosnia and Herzegovina	Poland
Bulgaria	Romania
Croatia	Slovakia
Czech Republic	Slovenia
Hungary	Yugoslavia

X. FSU Europe

Armenia	Latvia
Azerbaijan	Lithuania
Belarus	Moldova
Estonia	Russian Federation
Georgia	Ukraine

Thirteen World Regions (continued)

XI. Western Europe

Andorra	Ireland
Austria	Isle of Man
Azores	Italy
Belgium	Liechtenstein
Canary Islands	Luxembourg
Channel Islands	Madeira
Cyprus	Malta
Denmark	Monaco
Faeroe Islands	Netherlands
Finland	Norway
France	Portugal
Germany	Spain
Gibraltar	Sweden
Greece	Switzerland
Greenland	Turkey
Iceland	United Kingdom

XII. Latin America

Antigua & Barbuda	Guatemala
Argentina	Guyana
Bahamas	Haiti
Barbados	Honduras
Belize	Jamaica
Bermuda	Martinique
Bolivia	Mexico
Brazil	Netherlands Antilles
Chile	Nicaragua
Colombia	Panama
Costa Rica	Paraguay
Cuba	Peru
Dominica	St. Kitts & Nevis
Dominican Republic	St. Lucia
Ecuador	St. Vincent
El Salvador	Surinam
French Guiana	Trinidad & Tobago
Grenada	Uruguay
Guadeloupe	Venezuela

XIII. North America

Canada	Virgin Islands
Guam	United States of America
Puerto Rico	

Six Aggregated World Regions

Africa
  North Africa
  Sub-Saharan Africa

Asia–East
  China region
  Pacific Asia
  Pacific OECD

Asia–West
  Central Asia
  Middle East
  South Asia

Europe
  Eastern Europe
  FSU Europe
  Western Europe

Latin America

North America

Two Economic Regions

Industrialized region
  North America
  Western Europe
  Eastern Europe
  FSU Europe
  Pacific OECD

Developing region
  Latin America
  Central Asia
  Middle East
  North Africa
  Sub-Saharan Africa
  China region
  South Asia
  Pacific Asia

Appendix 2.2:
Assumed Matrix of Inter-regional Migration Flows (in Thousands)

From\To	North America	Western Europe	Pacific OECD[a]	Middle East	Total
Africa					
North Africa	90	250	20	15	375
Sub-Saharan Africa	115	150	40	5	310
Asia-East					
China region	270	50	50	–	370
Pacific Asia	400	50	100	10	560
Asia-West					
Central Asia	10	30	–	–	40
Middle East	15	30	10	–	55
South Asia	300	100	80	15	495
Europe					
Eastern Europe	50	100	–	–	150
FSU Europe[b]	50	150	25	–	225
Latin America	700	90	25	5	820
Total	2,000	1,000	350	50	3,400

[a]Organisation for Economic Co-operation and Development members in the Pacific region.
[b]European part of the former Soviet Union.
Note: In the simulations it was assumed that 80 percent of the cases lie between a matrix with all zeros and this high matrix, assuming a normal distribution. (The median of the assumed distribution is half the values given below. The 80 percent range goes from 0 to the stated values.)
Source: Lutz (1996a, p. 370).

Appendix 2.3:
Methods

Reprinted by permission from *Nature*. Lutz W, Sanderson W & Scherbov S (2001). The end of world population growth. *Nature*, vol. 412, 2 August 2001:543–545. Copyright © 2001 MacMillan Publishers Ltd.

Documentation and Sensitivity Analyses
for "The End of World Population Growth"
Wolfgang Lutz, Warren Sanderson, and Sergei Scherbov

The central finding of this study is that there is a high probability that the world's population growth will come to an end in this century. In Section 1, we state the statistical model that we use. In Section 2, we discuss different possible correlations (autocorrelation, correlations between deviations in fertility and life expectancy and correlations across regions) and show the results of sensitivity analyses and their implications on our central finding. In Section 3 we deal with the issue of possible baseline errors in both the size of the starting population and the starting level of fertility.

1. The Statistical Model

It is accepted procedure to create population forecasts from an initial distribution of the population by age and sex and forecasts of total fertility rates (TFR), life expectancies at birth, and net migration. Probabilistic population forecasts differ from deterministic forecasts in that they deal with the uncertainty of the course of future rates and therefore must specify future total fertility rates, life expectancies, and net migration as distributions and not as points. Distributions can also be used to deal with other uncertainties such as those relating to the base population size.

In order to generate the required distributions, let v be the total fertility rate, the change in life expectancy at birth, or net migration to be forecasted for periods 1 through T and v_t be its forecasted value at time t. We express v_t as the sum of two terms, its mean at time t, $\bar{v}_t$ and its deviation from the mean at time t, ε_t. In other words, $v_t = \bar{v}_t + \varepsilon_t$. The $\bar{v}_t$ are chosen based on the arguments given in the text of the paper. The ε_t term is assumed to be a normally distributed random variable with mean zero and standard deviation $\sigma(\varepsilon_t)$. The $\sigma(\varepsilon_t)$ are also based on arguments in the text.

Because of the persistence of the factors represented by the ε_t, we would generally expect them to be autocorrelated. One of the most commonly used methods of specifying how the ε_t term evolves over time is the simple autoregressive formation (AR(1)), where $\varepsilon_t = \alpha \cdot \varepsilon_{t-1} + u_t$, where u_t is an independently distributed normal random variable with mean zero and standard deviation $\sigma(u)$. Another commonly used method is the moving average formation of order q, MA(q) where q is the number of lagged terms in the moving average. We use the following moving average specification: $\varepsilon_t = \sum_{i=0}^{q} \alpha_i \cdot u_{t-i}$, where u_{t-i} are independently distributed standard normal random variables. To ensure that the standard deviation of ε_t is equal to its pre-specified value, we set the $\alpha_i = \frac{\sigma(\varepsilon_t)}{\sqrt{q+1}}$. Note that ε_t depends on $q + 1$ random terms.

The choice between AR(1) and MA(q) does not have to do with estimation, but rather with representation. Data do not exist that would allow the estimation of the parameters of either specification at the regional level required in the paper. Neither is more theoretically correct than the other. Both are just approximations to a far more complex reality. When comparably parameterized, they produce very similar distributions of ε_t (see *Figures 1* and 2).

The choice between the two, therefore, rests on which more accurately reflects arguments concerning the future. From our perspective, the moving average approach has the advantage that the $\sigma(\varepsilon_t)$ terms appear explicitly making it easier to translate ideas about the future into that specification.

We generate correlated random numbers for each forecast year. Fertility and life expectancy change deviations (ε_t) from pre-specified mean paths can be correlated across regions or fertility and life expectancy change deviations can be correlated with one another within a region. Suppose that we were interested in R correlated states (regions or vital rates). Let $e_t(e_{t,1}, \ldots, e_{t,R})$ be a column vector of the R autocorrelated values of e at time t generated as above, but under the assumption that $\sigma(e_{t,j})$ is 1.0. Let V be the assumed variance-covariance matrix for the R states. We call the Cholesky decomposition of V, C. We compute a column vector $\varepsilon_t(\varepsilon_{t,1}, \ldots, \varepsilon_{t,R})$ from the equation $\varepsilon_t = C' \cdot e_t$.

2. Sensitivity Analysis of the Implications of Various Correlations

The future levels of vital rates that enter the simulations can be correlated in different ways. Most important are (a) the correlations between deviations from assumed average trends in fertility and life expectancy, (b) the autocorrelation of deviations within each series of vital rates and (c) the correlations among the deviations from the average vital rate trends in different world regions.

Since the assumed signs and degrees of correlations do influence the results to varying degrees it is important to explicitly address the issue and discuss the implications for the validity of our central findings.

2.a Correlations Between Fertility and Life Expectancy Deviations

In our earlier work,[1] we discussed the impact of two different intraregional correlations over time between fertility deviations and deviations in the change in life expectancy at birth on the assumption of zero correlation both between the deviations in fertility levels and between the deviations in changes in life expectancies across regions. In the terminology of that paper, we considered correlations between fertility and mortality deviations of 0.0 and 1.0. In the terminology of the current paper, where we consider correlations between total fertility rates deviations and life expectancy change deviations, the correlations are 0.0 and −1.0. Compared to a correlation of 0.0, the correlation of −1.0 between fertility and life expectancy change deviations produced relatively small decreases in the means of the world population size distributions and relatively large decreases in the standard deviations. This is because high fertility combined with low life expectancies partially offset each other in terms of population size.

It is difficult to do an empirical analysis of past correlations between fertility and life expectancy deviations for our 13 regions. We did an approximate calculation using United Nations data by taking, where possible, a large country in each of our regions. We took United Nations vital rate assumptions from the 1988 assessment[2] and used them as the trend and calculated deviations from the trend for 1995–2000 using data from the 2000 assessment.[3] The thirteen countries are Egypt, Nigeria, China, Indonesia, Japan, Pakistan, Iran, India, Poland, France, Brazil, United States, and Bulgaria. The correlation between deviations in the total fertility rate and life expectancy at birth was 0.259, which is not statistically significantly different from zero (95 percent level of confidence, two-tailed test). On theoretical grounds there is no clear expectation as to what correlation should be expected in the future. That is why we chose 0.0, but also performed sensitivity analyses to see how our results would be affected by possible deviations from this assumption.

The sensitivity analysis presented here is at the level of one region, North Africa. This region was chosen because the quality of the demographic data in the region is quite good and because its population has a relatively low probability of reaching a peak within the century. The relatively low probability provides room for both upward and downward movements. If we were to present the results at the world level, we would have somewhat different results depending on the interregional correlations that we chose. Considering a single region allows us to present the effects more clearly. To further simplify matters, we have used only the female population. This, in no way, affects the generality of our findings.

Our results are presented in *Table 1* and *Figure 3*. *Table 1* shows the same phenomenon that we observed in our earlier work. The main effect of changing the correlation between fertility and life expectancy is on the variance of the distribution of future population sizes. For example, in 2100 when the correlation is –0.9 the 80 percent prediction interval is 123.6 million people wide, while when it is 0.9 it is 172.9 million people wide.

Figure 3 shows the probability of the female population reaching a peak for each year of the century for five different correlations between fertility and life expectancy, –0.9, –0.5, 0.0, 0.5, and 0.9 and for the 31 term moving average specification. By the end of the century, the five lines are so close to one another that they are barely distinguishable. In 2100, when the correlation is 0.0, the probability of the peak population being reached by the end of the century is 75.9 percent. If the correlation was 0.5, the probability would be 76.2 percent and if it was –0.5, it would be 74.5 percent. Therefore, if the correlation was somewhere between –0.5 and 0.5 and we supposed it to be 0.0, the maximum error in the probability of the peak being reached by the end of the century would be 1.4 percentage points. Indeed, if the true correlation was somewhere between –0.9 and 0.9 and we assumed it to be equal to zero, the maximum possible error that we could make in the probability of the peak being reached by the end of the century would be 3 percentage points. The results are similar for all regions.

The dataset with 1,000 simulations for the female population of North Africa for the case of the correlation –0.9 is in the file "nature_dataset_1a.xls." A similar dataset based on the assumption of a correlation of 0.9 is in "nature_dataset_1b.xls." [These datasets can be accessed via the "Download the IIASA-2001-projections-data" link on the Population Project's Web page at www.iiasa.ac.at/Research/POP/proj01/index.html. *Eds.*]

2.b Autocorrelation

For clarity, we also consider differences in first-order autocorrelation only for females in North Africa. *Figure 4* is similar to *Figure 3* except that it assumes zero correlation between fertility and life expectancy change deviations and considers three different numbers of terms in the moving average specification, 21, 31, and 41. The three lines are quite close to one another. The probabilities of reaching a peak by the end of the century are 78.9, 75.9, and 73.3 percent, respectively. In the text, our findings are based on a moving average specification with 31 terms. If the correct specification were somewhere between 21 and 41 terms, the maximum error that we would make in the probability of a peak being reached by the end of the century would be 3 percentage points upwards or 2.6 percentage points downward. A similar clustering occurs when this sensitivity analysis is carried out assuming the other four correlations between fertility and life expectancy change deviations discussed in the previous section. The autocorrelation coefficient for our 31-term case is 0.9677.

There are not enough time periods to make a useful empirical analysis of autocorrelation even from United Nations data. Our choice is consistent with Lee[4] (p. 161), which reports that the first-order correlation for the total fertility rate during the twentieth century in the United States was 0.96. Further, 31 years is close to the length of a generation and one way of interpreting Lee's finding is that there were influences on fertility that operated on generational scale.

2.c Correlations Across Regions

Due to rapidly increasing globalisation of medical technology as well as of new threats to life, it is assumed that the interregional correlations of the deviations from the expected trends in life expectancy improvements are very high. For fertility increasing globalisation of media (transmission of norms and fashions with respect to fertility relevant life styles) as well as reproductive technology is also likely to result in high global correlations. But due to the fact that fertility is much more strongly embedded in regional norms, traditions and religions the correlation is assumed to be somewhat lower than in the case of life expectancy.

For the results presented in the main text interregional correlations in the deviations from expected trends were assumed to be 0.9 in the case of life expectancy and 0.7 in the case of fertility. Under these assumptions, the probability that world population growth would come to an end during this century is 86 percent. We did two other computations, one in which the interregional correlation for life expectancy was lowered to 0.7 and the one for fertility was decreased to 0.5, and another with correlations 0.7 and 0.0, respectively. The probability that the world's population growth would end by 2100 remains virtually constant in all three cases with differences only visible around the middle of the century (see *Figure 5*).

Table 2 gives the median world population size and the 80 percent prediction intervals for the years 2000, 2025, 2050, 2075, and 2100. The table shows that median world population sizes are hardly affected by changing the correlation structure, but that the 80 percent prediction interval is. For example, in 2100 the 80 percent prediction interval for the interregional fertility correlation of 0.7 and the interregional life expectancy correlation of 0.9 is 6.54 billion people. In the case of fertility correlation of 0.0 and life expectancy correlation of 0.7, the 80 percent prediction interval is only 4.03 billion people wide. But as shown above, this does not significantly affect the probability of world population peaking by the end of this century.

The dataset incorporating 2,000 simulations at intervals of five years for our base case with interregional fertility correlation of 0.7 and interregional life expectancy correlation of 0.9 appears in file "nature_dataset_2.xls." [These datasets can be accessed via the "Download the IIASA-2001-projections-data" link on the Population Project's Web page at www.iiasa.ac.at/Research/POP/proj01/index. html. *Eds.*]

3. Baseline Errors

Errors in the baseline data of a population projection are a significant source of error of the projected population especially in the nearer term future. In the longer run errors in the assumed trends dominate. The analysis of these issues in the U.S. National Research Council (NRC) report,[5] which was based on earlier important work by Alho[6] and Keilman,[7] has recently been further developed by Bulatao[8] who distinguishes between the errors in the baseline population size, the errors in the assumed starting levels in fertility and mortality and the errors due to wrong assumption on the trends. His decomposition of the errors for selected UN and World Bank forecasts since 1973 attributes a smaller proportion of the total error to baseline errors than the NRC report did. Studying the errors at different levels of regional aggregation he concludes that world errors tend to be much smaller than the error for the average country because country errors have tended to offset.

What do these findings from past projections imply for the uncertainty ranges of future population trends presented here? In the following we will discuss (a) the sensitivity of assumed serious errors in the baseline population on our main results and (b) how assumed changes in the starting level of fertility (using the recently announced UN projections[3] as an example) impact our main conclusion.

3.a Errors in Baseline Population Size

We did calculations assuming that the true population of sub-Saharan Africa in 2000 was 5 percent and 10 percent higher than our figure. These are very high baseline errors for a world region by any standards. The consequence of this was that the probability of the world's population reaching a peak by 2100 was reduced by one-tenth of one percentage point (for both the 5 and 10 percent changes). The mean of the world's population distribution would be around 173 million people or roughly 2 percent higher in 2100 than we forecast, if the true population of sub-Saharan Africa in 2000 were 10 percent higher than our figure. The effect of an error in initial population size will be larger in sub-Saharan Africa than in other regions because of the still rapid population growth there. In the opposite case of overestimating the population of sub-Saharan Africa in 2000, the probability of world population growth ending during this century would be slightly higher than our figure. This sensitivity analysis shows that plausible errors in initial population sizes will have virtually no impact on our conclusion that the world population growth is likely to end in the current century.

3.b Errors in Baseline Total Fertility Rates

By using the recently released UN[3] population forecasts we can assess the effects of plausible changes in baseline total fertility estimates. Between 1999 and 2001 the UN has reassessed its estimates of fertility levels for 1995–2000 and increased fertility figures for some large countries in sub-Saharan Africa and South Asia. This change in baseline fertility is one of the sources (along with changed assumptions about trends) of an increase in projected world population sizes from UN[9] (1999) to UN[3] (2001).

Here we study the sensitivity of our findings to the changed UN baseline fertility assumptions. Our results are presented in *Tables 3* and *4*, where we utilise all the assumptions in our paper, except that we adjust our total fertility rates in the initial year according to the differences in estimates of 1995–2000 fertility between UN[9] (1999) and UN[3] (2001). In *Table 3*, we show the probability of a peak in population size being reached for the world and for our 13 regions for 25-year intervals from 2000 to 2100 using both total fertility rate sets as starting values. Using the higher total fertility rates, the probability that the world's population would peak during the century is 85.7 percent, compared to 86.0 percent using our original total fertility rates. The effect of this plausible increase in baseline total fertility rates has a negligible effect on the probability of reaching a peak in all regions of the world as shown in *Table 3*.

Table 4 shows the median population size and 80 percent prediction interval for the world's population and the population of our 13 regions by 25-year intervals from 2000 to 2100. It is the analogue of *Table 1* in the main text but based on higher initial total fertility rates. Using the lower total fertility rates, the world's median population size in 2100 is 8.41 billion with an 80 percent prediction interval between 5.58 and 12.12 billion people. With the higher total fertility rates, the world's median population size in 2100 is 8.45 billion with an 80 percent prediction interval between 5.57 and 12.22 billion. It is clear that adjusting the baseline total fertility rates higher has little effect on the distribution of future world population sizes in 2100.

4. Conclusion

The main finding of our paper is that there is a high probability, around 85 percent, that the population of the world will reach a peak sometime during the current century. We have considered the sensitivity of this finding to a number of uncertain parameters. The evidence strongly supports the conclusion that our main finding is not sensitive to plausible changes in those parameters.

5. References

1. Lutz, W., Sanderson, W. & Scherbov, S. Probabilistic population projections based on expert opinion. In *The Future Population of the World: What Can We Assume Today?* (ed. Lutz, W.) 397–385 (Earthscan, London, rev. ed., 1996).
2. United Nations. *World Population Prospects 1988* (United Nations, New York, ST/ESA/SER.A/106, 1989).
3. United Nations. 2000 Assessment (United Nations, New York, 2001). Web site http://www.un.org/esa/population.
4. Lee, R. D. Probabilistic approaches to population forecasting. In *Frontiers of Population Forecasting* (eds. Lutz, W., Vaupel, J. W. & Ahlburg, D. A.), a supplement to *Population and Development Review* **24** (1998), 156–190 (1999).
5. Bongaarts, J. & Bulatao, R. A., Eds, *Beyond Six Billion. Forecasting the World's Population.* (National Academy Press, Washington, DC, 2000).
6. Alho, J. M. The magnitude of error due to different vital processes in population forecasts. *International Journal of Forecasting* **8**, 301–314 (1992).
7. Keilman, N. How accurate are the United Nations world population projections? In *Frontiers of Population Forecasting* (eds. Lutz, W., Vaupel, J. W. & Ahlburg, D. A.), a supplement to *Population and Development Review* **24** (1998), 15–41 (1999).
8. Bulatao, R. A. Visible and Invisible Sources of Error in World Population Projections. Paper presented at the Annual Meeting of the Population Association of America, Washington, DC, 29–31 March 2001.
9. United Nations. *Long-Range World Population Projections: Based on the 1998 Revision* (United Nations, New York, ESA/P/WP.153, 1999).

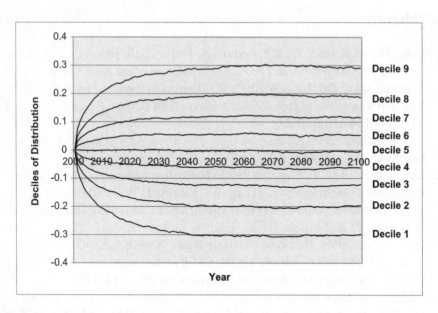

Figure 1. AR(1), $\alpha = 0.9677$, $\sigma(u) = 0.05896$, $v(0) = 0$, 10,000 simulations.

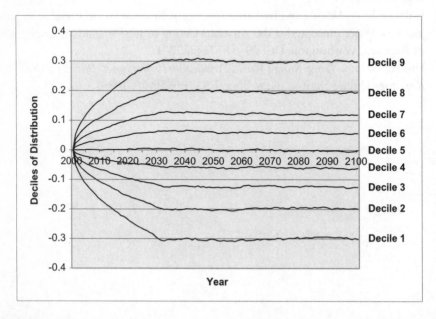

Figure 2. MA 30(31 terms), $\sigma(\varepsilon_t) = 0.234$, 31 initial values of $u = 0$, 10,000 simulations.

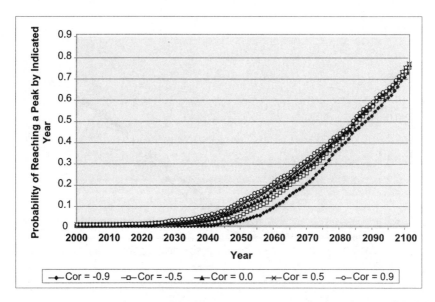

Figure 3. Probability of the female population of North Africa reaching a peak by indicated year using 31-term moving average specification for correlations between total fertility rate of female life expectancy at birth of –0.9, –0.5, 0.0, 0.5, and 0.9.

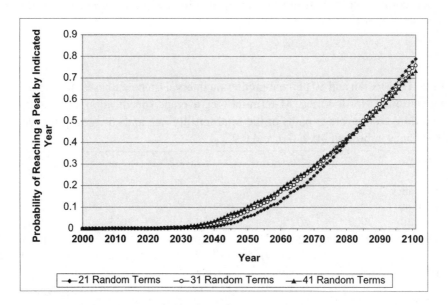

Figure 4. Probability of the female population of North Africa reaching a peak by indicated year using correlation of 0.0 between total fertility rate and female life expectancy at birth for moving average specifications of 21, 31, and 41 terms.

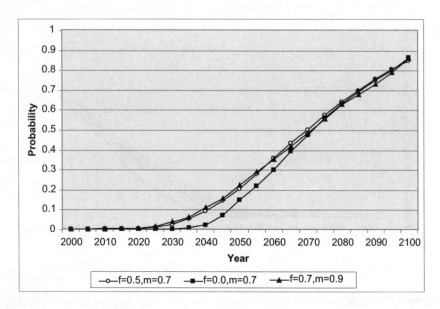

Figure 5. Probability that the peak in population size is reached before the indicated date for three different structures of interregional correlations. f = interregional correlation in total fertility rates; m = interregional correlation in life expectancies at birth.

Table 1. Median and 80 percent prediction interval (in parentheses) for the female population of North Africa, 31-term moving average specification, correlations of deviations from average paths of the total fertility rate and changes in female life expectancy at birth of –0.9, 0.0, and 0.9.

Fertility – Life Expectancy Deviation Correlation	2000	2025	2050	2075	2100
–0.9	85.8	129.5 (116.3–141.7)	160.9 (133.1–187.9)	178.6 (132.7–224.3)	174.3 (119.3–242.9)
0.0	85.8	129.0 (114.6–144.2)	161.1 (127.7–196.5)	177.3 (122.9–235.4)	176.3 (107.8–260.5)
0.9	85.8	129.8 (113.2–145.4)	160.1 (126.2–202.1)	174.4 (117.6–247.0)	175.0 (100.9–273.8)

Table 2. Median world population size and 80 percent prediction intervals (in parentheses) for three sets of interregional correlations of deviations from average paths of total fertility rates and changes in life expectancies at birth.

	2000	2025	2050	2075	2100
Fertility Corr. = 0.7, Life Exp. Corr. = 0.9	6.06	7.83 (7.22–8.46)	8.80 (7.35–10.44)	8.95 (6.64–11.65)	8.41 (5.58–12.12)
Fertility Corr. = 0.5, Life Exp. Corr. = 0.7	6.06	7.80 (7.23–8.38)	8.78 (7.41–10.20)	8.83 (6.78–11.22)	8.35 (5.73–11.42)
Fertility Corr. = 0.0, Life Exp. Corr. = 0.7	6.06	7.80 (7.46–8.16)	8.78 (7.97–9.71)	8.89 (7.45–10.49)	8.43 (6.51–10.54)

Table 3. Probability that population will reach a peak before the given date using total fertility rates based on the assumptions used in the text and those with higher baseline fertility following the UN[3] (2001) assessment.

	2075		2100	
Region	TFR Used in paper fertility	TFR Higher baseline	TFR Used in paper fertility	TFR Higher baseline
World	0.557	0.557	0.860	0.857
European Former Soviet Union	0.935	0.949	0.973	0.979
Eastern Europe	0.928	0.933	0.972	0.972
Western Europe	0.782	0.777	0.939	0.935
Pacific OECD	0.839	0.837	0.959	0.957
Pacific Asia	0.592	0.588	0.869	0.866
China Region	0.814	0.810	0.937	0.932
South Asia	0.681	0.680	0.924	0.923
Middle East	0.313	0.323	0.715	0.712
Central Asia	0.379	0.382	0.754	0.751
Latin America	0.324	0.324	0.666	0.659
North America	0.367	0.373	0.703	0.699
Sub-Saharan Africa	0.337	0.339	0.734	0.729
North Africa	0.363	0.385	0.753	0.750

Table 4. Median population sizes and 80 percent prediction intervals (in parentheses) using all the same assumptions as *Table 1* in the main text but with total fertility adjusted upwards according to the differences between UN[9] (1999) and UN[3] (2001).

Region	2000	2025	2050	2075	2100
World (billions)	6.06	7.86 (7.23–8.50)	8.84 (7.36–10.50)	9.00 (6.65–11.71)	8.45 (5.57–12.22)
European Former Soviet Union (millions)	235.64	215.45 (199.26–231.07)	182.28 (148.57–219.53)	152.35 (104.33–209.96)	134.13 (79.63–209.97)
Eastern Europe (millions)	121.19	116.54 (108.12–124.58)	102.56 (84.54–123.01)	85.24 (59.17–117.17)	72.94 (42.54–113.65)
Western Europe (millions)	455.63	477.86 (445.30–509.51)	470.37 (398.55–551.28)	434.10 (321.26–563.53)	391.10 (255.75–569.63)
Pacific OECD (millions)	149.93	154.70 (143.61–165.58)	148.40 (124.42–174.50)	135.38 (99.70–175.83)	122.45 (78.54–172.50)
Pacific Asia (millions)	476.43	626.34 (568.23–683.40)	701.60 (573.37–844.29)	702.05 (507.59–938.20)	652.33 (407.92–947.95)
China Region (billions)	1.41	1.61 (1.49–1.72)	1.58 (1.30–1.86)	1.42 (1.00–1.89)	1.25 (0.76–1.88)
South Asia (billions)	1.37	1.95 (1.74–2.16)	2.26 (1.80–2.79)	2.25 (1.54–3.10)	1.97 (1.19–3.04)
Middle East (millions)	172.12	284.60 (251.38–317.63)	367.39 (299.58–443.60)	411.97 (294.99–541.89)	410.02 (258.15–592.87)
Central Asia (millions)	55.88	81.28 (72.65–90.01)	99.64 (79.31–120.96)	106.82 (75.20–144.89)	105.42 (65.73–159.17)
Latin America (millions)	515.27	708.86 (641.17–776.57)	840.11 (677.68–1006.83)	904.47 (644.97–1202.10)	933.11 (583.87–1385.09)
North America (millions)	313.67	379.54 (350.77–410.72)	422.46 (357.84–498.40)	440.46 (342.93–566.49)	452.61 (311.39–630.19)
Sub-Saharan Africa (millions)	611.19	1000.76 (874.92–1126.09)	1358.10 (1039.89–1747.53)	1569.20 (1058.01–2253.84)	1542.84 (901.33–2515.01)
North Africa (millions)	173.26	253.49 (224.62–281.40)	305.07 (243.26–372.08)	327.05 (231.14–434.54)	323.90 (207.67–471.19)

References

Bongaarts J (2002). The end of the fertility transition in the developed world. *Population and Development Review* **28**:419–443.

Bucht B (1996). Mortality trends in developing countries: A survey. In *The Future Population of the World. What Can We Assume Today?*, Revised Edition, ed. Lutz W, pp. 133–148. London, UK: Earthscan.

Casterline JB (2001). The pace of fertility transition: National patterns in the second half of the twentieth century. In *Global Fertility Transition*, eds. Bulatao RA & Casterline JB, pp. 17–52. Supplement to *Population and Development Review*, 2001, **27**. New York, NY, USA: The Population Council.

CPIRC (1998). *Data on the Survey of Reproduction Health*. Beijing, China: China Population Information and Research Center.

CPIRC (2001). http://www.cpirc.org.cn (downloaded on 6 April 2001). Beijing, China: China Population Information and Research Center.

Day L (1991). Upper-age longevity in low-mortality countries: A dissenting view. In *Future Demographic Trends in Europe and North America. What Can We Assume Today?*, ed. Lutz W, pp. 117–128. New York, NY, USA: Academic Press.

Duchêne J & Wunsch G (1991). Population aging and the limits to human life. In *Future Demographic Trends in Europe and North America. What Can We Assume Today?*, ed. Lutz W, pp. 27–40. New York, NY, USA: Academic Press.

Feeney G (1996). Fertility in China: Past, present, prospects. In *The Future Population of the World. What Can We Assume Today?*, Revised Edition, ed. Lutz W, pp. 102–130. London, UK: Earthscan.

Frejka T & Calot G (2001). Cohort reproductive patterns in low fertility countries. *Population and Development Review* **27**:103–132.

Jeffrey R (2002). *Subjective Probability: The Real Thing*. Princeton, NJ, USA: Princeton University Press.

Keilman N (1999). How accurate are the United Nations world population projections? In *Frontiers of Population Forecasting*, eds. Lutz W, Vaupel JW & Ahlburg DA, pp. 15–41. Supplement to *Population and Development Review*, 1998, **24**. New York, NY, USA: The Population Council.

Keyfitz N (1981). The limits of population forecasting. *Population and Development Review* **7**:579–593.

Kohler HP & Philipov D (2001). Variance effects in the Bongaarts–Feeney formula. *Demography* **38**:1–16.

Lee RD (1999). Probabilistic approaches to population forecasting. In *Frontiers of Population Forecasting*, eds. Lutz W, Vaupel JW & Ahlburg DA, pp. 156–190. Supplement to *Population and Development Review*, 1998, **24**. New York, NY, USA: The Population Council.

Lutz W (1996a). *The Future Population of the World. What Can We Assume Today?*, Revised Edition. London, UK: Earthscan.

Lutz W (1996b). Future reproductive behavior in industrialized countries. In *The Future Population of the World. What Can We Assume Today?*, Revised Edition, ed. Lutz W, pp. 253–277. London, UK: Earthscan.

Lutz W & Ren Q (2002). Determinants of human population growth. *Philosophical Transactions of the Royal Society of London B* **357**:1197–1210.

Lutz W & Scherbov S (2003). Toward Structural and Argument-based Probabilistic Population Projections in Asia: Endogenizing the Education–Fertility Links, Interim Report IR-03-014. Laxenburg, Austria: International Institute for Applied Systems Analysis.

Lutz W, Saariluoma P, Sanderson WC & Scherbov S (2000). New Developments in the Methodology of Expert- and Argument-Based Probabilistic Forecasting. Interim Report IR-00-020. Laxenburg, Austria: International Institute for Applied Systems Analysis.

Lutz W, Sanderson W & Scherbov S (2001). The end of world population growth. *Nature* **412**:543–545.

Manton KG (1991). New biotechnologies and the limits to life expectancy. In *Future Demographic Trends in Europe and North America. What Can We Assume Today?*, ed. Lutz W, pp. 97–116. New York, NY, USA: Academic Press.

Manton KG, Stallard E & Tolley HD (1991). Limits to human life expectancy. *Population and Development Review* **17**:603–637.

Mesle F (1993). The future of mortality rates. In *The Future of Europe's Population: A Scenario Approach*, ed. Cliquet R, pp. 45–66. Strasbourg, France: The Council of Europe, European Population Committee.

National Research Council (2000). *Beyond Six Billion: Forecasting the World's Population*. Panel on Population Projections (eds. Bongaarts J & Bulatao RA). Committee on Population, Commission on Behavioral and Social Sciences and Education. Washington, DC, USA: National Academy Press.

Oeppen J & Vaupel JW (2002). Broken limits to life expectancy. *Science* **296**:1029–1031.

Olshansky SJ, Carnes BA & Cassel C (1990). In search of Methuselah: Estimating the upper limits of human longevity. *Science* **ii**:634–640.

Preston S (2001). *Demographic Surprises*. Keynote lecture delivered at the IUSSP General Conference 2001 in Salvador, Brazil. Unpublished.

Rogers A & Castro L (1981). *Model Migration Schedules*. Research Report RR-81-30. Laxenburg, Austria: International Institute for Applied Systems Analysis.

United Nations (1981). *Long-range Global Population Projections, Based on Data as Assessed in 1978*. ESA/P/WP.75. New York, NY, USA: United Nations, Population Division.

United Nations (1998). *World Population Prospects. The 1996 Revision*. ST/ESA/SER.A/167. New York, NY, USA: United Nations, Department of Economic and Social Affairs, Population Division.

United Nations (2001). *World Population Prospects: The 2000 Revision*, CD-ROM. New York, NY, USA: United Nations.

United Nations (2003a). *World Population Prospects: The 2002 Revision. Highlights.* New York, NY, USA: United Nations. (www.un.org/esa/population)

United Nations (2003b). *World Population in 2300. Highlights.* ESA/P/WP.187. Draft. New York, NY, USA: United Nations. (www.un.org/esa/population/publications/longrange2/longrange2.html)

US Census Bureau (2003). *US Bureau of the Census, International Data Base.* Washington, DC, USA: US Census Bureau. (www.census.gov/ipc/www/idbnew.html; data updated July, 17, 2003)

Vaupel JW & Lundström H (1996). The future of mortality at older ages in developed countries. In *The Future Population of the World. What Can We Assume Today?*, Revised Edition, ed. Lutz W, pp. 278–295. London, UK: Earthscan.

Vaupel JW, Carey JR, Christensen K, Johnson TE, Yashin AI, Holm NV, Iachine IA, Kannisto V, Khazaeli AA, Liedo P, Longo VD, Zeng Y, Manton KG & Curtsinger JW (1998). Biodemographic trajectories of longevity. *Science* **280**:855–860.

Vishnevsky A (1991). Demographic revolution and the future of fertility: A systems approach. In *Future Demographic Trends in Europe and North America. What Can We Assume Today?*, ed. Lutz W, pp. 257–270. New York, NY, USA: Academic Press.

World Bank (2002). *The 2002 World Development Indicators*, CD-ROM. Washington DC, USA: International Bank for Reconstruction and Development, The World Bank.

Zhai Z, Liu S, Chen W & Duan CR (2000). Stabilizing China's low fertility: Concepts, theories and strategies. *Population Research* **24**:1–17.

Zlotnik H (1996). Migration to and from developing regions: A review of past trends. In *The Future Population of the World. What Can We Assume Today?*, Revised Edition, ed. Lutz W, pp. 299–335. London, UK: Earthscan.

Chapter 3

Applications of Probabilistic Population Forecasting

Warren C. Sanderson, Sergei Scherbov, Wolfgang Lutz, and Brian C. O'Neill

In Chapter 2, we present probabilistic forecasts for the population of the world and 13 regions from 2000 to 2100. A key element of our approach is making forecasts that are not just single numbers, but distributions of possibilities at future dates. These distributions allow us to develop new forecasting applications and to explore older ones in a new light. In this chapter, we look at three sorts of applications: the probabilistic analysis of age structures, conditional probabilistic forecasting, and probabilistic forecasting with future jump-off dates.

Although probabilistic population forecasting originally focused on population size, it is increasingly used in the analysis of future patterns of age structure. The issue that motivates this study is the viability of national pension systems. Policy makers need to know the likelihood that pension systems will remain within certain financial limits in the future. This depends not only on the number and age distribution of future pensioners, but on the age distribution of those who contribute to the system as well. Since fertility, mortality, and migration are all uncertain in themselves, they generate patterns of uncertainty in the ratio of pensioners to contributors that are impossible to predict without probabilistic population forecasts. We present information on six aspects of aging:

- Proportion of the population aged 60 and older.
- Proportion of the population aged 80 and older.

- Ratio of the population aged 60 and older to those aged 20–59.
- Proportion of the population younger than 20.
- Ratios of the numbers of people aged 60 and older and 80 and older to the number of people younger than 20.
- Median age of the voting population.

We then move to the second of our applications, conditional probabilistic forecasting. We have already informally introduced the idea of conditional forecasting in Chapter 2, where we look at the distribution of the world's population by region conditional on its being either below 6 billion or above 12 billion in 2100. Here we take a more systematic look at conditional forecasting. Such conditional forecasts are particularly important for policy considerations. Policy makers might want to know the consequences of, for example, alternative fertility paths. Traditionally, such questions have been addressed through alternative scenarios. Here, we show how the scenario approach can be integrated into the broader context of probabilistic forecasting.

In the final section, we discuss probabilistic forecasts that start some time in the future. Population forecasts made in the future will be different from those made today because of the observations made between now and then. We can predict today what our future forecasts will be, conditional on those observations. This allows us to tell policy makers not only what distributions of outcomes to expect on the basis of today's information, but also how those distributions are likely to change as we gather more observations with the passage of time.

3.1   Massive Population Aging

The introduction to this book begins with the statement that, while the 20th century was the century of population growth, the 21st century will be the century of population aging. In Chapter 2 we discuss the slowing of population growth rates; in this chapter we show that the population of the world and of each of our 13 regions will grow significantly older. Data on the first decile, median, ninth decile, and the uncertainty measure for the proportion of the population aged 60 and older are given in *Table 3.1* for the world at 25-year intervals from 2000 to 2100. The uncertainty measure that we use here is the relative interdecile range (RIDR). It is simply the interdecile range (the ninth decile minus the first decile) divided by the median. In 2000, 10 percent of the world's population was aged 60 and older. According to our median forecast, this proportion will grow to around one-third by 2100. The interdecile range in 2100 is between 24 and 44 percent. The aging of the world's population will happen gradually, but regularly, over the 21st century. The median proportion that is aged 60 and older increases by around 12 percentage points from

Table 3.1. Distribution of forecast proportions of world population aged 60 and older and RIDR, at 25-year intervals from 2000 to 2100.

Year	1st decile	Median	9th decile	RIDR[a]
2000	0.100	0.100	0.100	–
2025	0.134	0.148	0.162	0.191
2050	0.173	0.217	0.266	0.430
2075	0.208	0.277	0.359	0.543
2100	0.243	0.336	0.437	0.578

[a]The relative interdecile range (RIDR) is the difference between the ninth decile of the distribution and the first decile divided by the median.
Source: Authors' calculations.

2000 to 2050, and then by another 12 percentage points from 2050 to 2100. In terms of population growth, the first half of the 21st century will be far different from the second half, but in terms of aging, the two halves are almost identical.

Table 3.2 shows the same sort of information for our regions. In 2100, sub-Saharan Africa will have the lowest proportion of its population aged 60 and older, with only 20 percent in the category according to the median forecast. This is around the same proportion of people aged 60 and older that we find in the Pacific OECD,[1] Western Europe, Eastern Europe, and FSU Europe[2] today. The aging of the sub-Saharan African population will be much slower than for the world as a whole in the first half of the 21st century, after which it will become much faster. According to the median forecast, the proportion aged 60 and older rises from 5 percent of the population in 2000 to only 7 percent in 2050, and then rises much more rapidly to 20 percent in 2100.

The Pacific OECD is at the other end of the spectrum. In 2000, 22 percent of its population was already aged 60 and older. This proportion is expected to rise rapidly during the first half of the 21st century to 39 percent in 2050 (according to the median forecast) and then somewhat more slowly to 49 percent in 2100. Its interdecile range in 2100 is between 36 and 62 percent of the population.

North America, Western Europe, and Eastern Europe are expected to follow the same pattern as the Pacific OECD, but at somewhat lower proportions. In Western Europe, for example, the proportion aged 60 and older is expected to rise from 20 percent in 2000, to 35 percent in 2050, and to 45 percent at the end of the 21st century. The surprise in *Table 3.2* comes when we look at FSU Europe. Like the Pacific OECD, North America, Western Europe, and Eastern Europe, rapid aging occurs in FSU Europe in the first half of the 21st century, but then, quite in contrast to those other regions, it virtually comes to an end for the next 50 years. FSU Europe, which began the 21st century with proportions aged 60 and older like those

---

[1]Organisation for Economic Co-operation and Development members in the Pacific region.
[2]European part of the former Soviet Union.

Table 3.2. Distribution of forecast proportions of regional populations aged 60 and older and RIDR, at 25-year intervals from 2000 to 2100.

Region	1st decile	Median	9th decile	RIDR[a]
North Africa				
2000	0.061	0.061	0.061	–
2025	0.091	0.102	0.115	0.242
2050	0.147	0.190	0.238	0.483
2075	0.201	0.272	0.358	0.576
2100	0.225	0.322	0.431	0.641
Sub-Saharan Africa				
2000	0.046	0.046	0.046	–
2025	0.044	0.049	0.056	0.251
2050	0.050	0.068	0.089	0.576
2075	0.091	0.133	0.187	0.727
2100	0.138	0.196	0.267	0.660
North America				
2000	0.164	0.164	0.164	–
2025	0.231	0.254	0.279	0.189
2050	0.231	0.295	0.364	0.452
2075	0.255	0.347	0.450	0.561
2100	0.279	0.400	0.519	0.602
Latin America				
2000	0.079	0.079	0.079	–
2025	0.117	0.132	0.147	0.225
2050	0.171	0.220	0.277	0.479
2075	0.202	0.283	0.379	0.623
2100	0.222	0.326	0.441	0.672
Central Asia				
2000	0.083	0.083	0.083	–
2025	0.103	0.117	0.131	0.241
2050	0.149	0.194	0.248	0.508
2075	0.202	0.279	0.367	0.593
2100	0.238	0.340	0.453	0.633
Middle East				
2000	0.056	0.056	0.056	–
2025	0.076	0.087	0.100	0.264
2050	0.139	0.179	0.226	0.486
2075	0.213	0.285	0.368	0.543
2100	0.244	0.350	0.465	0.634
South Asia				
2000	0.070	0.070	0.070	–
2025	0.092	0.104	0.118	0.243
2050	0.136	0.177	0.226	0.506
2075	0.201	0.271	0.357	0.574
2100	0.248	0.351	0.469	0.629

[a]The relative interdecile range (RIDR) is the difference between the ninth decile of the distribution and the first decile divided by the median.
Source: Authors' calculations.

Table 3.2. Continued.

	1st decile	Median	9th decile	RIDR[a]
China region				
2000	0.099	0.099	0.099	–
2025	0.172	0.188	0.205	0.176
2050	0.242	0.303	0.370	0.424
2075	0.254	0.350	0.462	0.594
2100	0.268	0.393	0.530	0.665
Pacific Asia				
2000	0.076	0.076	0.076	–
2025	0.122	0.136	0.151	0.210
2050	0.177	0.227	0.285	0.476
2075	0.210	0.290	0.386	0.608
2100	0.252	0.360	0.485	0.649
Pacific OECD[b]				
2000	0.220	0.220	0.220	–
2025	0.290	0.319	0.350	0.188
2050	0.313	0.390	0.470	0.402
2075	0.313	0.427	0.545	0.544
2100	0.356	0.491	0.619	0.535
Western Europe				
2000	0.199	0.199	0.199	–
2025	0.249	0.274	0.299	0.181
2050	0.281	0.353	0.429	0.418
2075	0.288	0.396	0.510	0.560
2100	0.314	0.448	0.585	0.605
Eastern Europe				
2000	0.177	0.177	0.177	–
2025	0.240	0.263	0.287	0.181
2050	0.300	0.377	0.459	0.422
2075	0.279	0.397	0.527	0.625
2100	0.287	0.422	0.569	0.668
FSU Europe[c]				
2000	0.187	0.187	0.187	–
2025	0.241	0.263	0.286	0.168
2050	0.287	0.360	0.439	0.423
2075	0.252	0.360	0.487	0.653
2100	0.245	0.367	0.503	0.701

[a]The relative interdecile range (RIDR) is the difference between the ninth decile of the distribution and the first decile divided by the median.
[b]Organisation for Economic Co-operation and Development members in the Pacific region.
[c]European part of the former Soviet Union.
Source: Authors' calculations.

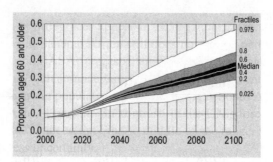

Figure 3.1. Evolution of the distribution of the proportion of the population aged 60 and older in Pacific Asia. *Source*: Authors' calculations.

seen in the rest of Europe, ends it with proportions more like those in Pacific Asia, the China region, the Middle East, Central Asia, and Latin America.

The main reason for this anomalous behavior has to do with fertility. Fertility currently is extremely low in FSU Europe, but we do not expect that it will stay so low over the entire 21st century. Indeed, we assume that in the long run fertility in FSU Europe will be roughly the same as in North America. The low proportion aged 60 and older in the second half of the 21st century arises in part because of the relatively low fertility early in the century and the considerably higher fertility during the second half. Not only is the median proportion aged 60 and older in FSU Europe relatively low in 2100, but it is also the most uncertain of all the regional proportions. The interdecile range is between 25 and 50 percent.

There is some concern in political circles in Europe that North America, with its higher fertility and higher migration rate, will have an economic advantage over Europe because of its younger population. In this regard, it is interesting to compare the proportions aged 60 and older in Western Europe and North America. In 2000, the proportion was around 4 percentage points higher in Western Europe, 20 percent compared with 16 percent in North America. *Table 3.2* shows that, as the century progresses, the difference in proportions remains quite constant. In 2100, according to the median forecast, the difference is only 5 percentage points, 45 percent in Western Europe and 40 percent in North America.

Pacific Asia is a good representative of regions that are not at the extremes. *Figure 3.1* shows how the distribution of these proportions changes over time. In 2000, 8 percent of the population was aged 60 and older. A half-century later, the median proportion rises to 23 percent and then to slightly over one-third at the end of the 21st century. The evolution of the proportion aged 60 and older in Pacific Asia and its uncertainty shown in *Figure 3.1* are typical of many of our regions.

Let us move now from the proportion aged 60 and older to the proportion aged 80 and older. *Table 3.3* shows the data for the world. In 2000 only around 1 percent

Table 3.3. Distribution of forecast proportions of world population aged 80 and older and RIDR, at 25-year intervals from 2000 to 2100.

Year	1st decile	Median	9th decile	RIDR[a]
2000	0.011	0.011	0.011	–
2025	0.014	0.017	0.020	0.401
2050	0.023	0.040	0.064	1.024
2075	0.028	0.068	0.125	1.431
2100	0.039	0.108	0.199	1.480

[a]The relative interdecile range (RIDR) is the difference between the ninth decile of the distribution and the first decile divided by the median.
Source: Authors' calculations.

of the world's population was aged 80 and older. By 2050, according to the median forecast, that fraction will climb to 4 percent, and then to 11 percent in 2100. To put this 11 percent figure into some perspective, we should remember that this is slightly higher than the proportion of the population aged 60 and older in 2000.

The proportions aged 80 and older are extremely uncertain because we must allow for such an enormous variety of possibilities concerning life expectancy a century in the future. The interdecile range around the 11 percent figure lies between a low of 4 percent and a high of 20 percent. The uncertainty measure, RIDR, for the proportion aged 60 and older in 2050 is 0.430. The analogous figure for the proportion aged 80 and older is 1.024. In 2100, the two uncertainty figures are 0.578 and 1.480, respectively. We must be very cautious, therefore, in discussing what the proportion of the population aged 80 and older will be, especially after 2050. We can meaningfully talk about those proportions only in terms of wide intervals.

Regional forecasts of the proportion of the population aged 80 and older are shown in *Table 3.4*. The Pacific OECD has the highest proportion of its population aged 80 and older. *Figure 3.2* shows how the distribution of this proportion develops. In 2000 it was around 4 percent. According to the median forecast, it rises to 13 percent in 2050 and then to 26 percent in 2100. In comparison, the proportion of the population in that region aged 60 and older was 22 percent in 2000. In addition to having a considerably smaller population in 2100, the Pacific OECD could have a greater proportion aged 80 and older than it has aged 60 and older today. Although the uncertainty of the proportion aged 80 and older is smallest in the Pacific OECD region, it is still considerable. The interdecile range (not shown in the figure) is from 10 to 40 percent.

A world in which 40 percent of the population is aged 80 and older would certainly be an extremely different world from the one we inhabit today. The Pacific OECD region is not alone in this respect. In Western Europe, the upper end of the interdecile range in 2100 is around 36 percent. If extremely large increases in the

Table 3.4. Distribution of forecast proportions of regional populations aged 80 and older and RIDR, at 25-year intervals from 2000 to 2100.

	1st decile	Median	9th decile	RIDR[a]
North Africa				
2000	0.005	0.005	0.005	–
2025	0.007	0.008	0.010	0.360
2050	0.013	0.024	0.040	1.143
2075	0.018	0.055	0.110	1.675
2100	0.026	0.097	0.198	1.774
Sub-Saharan Africa				
2000	0.003	0.003	0.003	–
2025	0.003	0.003	0.003	0.253
2050	0.003	0.005	0.006	0.600
2075	0.005	0.010	0.017	1.214
2100	0.005	0.023	0.053	2.080
North America				
2000	0.032	0.032	0.032	–
2025	0.029	0.037	0.048	0.518
2050	0.042	0.087	0.143	1.166
2075	0.051	0.126	0.220	1.337
2100	0.073	0.186	0.308	1.267
Latin America				
2000	0.009	0.009	0.009	–
2025	0.011	0.013	0.016	0.415
2050	0.020	0.037	0.061	1.115
2075	0.024	0.070	0.139	1.639
2100	0.031	0.111	0.217	1.675
Central Asia				
2000	0.008	0.008	0.008	–
2025	0.008	0.009	0.011	0.405
2050	0.014	0.028	0.048	1.174
2075	0.022	0.064	0.125	1.615
2100	0.035	0.110	0.213	1.621
Middle East				
2000	0.005	0.005	0.005	–
2025	0.006	0.007	0.009	0.429
2050	0.012	0.023	0.039	1.180
2075	0.023	0.063	0.122	1.568
2100	0.038	0.121	0.232	1.610
South Asia				
2000	0.006	0.006	0.006	–
2025	0.007	0.009	0.010	0.314
2050	0.012	0.020	0.032	1.001
2075	0.017	0.046	0.092	1.643
2100	0.023	0.088	0.190	1.908

[a]The relative interdecile range (RIDR) is the difference between the ninth decile of the distribution and the first decile divided by the median.
Source: Authors' calculations.

Table 3.4. Continued.

	1st decile	Median	9th decile	RIDR[a]
China region				
2000	0.009	0.009	0.009	–
2025	0.015	0.018	0.022	0.379
2050	0.035	0.062	0.100	1.059
2075	0.037	0.100	0.193	1.549
2100	0.042	0.143	0.280	1.661
Pacific Asia				
2000	0.006	0.006	0.006	–
2025	0.010	0.012	0.015	0.355
2050	0.019	0.035	0.058	1.100
2075	0.021	0.066	0.133	1.699
2100	0.030	0.111	0.225	1.753
Pacific OECD[b]				
2000	0.035	0.035	0.035	–
2025	0.057	0.075	0.095	0.514
2050	0.069	0.129	0.200	1.021
2075	0.073	0.179	0.307	1.307
2100	0.112	0.258	0.399	1.111
Western Europe				
2000	0.033	0.033	0.033	–
2025	0.036	0.047	0.060	0.499
2050	0.056	0.106	0.167	1.055
2075	0.058	0.148	0.263	1.384
2100	0.081	0.214	0.358	1.291
Eastern Europe				
2000	0.019	0.019	0.019	–
2025	0.031	0.038	0.047	0.418
2050	0.044	0.083	0.136	1.095
2075	0.051	0.142	0.265	1.504
2100	0.058	0.176	0.326	1.519
FSU Europe[c]				
2000	0.020	0.020	0.020	–
2025	0.027	0.033	0.039	0.375
2050	0.040	0.071	0.115	1.059
2075	0.040	0.117	0.226	1.592
2100	0.037	0.132	0.263	1.710

[a]The relative interdecile range (RIDR) is the difference between the ninth decile of the distribution and the first decile divided by the median.
[b]Organisation for Economic Co-operation and Development members in the Pacific region.
[c]European part of the former Soviet Union.
Source: Authors' calculations.

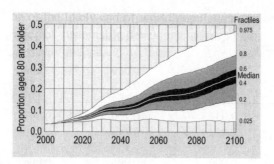

Figure 3.2. Evolution of the distribution of the proportion of the population aged 80 and older in the Pacific OECD region. Note the wide uncertainty by 2100. *Source*: Authors' calculations.

proportion aged 80 and older are to occur in the future, they will do so only during the second half of the 21st century, and this development will be slow enough to give plenty of time to plan and adjust.

Sub-Saharan Africa is forecast to have by far the lowest proportion aged 80 and older in 2100. The median forecast yields a proportion only of around 2 percent, with an interdecile range between nearly 0 percent and 5 percent. This low proportion results in part from the HIV/AIDS pandemic, which will kill children and young mothers for at least the next decade, and so reduce the number of people surviving to age 80 in 2100. However, it also results from a combination of relatively high fertility and relatively low life expectancy for reasons other than HIV/AIDS.

Many regions with only a small percentage of their populations aged 80 and older in 2000 will have around 10 percent in that age group in 2100. These include North Africa, Latin America, Central Asia, the Middle East, South Asia, and Pacific Asia. Clearly, the world's population will be aging considerably during the 21st century. As with the proportions aged 60 and older, the differences between North America and Western Europe in terms of proportions of the population aged 80 and older are small and extremely uncertain. When people think about the increased proportion elderly in 2100, they often have in mind the examples of the elderly people that they know today. But the elderly in 2100 will be much more educated than today's older population. An 80-year-old in 2100 will have been born in 2020 and will graduate secondary school in around 2038. By the time those born in 2020 go to school, enrollment rates will be much higher than they were when today's 80-year-olds were being educated. For more information about the likely educational attainments of populations in the future, see Chapters 4, 7, and 8.

Another perspective on the aging question, however, can be obtained by looking at the old-age dependency ratio. This figure is the ratio of the population aged 60 and older to the population aged 20–59. If people all retired at age 60 and

Table 3.5. Distribution of forecast old-age dependency ratios and RIDR for world population, at 25-year intervals from 2000 to 2100.

Year	1st decile	Median	9th decile	RIDR[a]
2000	0.196	0.196	0.196	–
2025	0.260	0.278	0.298	0.135
2050	0.324	0.418	0.530	0.493
2075	0.375	0.562	0.804	0.765
2100	0.429	0.717	1.088	0.920

[a]The relative interdecile range (RIDR) is the difference between the ninth decile of the distribution and the first decile divided by the median.
Source: Authors' calculations.

all worked from age 20–59, the old-age dependency ratio would be the ratio of retirees to workers. Data on that ratio for the world are given in *Table 3.5*. We need to recognize that people aged 60 and older are not necessarily "dependent." The term "dependency ratio" is archaic, but it is commonly used in the literature, and to employ any other term here would be needlessly confusing.

Table 3.5 shows the first, median, and ninth deciles of the distributions of dependency ratios as well as the RIDR for the world for the years 2000, 2025, 2050, 2075, and 2100. Two general observations can be drawn immediately from *Table 3.5*. First, dependency ratios increase rapidly as the 21st century progresses and, second, the amount of uncertainty about those ratios is considerable, especially later in the century.

For the world as a whole, the dependency ratio increases from 20 percent in the year 2000 to 42 percent in 2050 and then to 72 percent in 2100 (median forecast). In other words, relative to the number of people aged 20–59, the total number of older people will increase more than 3.5-fold over the century. However, that 72 percent figure is very unsure, with an interdecile range of between 43 and 109 percent. To put this in other terms, in the world as a whole in 2000 there were about five people aged 20–59 for every person aged 60 and older. We expect that number to decline to around 2.5 by 2050, and to only around 1.4 by 2100. The prediction interval in 2100 is from nearly 2 people aged 20–59 for each person aged 60 and older to 0.9 people (less than one working-age person) for every person aged 60 and older.

Let us continue our discussion about the demographic differences between North America and Western Europe. The figures for regional dependency rates are shown in *Table 3.6*. The old-age dependency ratio in Western Europe in 2000 was 36 percent. In North America it was 30 percent. By mid-century the median ratio in Western Europe grows to 77 percent, while in North America it increases to only 61 percent. For each person in Western Europe aged 60 and older, there will be 1.3 people aged 20–59. In North America, that figure will be 1.6 people. The interdecile range for the old-age dependency ratio in Western Europe in 2050 is from 55 to 102 percent. In North America, the range covers the interval from 44 to 81 percent. Clearly, there is so much overlap in these intervals that we cannot make a firm prediction that in 2050 the old-age dependency ratio will be considerably lower in North America than in Western Europe. In 2100, the median forecast of the ratio is 114 percent in Western Europe and 99 percent in North America. In the current forecasts there is such a wide overlap in the interdecile ranges for 2100 that there can be no firm conclusion that the difference in the ratios will be economically significant.

As expected, the Pacific OECD region had the highest dependency ratio in 2000 and continues to top the table in 2100. In 2000, the dependency ratio was 39 percent. The median dependency ratio in 2100 is 134 percent. To put this somewhat differently, for every 100 people aged 20–59 in 2100, we expect there to be 134 people aged 60 and older. The interdecile range for this number is between 63 and 222 elderly per 100 persons of working age. Thus, although it is clear that the dependency ratio will increase over the 21st century in the Pacific OECD, it is unclear whether in 2100 it will be only twice as large as in 2000 or five times as large.

The dependency ratio changes very differently in sub-Saharan Africa. In 2000 it is 12 percent, and the median figure for 2050 is only 13 percent. Over the second half of the 21st century, the median increases to 36 percent, far lower than in any other region in the world. Even the uncertainty regarding the future distribution of the dependency ratio is lower for sub-Saharan Africa. The interdecile range for the year 2100 is between 23 and 53 percent.

It is interesting to compare the interdecile ranges in 2100 for Latin America and FSU Europe. The lower end of the interval is 38 percent in Latin America and a marginally higher 39 percent in FSU Europe. The upper bounds on those intervals, however, are very different: 117 percent for Latin America and 147 percent in FSU Europe. These interdecile ranges take into account the complex interactions between fertility, mortality, and migration paths and the initial age structure of the population. Depending on these interactions, the interdecile ranges can have similar lower bounds and different upper bounds, as in this case. These uncertainty distributions provide useful information for policy makers, but are impossible to predict without probabilistic forecasting.

We turn now to the other end of the age distribution. *Table 3.7* shows the proportions of the world's population younger than 20. In 2000, around 39 percent of the world's population was in that age group. The proportion decreases to about 27 percent in 2050 and to 19 percent in 2100 in the median scenario. Let us try to put this last figure into perspective. Imagine a world in which the number of births is constant and everyone lives exactly 100 years. In this world, we would not have an age pyramid, but an age rectangle, with the same number of people in each age

Table 3.6. Distribution of forecast old-age dependency ratios and RIDR for regional populations, at 25-year intervals from 2000 to 2100.

	1st decile	Median	9th decile	RIDR[a]
North Africa				
2000	0.130	0.130	0.130	–
2025	0.180	0.192	0.205	0.129
2050	0.266	0.351	0.456	0.541
2075	0.356	0.554	0.811	0.822
2100	0.372	0.688	1.112	1.076
Sub-Saharan Africa				
2000	0.116	0.116	0.116	–
2025	0.109	0.111	0.113	0.041
2050	0.103	0.129	0.160	0.438
2075	0.157	0.243	0.359	0.830
2100	0.230	0.356	0.530	0.843
North America				
2000	0.297	0.297	0.297	–
2025	0.456	0.505	0.557	0.199
2050	0.439	0.609	0.813	0.613
2075	0.484	0.789	1.170	0.870
2100	0.528	0.987	1.548	1.034
Latin America				
2000	0.156	0.156	0.156	–
2025	0.225	0.243	0.261	0.149
2050	0.322	0.429	0.557	0.547
2075	0.360	0.590	0.899	0.913
2100	0.379	0.717	1.165	1.096
Central Asia				
2000	0.178	0.178	0.178	–
2025	0.206	0.220	0.235	0.133
2050	0.274	0.366	0.480	0.562
2075	0.358	0.568	0.835	0.841
2100	0.410	0.738	1.169	1.027
Middle East				
2000	0.127	0.127	0.127	–
2025	0.155	0.166	0.179	0.141
2050	0.250	0.330	0.425	0.533
2075	0.386	0.583	0.833	0.767
2100	0.424	0.773	1.224	1.036
South Asia				
2000	0.146	0.146	0.146	–
2025	0.183	0.193	0.205	0.117
2050	0.241	0.318	0.414	0.544
2075	0.342	0.524	0.765	0.808
2100	0.397	0.724	1.181	1.083

[a]The relative interdecile range (RIDR) is the difference between the ninth decile of the distribution and the first decile divided by the median.
Source: Authors' calculations.

Table 3.6. Continued.

	1st decile	Median	9th decile	RIDR[a]
China region				
2000	0.175	0.175	0.175	–
2025	0.306	0.329	0.354	0.145
2050	0.457	0.614	0.803	0.564
2075	0.440	0.757	1.197	0.999
2100	0.418	0.905	1.581	1.285
Pacific Asia				
2000	0.144	0.144	0.144	–
2025	0.230	0.246	0.263	0.135
2050	0.327	0.438	0.571	0.558
2075	0.350	0.581	0.897	0.941
2100	0.415	0.783	1.280	1.105
Pacific OECD[b]				
2000	0.392	0.392	0.392	–
2025	0.578	0.649	0.722	0.222
2050	0.642	0.908	1.206	0.621
2075	0.579	1.037	1.648	1.031
2100	0.626	1.340	2.222	1.191
Western Europe				
2000	0.360	0.360	0.360	–
2025	0.478	0.528	0.581	0.195
2050	0.553	0.770	1.022	0.609
2075	0.530	0.926	1.431	0.972
2100	0.548	1.141	1.929	1.210
Eastern Europe				
2000	0.316	0.316	0.316	–
2025	0.448	0.488	0.534	0.176
2050	0.604	0.848	1.140	0.632
2075	0.466	0.919	1.555	1.184
2100	0.445	1.027	1.846	1.364
FSU Europe[c]				
2000	0.342	0.342	0.342	–
2025	0.454	0.489	0.528	0.151
2050	0.580	0.791	1.062	0.610
2075	0.416	0.810	1.365	1.172
2100	0.393	0.838	1.466	1.280

[a]The relative interdecile range (RIDR) is the difference between the ninth decile of the distribution and the first decile divided by the median.
[b]Organisation for Economic Co-operation and Development members in the Pacific region.
[c]European part of the former Soviet Union.
Source: Authors' calculations.

Table 3.7. Distribution of forecast proportions of world population younger than 20 and RIDR, at 25-year intervals from 2000 to 2100.

Year	1st decile	Median	9th decile	RIDR[a]
2000	0.389	0.389	0.389	–
2025	0.274	0.323	0.366	0.287
2050	0.212	0.266	0.315	0.387
2075	0.176	0.227	0.274	0.431
2100	0.145	0.194	0.248	0.531

[a]The relative interdecile range (RIDR) is the difference between the ninth decile of the distribution and the first decile divided by the median.
Source: Authors' calculations.

group. In that hypothetical world, 20 percent of the population would be in the 0–19 age group, almost exactly the proportion that is projected for 2100. The 0–19 age group covers one-fifth of all the ages from 0 through 99 and in 2100 would have about one-fifth of the world's population.

In 2100, the interdecile range for the proportion under 20 spans the interval from around 15 percent to around 25 percent. Even the larger figure is considerably lower than the proportion in 2000. In 2025, there is more uncertainty about the proportion under 20 than there is about the proportion aged 60 and older. This is because none of the people in the under-20 age group were alive when the forecast was made, but all of those aged 60 and older were. By 2100, the uncertainties in the numbers of people in the two age groups converge (see *Tables 3.1* and *3.7*).

Table 3.8 shows the proportions of the population younger than 20 for our regions. In Latin America, 42 percent of the population was 20 or younger in 2000. According to the median forecast, that proportion is expected to fall rapidly over the first half of the 21st century to 26 percent in 2050, and then to 22 percent in 2100. In North America, the proportion in 2000 was 28 percent, and it falls much more slowly than that in Latin America, reaching 22 percent in 2050 and 19 percent in 2100. Thus, although they start at different levels, after 2050 the proportions of young people in the population are forecast to be roughly the same in Latin America and in North America.

Seven of our 13 regions have median proportions younger than 20 years in 2100 that are above 19 percent. This very heterogeneous group comprises North Africa, sub-Saharan Africa, North America, Latin America, Central Asia, the Middle East, and FSU Europe. Six regions have lower proportions: South Asia, the China region, Pacific Asia, the Pacific OECD, Western Europe, and Eastern Europe. This regional grouping is mainly the result of our assumption about long-run fertility levels (see Chapter 2). Simply put, we believe that, in the long run, fertility will be higher in regions with lower population density.

Table 3.8. Distribution of forecast proportions of regional populations younger than 20 and RIDR, for 2000, 2025, 2050, and 2100.

	1st decile	Median	9th decile	RIDR[a]
North Africa				
2000	0.468	0.468	0.468	–
2025	0.298	0.365	0.419	0.332
2050	0.220	0.274	0.323	0.376
2100	0.156	0.212	0.266	0.517
Sub-Saharan Africa				
2000	0.553	0.553	0.553	–
2025	0.447	0.506	0.554	0.211
2050	0.329	0.408	0.471	0.348
2100	0.198	0.257	0.313	0.446
North America				
2000	0.282	0.282	0.282	–
2025	0.203	0.241	0.281	0.327
2050	0.173	0.221	0.270	0.436
2100	0.137	0.192	0.255	0.615
Latin America				
2000	0.416	0.416	0.416	–
2025	0.269	0.327	0.376	0.328
2050	0.205	0.264	0.318	0.428
2100	0.160	0.218	0.278	0.538
Central Asia				
2000	0.450	0.450	0.450	–
2025	0.291	0.355	0.408	0.331
2050	0.215	0.273	0.327	0.409
2100	0.142	0.196	0.254	0.571
Middle East				
2000	0.503	0.503	0.503	–
2025	0.320	0.391	0.444	0.317
2050	0.226	0.278	0.326	0.359
2100	0.142	0.193	0.249	0.555
South Asia				
2000	0.450	0.450	0.450	–
2025	0.289	0.357	0.410	0.338
2050	0.206	0.265	0.317	0.420
2100	0.109	0.163	0.218	0.666

[a]The relative interdecile range (RIDR) is the difference between the ninth decile of the distribution and the first decile divided by the median.

Source: Authors' calculations.

Table 3.8. Continued.

	1st decile	Median	9th decile	RIDR[a]
China region				
2000	0.336	0.336	0.336	–
2025	0.196	0.243	0.284	0.363
2050	0.148	0.204	0.257	0.532
2100	0.112	0.170	0.234	0.715
Pacific Asia				
2000	0.398	0.398	0.398	–
2025	0.255	0.310	0.359	0.337
2050	0.199	0.254	0.303	0.409
2100	0.115	0.173	0.232	0.676
Pacific OECD[b]				
2000	0.218	0.218	0.218	–
2025	0.149	0.188	0.227	0.412
2050	0.127	0.179	0.225	0.545
2100	0.088	0.140	0.198	0.788
Western Europe				
2000	0.250	0.250	0.250	–
2025	0.166	0.210	0.247	0.385
2050	0.138	0.188	0.236	0.525
2100	0.101	0.156	0.218	0.754
Eastern Europe				
2000	0.264	0.264	0.264	–
2025	0.153	0.202	0.241	0.439
2050	0.123	0.177	0.234	0.626
2100	0.100	0.162	0.228	0.792
FSU Europe[c]				
2000	0.268	0.268	0.268	–
2025	0.154	0.201	0.244	0.447
2050	0.133	0.188	0.241	0.575
2100	0.134	0.194	0.260	0.649

[a]The relative interdecile range (RIDR) is the difference between the ninth decile of the distribution and the first decile divided by the median.
[b]Organisation for Economic Co-operation and Development members in the Pacific region.
[c]European part of the former Soviet Union.
Source: Authors' calculations

Perhaps the biggest surprise in *Table 3.8* is provided by the RIDRs. We are more certain about the proportion younger than 20 in sub-Saharan Africa than in the Pacific OECD region. The main reason for this difference is the interaction between differences in age structures and mortality variability. Mortality uncertainty, especially by 2100, is very large. When this uncertainty is combined with a very old population, such as that in the Pacific OECD, considerable uncertainty in population size is generated. This uncertainty is important here because we are considering the proportion of the total population younger than 20. Uncertainty about the size of the total population is translated into uncertainty about that proportion. In sub-Saharan Africa, however, while mortality is even more uncertain, the population is so young that even large variations in mortality rates do not cause such large differences in population size.

In *Table 3.9* we show the ratio of the number of people aged 60 and older and the ratio of the number of people aged 80 and older to the number of people aged 0–19 for our 13 regions. Instead of distributions, in *Table 3.9* we give ratios of the median forecasts only. Let us begin with the Pacific OECD again. In 2000, for every 100 people aged 0–19 there were 101 people aged 60 and older, and 16 people aged 80 and older. By 2050, the forecast says that for every 100 people aged 0–19 there will be 219 people aged 60 and older, and 72 people aged 80 and older. By 2100, for every 100 people aged 0–19 there is expected to be 352 people aged 60 and older, and 185 people aged 80 and older. In other words, there could be around 2 people aged 80 and older for each person aged 0–19. In 2100, the elderly will distinctly outnumber the young.

In *Table 3.9*, six regions besides the Pacific OECD show more than 200 people aged 60 and older for every 100 people aged 0–19 in 2100: North America, South Asia, the China region, Pacific Asia, Western Europe, and Eastern Europe. In Asia, only Central Asia has fewer than 200 (in fact, 174) people aged 60 and older for every 100 people aged 0–19. In Europe, only FSU Europe has a figure lower than 200, which in 2100 is 189 people aged 60 and older for every person aged 0–19. In Chapter 10, we introduce a new concept that deals with relationships between the welfare of people and age structures. The unbalanced age structures foreseen here were one of the motivating factors behind the development of this new concept.

Sub-Saharan Africa is the only region that in 2100 is expected to have fewer people aged 60 and older than it has people aged 0–19. For every 100 young people there are expected to be only 76 people aged 60 and older, and 9 people aged 80 and older. The age structure of sub-Saharan Africa is currently very different from those of more developed regions. By 2100, we expect it to be vastly different from the age structure of every other region in the world.

We conclude our consideration of the probabilistic forecasting of age structures with some political considerations. It is natural to imagine that political power in

Table 3.9. Ratios of populations aged 60 and older and 80 and older to those aged 19 and younger using median forecasts, for 13 regions for 2000, 2025, 2050, and 2100.

Region	Year	Ratio 60 and older to 19 and younger	Ratio 80 and older to 19 and younger
North Africa	2000	0.131	0.010
	2025	0.281	0.022
	2050	0.693	0.088
	2100	1.522	0.458
Sub-Saharan Africa	2000	0.084	0.006
	2025	0.098	0.006
	2050	0.166	0.011
	2100	0.760	0.089
North America	2000	0.582	0.115
	2025	1.057	0.155
	2050	1.334	0.393
	2100	2.081	0.967
Latin America	2000	0.189	0.021
	2025	0.403	0.040
	2050	0.836	0.139
	2100	1.495	0.509
Central Asia	2000	0.185	0.018
	2025	0.329	0.026
	2050	0.712	0.103
	2100	1.736	0.563
Middle East	2000	0.111	0.010
	2025	0.223	0.019
	2050	0.642	0.082
	2100	1.812	0.626
South Asia	2000	0.156	0.013
	2025	0.292	0.024
	2050	0.669	0.077
	2100	2.147	0.538
China region	2000	0.293	0.027
	2025	0.771	0.074
	2050	1.488	0.305
	2100	2.315	0.844
Pacific Asia	2000	0.191	0.015
	2025	0.438	0.040
	2050	0.893	0.139
	2100	2.086	0.643
Pacific OECD[a]	2000	1.008	0.161
	2025	1.695	0.397
	2050	2.187	0.723
	2100	3.517	1.851
Western Europe	2000	0.795	0.134
	2025	1.302	0.225
	2050	1.880	0.563
	2100	2.878	1.376
Eastern Europe	2000	0.670	0.070
	2025	1.302	0.189
	2050	2.126	0.469
	2100	2.610	1.091
FSU Europe[b]	2000	0.697	0.074
	2025	1.307	0.162
	2050	1.912	0.379
	2100	1.892	0.683

[a]Organisation for Economic Co-operation and Development members in the Pacific region.
[b]European part of the former Soviet Union.
Source: Authors' calculations.

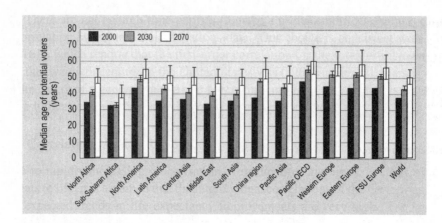

Figure 3.3. Median age of potential voters (18 and older) for the world and the 13 regions for the years 2000, 2030, and 2070 (intervals superimposed on the bars give interdecile ranges). *Source*: Authors' calculations.

democratic countries will shift toward the groups that become more numerous. For an initial view of this issue, we computed the distributions of the median ages of the populations aged 18 and older. We call this population "potential voters," even though there are a variety of minimum voting ages in the world, and even though voting is still uncommon in some of the regions.

Figure 3.3 shows three bars for each region, one each for the years 2000, 2030, and 2070. The heights of the bars for 2030 and 2070 show the median forecast of the median age of potential voters; the intervals shown at the tops of these bars indicate the interdecile ranges.

In 2000, the median age of the world's potential voters was 38; by 2030 it rises to 43, and then to 50 by 2070. In 2070, the interdecile range spans the interval from 46 to 55 years of age. In North America, the median age of potential voters increases from 44 to 55 from 2000 to 2070. In Latin America, the median age changes more rapidly, going from 36 in 2000 to 51 in 2070. A change of the same magnitude is likely to occur in the Middle East, where the median age changes from 34 to 50 over the 70-year period.

In six of the 13 regions—North America, the China region, the Pacific OECD, Western Europe, Eastern Europe, and FSU Europe—there is over a 10 percent chance that the median age of potential voters will be above 60 in 2070. It is interesting that the ninth decile of the median age distribution is slightly higher in the China region, at 62 years, than it is in North America, at 61 years. For comparison, the ninth decile for Western Europe is 66 years; for the Pacific OECD it is 69 years.

Aging will produce profound changes in our societies as the 21st century unfolds. Some of these changes will undoubtedly occur in political systems as the mean age of the voting population approaches and possibly surpasses the (current) mean age at retirement from the labor force. Even with all the uncertainties involved, we can say with assurance that significant aging will occur in all the regions of the world as the century progresses. Since we can foresee these changes, we can plan for them. What we have done here is to provide policy makers with the uncertainties associated with our forecasts. Knowledge of these uncertainties is crucial to forming an appropriate forward-looking policy, because it provides information about the range of likely outcomes for which robust policies need to be designed.

3.2 Conditional Probabilistic Forecasting[3]

In the past, when demographers wanted to communicate the uncertainties inherent in their forecasts they used scenarios. Scenario analysis is still very popular in many different disciplines that need to study possible future trends. In population forecasting, scenarios typically are clear "if-then" statements in which the implications of a certain set of assumptions on fertility, mortality, and migration are demonstrated (Lutz 1995). Such scenarios can illustrate the laws of population dynamics, but do not give the user any information about the likelihood of the described path. For instance, an immediate replacement fertility scenario merely shows what would happen if fertility were to immediately jump to the replacement level without saying that this is a likely or even plausible path. For policy makers who want to know the long-term consequences of, for example, alternative fertility trends that result from alternative policies, such scenarios are quite useful. Conditional probabilistic forecasting is a way of posing and answering this type of question within a probabilistic framework.

Figure 3.4 shows the distribution of the world's population in 2050 conditional on average fertility and mortality levels over the period from 2000 to 2050. The *x*-axis is divided into three ranges labeled "low," "medium," and "high" fertility. Low fertility includes all of our 2,000 simulated futures in which the average total fertility rate in 2000–2050 was below 1.6; medium fertility includes those paths in which the average total fertility rate was between 1.6 and 1.8; and high fertility includes paths in which the average total fertility rate (over the whole projection period) was above 1.8.

Within each of the three panels are three lines that have different symbols near their centers. The lines with the diamonds near their centers refer to paths in which the average life expectancy at birth in 2000–2050 was below 68 years; the lines with

---

[3]Sections 3.2 and 3.3 were written simultaneously with Sanderson *et al*. (forthcoming). Therefore, some of the tables and figures are identical and some of the text is the same.

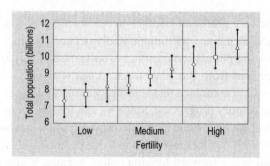

Figure 3.4. Median and interdecile ranges for world population sizes in 2050 conditional on three alternative fertility and mortality levels. Diamonds = median population sizes, low life expectancy. Squares = median population sizes, medium life expectancy. Triangles = median population sizes, high life expectancy. Circles = interdecile ranges. *Source*: Authors' calculations.

the squares refer to paths in which the average life expectancy was between 68 and 71 years; and the lines with triangles, to paths with average life expectancies over 71 years. The aggregations of the total fertility rates and life expectancies at birth were chosen so that one-third of the paths occurred in each group. The symbols are placed at the medians of the distributions. The circles at the endpoints of the lines indicate the interdecile ranges.

Now we are in the position to answer some "what if" questions. For example, what would be the effect on world population size in 2050 of high fertility outcomes versus low fertility outcomes over the coming decades, combined with medium levels of future mortality? We can immediately read the answer in *Figure 3.4*. With low fertility, the median population of the world in 2050 would be around 7.7 billion, with an interdecile range covering the area from 7.0 to 8.3 billion. With high fertility, the median population would be considerably higher, around 10.0 billion, with an interdecile range between 9.2 and 10.9 billion. The difference between the medians is 2.3 billion, which is quite large considering that the unconditional population is 8.8 billion. Clearly, the difference in fertility is very significant.

We can also use *Figure 3.4* to tell us about the influence of differences in life expectancies on future population size. We can do this easily by looking at the middle panel, labeled "medium" fertility. When life expectancies are in the low group, the median population size is 8.3 billion. When they are in the high group, the median population is 9.2 billion. The difference is 1.2 billion. Therefore, in 2050 the effect on population size of moving from low to high fertility, keeping life expectancy constant, is roughly twice that of moving from low to high life expectancy, keeping fertility constant.

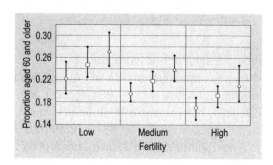

Figure 3.5. Median and interdecile ranges for global proportion aged 60 and older in 2050 conditional on three alternative fertility and mortality levels. Diamonds = median proportions over age 60, low life expectancy. Squares = median proportions over age 60, medium life expectancy. Triangles = median proportions over age 60, high life expectancy. Circles = interdecile ranges. *Source*: Authors' calculations.

Figure 3.5 is similar to *Figure 3.4*, except that it deals with the proportion aged 60 and older. As fertility increases, this age proportion decreases, but as life expectancy increases, this age proportion increases. Let us consider the difference in this age proportion caused by high fertility as opposed to low fertility, again assuming medium life expectancy. The median proportion aged 60 and older is 25 percent in 2050 when fertility is low and around 19 percent when it is high. Assuming medium fertility and varying mortality, we see that when mortality is low this age proportion is below 20 percent, compared with 24 percent when mortality is high. Thus, the effects of fertility and mortality are more similar in determining the proportion aged 60 and older than they are in determining population size.

Figures 3.6 and *3.7* show the distributions of forecasts of the proportion of the population aged 60 and older, conditional on fertility and the level of migration, for Western Europe and North America, respectively. In the case of migration, the paths to 2050 are again divided into thirds. In both regions, the effects of higher migration on the proportion of the population aged 60 and older are greater when fertility is low than when fertility is high. The effects of the different migration outcomes are limited. They are smaller in Western Europe than in North America, because the migration flows into Western Europe themselves are smaller. A more extensive and systematic analysis using conditional probabilistic forecasting is given in Lutz and Scherbov (2002), which asks whether immigration can compensate for Europe's low fertility.

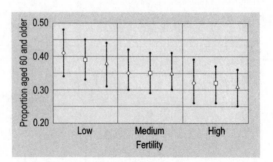

Figure 3.6. Median and interdecile ranges for proportion aged 60 and older in Western Europe in 2050 conditional on three alternative fertility and migration levels. Diamonds = median proportions over age 60, low migration. Squares = median proportions over age 60, medium migration. Triangles = median proportions over age 60, high migration. Circles = interdecile ranges. *Source*: Authors' calculations.

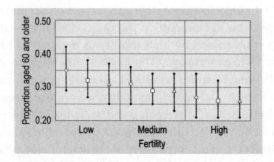

Figure 3.7. Median and interdecile ranges for proportion aged 60 and older in North America in 2050 conditional on three alternative fertility and migration levels. Diamonds = median proportions over age 60, low migration. Squares = median proportions over age 60, medium migration. Triangles = median proportions over age 60, high migration. Circles = interdecile ranges. *Source*: Authors' calculations.

The importance of the examples presented in this chapter is not solely in the results that we have reported. It is also important that we have established how probabilistic forecasts can be used to pose and answer "what if" questions.

3.3   Conditional Probabilistic Forecasts with Future Jump-Off Dates

We have shown that it is likely that world population growth will come to an end during the 21st century and that the second half of the century will probably be a period of roughly constant world population size. We have also presented a host of interesting results regarding future age structures. However, we already know that, with the passage of time, the future will look different from the rates we have just set out. Whenever forecasts are presented to policy makers, one question inevitably arises. The policy maker remembers that the previous set of forecasts was different from the current one and asks whether the next set will be different as well.

To answer this question, we need probabilistic forecasts that begin at future dates. These are, of course, conditional on what happens between the beginning of the current forecast period and the future jump-off date. For example, imagine that it is the year 2000 and we are forecasting the size of the world's population in 2050. We make the forecast and compute the distribution of population sizes in 2050. We might also be interested in how different our forecast distribution of population sizes in 2050 would be if we were to make our forecast in 2010 instead of 2000. Certainly, the users of our forecasts will be interested in this. They have to decide whether to take certain actions now or wait to learn more through the passage of time. Policy makers want to be confident that if they take some action based on the current set of forecasts, they will not look foolish when the next set of forecasts appears.

We learn through the passage of time, and what we learn changes the way we think about the future. In this section, we take some small first steps toward understanding how this learning process takes place, so that users of our forecasts are not surprised by the way forecasts are updated and so that policy makers can use our forecasts in the design of adaptive policies. In many environmental fields we come across the question, Should we act now or should we wait until we learn more? Population forecasting is a good field in which to discover what we will learn by waiting. Population is an important driver of some processes of environmental change, and population forecasts are simple enough to be able to determine what we will learn from the passage of time.

Time resolves uncertainties, and this leads to a new vision of the future. New forecasts make the old ones appear to be wrong because the forecasts were of particular numbers, not distributions. Probabilistic forecasting allows us to see how our forecasts could evolve. It is inevitable that a probabilistic forecast of the world's population in 2050 made, for example, in 2010 will have a different median value than one made in 2000, even if the earlier projection was correct probabilistically. A projection is correct probabilistically if it produces the correct future distributions of outcomes and the correct relationships between those distributions. The distribution of outcomes for 2050, for example, based on a forecast with a jump-off year of 2000 will generally be different from the distribution of outcomes for 2050 based on a forecast with a jump-off year of 2000 *and* knowledge of the true population in 2010. Rather than interpreting changes in forecasts made at different dates for a fixed future year as being a forecasting failure, we now see it as an essential and interesting part of the forecasting process. Unfortunately, we only have space here to present a very brief introduction to the subject of conditional probabilistic forecasts with future jump-off dates.

Probabilistic forecasts are very different from the deterministic forecasts made by the United Nations (UN) and other agencies. Imagine that the UN made a forecast in 2000 for a country with a population of 100 million and that the medium variant was 110 million for 2010 and 120 million for 2020. Suppose that in 2000 one envisioned the situation in which the population of the country did, indeed, turn out to be 110 million in 2010. What could we say in that case about the likely population of the country in 2020? The answer is that we could say almost nothing. The population of the country could have reached exactly 110 million in 2010 because of any number of different combinations of fertility, mortality, and migration paths, not just the set of assumptions made in the original forecast. Perhaps the correct population will be 112 million or 108 million. Thinking again from the perspective of the year 2000, it is hard to imagine exactly what we will have learned about the future after 2010 if the population of the country in 2010 is 108 or 112 million.

Probabilistic forecasts have built into them information about what will be learned from future observations. Of course, this assumes that the forecast is probabilistically correct. Using a probabilistic forecast with a jump-off date of 2000 we can ask, *in 2000*, what we expect the distribution of population sizes will be in 2020 conditional on the population of the country's being 108 million, for example, in 2010. Using probabilistic forecasting we can ask, in 2000, how much we would learn about the population in 2020 from observing the size of the population in 2010.

There are two types of learning, passive learning and active learning. Passive learning occurs simply through the resolution of uncertainties with time. Active learning, on the other hand, is the kind that leads to a better understanding of the processes that underlie change—in this case, demographic change. In Chapter 2, in the discussion of changes between the 1996 IIASA projections and the 2001 IIASA projections, we consider both kinds of learning. In this section, we deal only with passive learning, and we understand that it provides only a lower limit on what we will truly learn as time passes. The extent and nature of passive learning built into probabilistic forecasts are interesting to analyze and potentially useful in decision making.

If we were actually going to perform a technically correct passive learning exercise conditional on observations in 2010, we would need to take our 2,000 simulated outcomes for 2010 and, for each one of them, produce 2,000 more random paths for the period after 2010. This would require a total of four million simulations, far more than we can handle on our personal computers. To make this inquiry practical, we use a far simpler approach. Instead of observing exact population characteristics, we assume that we can only observe whether or not the outcomes are above or below the medians of their distributions. There is nothing theoretically attractive in this division of our observations into only two groups in 2010. We do this here to make this introduction to passive demographic learning as simple as possible.

Table 3.10 consists of two panels. Panel A provides the distributions of future world population size expressed in the following intervals: below 6 billion, 6–7 billion, 7–8 billion, and so on, with the uppermost interval being above 12 billion. The numbers in the cells are the percentages of our 2,000 simulated future population paths. The final two columns give, respectively, median population sizes and the uncertainty measure, RIDR (the size of the interdecile range divided by the median).

Panel B of *Table 3.10* is based on a division of the 2010 distribution into population paths that are above the median in that year and those that are below it, with 1,000 observations in each subgroup. These population paths are those predicted from our population forecast that begins in 2000. There are two rows in panel B for each decade after 2010, one labeled with an "L" and the other with an "H." The "L" rows are the population distributions at the indicated date for the observations below the median in 2010, and the "H" rows are from the paths above the median in 2010. Panel B has an additional column, which gives a persistence measure. For every future decade or, alternatively, for every pair of "L" and "H" observations, there is only one persistence figure.

The persistence measure tells us the extent to which the information we obtained by noting whether we were in the upper or lower half of the distribution in 2010 remains useful for forecasts of the future. In this particular case, where we divide the observations in 2010 into two parts, there is a particularly simple persistence measure that we can use. This is the difference between the proportion of paths above the median in any given year (in panel A) observed in the subpopulation that was above the median in 2010 and the same proportion in the subpopulation that was below the median in 2010. For example, suppose we considered the year 2050. The median population size for the world in 2050 is 8.8 billion people. If the proportion above 8.8 billion in 2050 from the subpopulation that was above the median in 2010 is 0.720, and the proportion above 8.8 billion from the subpopulation that was below the median in 2010 is 0.245, then the persistence measure

Table 3.10. Forecasted distribution of the world's population size. Panel A = unconditional forecasts beginning in 2000; panel B = forecasts made in 2000 and conditional on whether realized world population in 2010 was below (L) or above (H) the median population size forecast in 2000 for 2010.

Year	Population size intervals (billions)								Median (millions)	RIDR[a]	Persistence
	Below 6	6–7	7–8	8–9	9–10	10–11	11–12	Above 12			
Panel A: 2000 base											
2000	0.00	100.00	0.00	0.00	0.00	0.00	0.00	0.00	6,055	0.000	
2010	0.00	85.05	14.95	0.00	0.00	0.00	0.00	0.00	6,828	0.062	
2020	0.00	8.05	81.45	10.50	0.00	0.00	0.00	0.00	7,538	0.129	
2030	0.10	3.05	41.85	47.35	7.50	0.15	0.00	0.00	8,085	0.195	
2040	0.15	3.75	24.85	40.25	25.15	5.20	0.65	0.00	8,525	0.270	
2050	0.50	5.05	18.95	30.95	26.80	13.45	3.30	1.00	8,796	0.352	
2060	1.55	7.00	17.45	25.75	22.35	16.25	6.45	3.20	8,935	0.427	
2070	4.00	8.35	16.90	21.20	19.90	15.05	8.50	6.10	8,974	0.520	
2080	6.80	10.10	16.00	18.45	18.45	12.55	9.00	8.65	8,890	0.606	
2090	10.00	12.75	14.85	17.90	15.00	12.25	6.45	10.80	8,678	0.702	
2100	14.25	14.05	14.45	16.50	12.90	10.45	6.85	10.55	8,413	0.779	
Panel B: 2010 base											
2020/L	0.00	16.10	83.90	0.00	0.00	0.00	0.00	0.00	7,268	0.088	0.763
2020/H	0.00	0.00	79.00	21.00	0.00	0.00	0.00	0.00	7,787	0.081	
2030/L	0.20	6.10	70.30	23.40	0.00	0.00	0.00	0.00	7,704	0.147	0.627
2030/H	0.00	0.00	13.40	71.30	15.00	0.30	0.00	0.00	8,486	0.139	
2040/L	0.30	7.50	42.30	42.40	7.40	0.10	0.00	0.00	7,996	0.224	0.549
2040/H	0.00	0.00	7.40	38.10	42.90	10.30	1.30	0.00	9,083	0.216	
2050/L	1.00	9.90	31.10	36.60	17.90	3.20	0.30	0.00	8,152	0.294	0.475
2050/H	0.00	0.20	6.80	25.30	35.70	23.70	6.30	2.00	9,521	0.279	
2060/L	3.10	12.80	26.90	31.30	17.30	6.80	1.60	0.20	8,256	0.389	0.453
2060/H	0.00	1.20	8.00	20.20	27.40	25.70	11.30	6.20	9,760	0.352	
2070/L	7.80	13.60	23.90	25.20	17.40	8.70	1.90	1.50	8,213	0.485	0.399
2070/H	0.20	3.10	9.90	17.20	22.40	21.40	15.10	10.70	9,891	0.438	
2080/L	12.50	14.70	22.20	19.80	16.90	7.90	4.10	1.90	8,045	0.568	0.355
2080/H	1.10	5.50	9.80	17.10	20.00	17.20	13.90	15.40	9,816	0.536	
2090/L	16.10	18.00	18.50	18.30	13.30	9.40	3.60	2.80	7,888	0.641	0.315
2090/H	3.90	7.50	11.20	17.50	16.70	15.10	9.30	18.80	9,638	0.647	
2100/L	22.00	17.70	16.60	17.60	9.90	9.00	3.60	3.60	7,652	0.716	0.271
2100/H	6.50	10.40	12.30	15.40	15.90	11.90	10.10	17.50	9,328	0.734	

[a]The relative interdecile range (RIDR) is the difference between the ninth decile of the distribution and the first decile divided by the median.
Source: Authors' calculations.

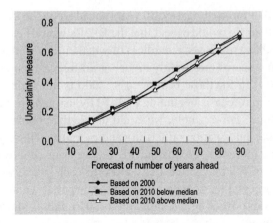

Figure 3.8. Comparison of RIDR (ninth decile minus first decile divided by median) for forecasts made for 10 through 90 years ahead starting from 2000 and starting from an observation either above the median or below the median in 2010. *Source*: Authors' calculations.

would be 0.475 (= 0.720 – 0.245), the figure in panel B. In the case of perfect persistence, in which all the observations above the median in 2010 are also above the median in 2050, this persistence measure is 1.0. When the information from 2010 is irrelevant, the persistence measure is 0.0.

One disadvantage of this very simplified example is that the forecasts with jump-off dates in 2000 and 2010 are not exactly comparable. The vital rate paths used in the 2000 forecasts all start at their observed values, while the paths in the forecasts that have the 2010 jump-off date have a distribution of starting values. One way to test the plausibility of this example is to consider the uncertainty of forecasts of various durations based on a jump-off date of 2000 and a jump-off date of 2010. Holding duration of forecast constant, the example would be questionable if the uncertainties were very different depending on whether the forecasts are made in 2000 or 2010.

If we begin in the year 2000 and forecast 10 years into the future, the RIDR is 0.062, which can be read off the row in panel A labeled 2010. If we were to forecast 10 years ahead based on being below the median in 2010, the RIDR would be 0.088. This can be read off the row in panel B labeled 2020/L. To test the plausibility of the example, we have computed the RIDRs for 10- through 90-year forecasts with a jump-off date in 2000 and the two subsamples assuming a jump-off date in 2010. These are shown in *Figure 3.8*. The results from the two 2010 groups track those from 2000 quite well, but are always slightly higher than the RIDRs computed from the forecasts with a jump-off date in 2000.

If we thought that forecasting, say, 50 years ahead would be as difficult in 2010 as it was in 2000, then we would expect that the RIDRs would be close to being the same for 50-year-ahead forecasts, regardless of whether they start at 2000 or 2010. That the uncertainty scores are slightly higher at all forecast lengths for forecasts beginning in 2010 than for those beginning in 2000 is not surprising. We could obtain more accurate forecasts beginning in 2010 by using more information than population size alone. For example, we could divide the population in 2010 into more groups and use information on fertility and mortality. However, dividing the population in 2010 into more groups quickly reduces our subgroup sizes. Since the RIDRs shown in *Figure 3.8* are quite close to each other, we conclude that our procedure is acceptable, as long as we remember that we are likely to learn somewhat more from observing the situation in 2010 than is shown in the tables and figures that follow.

The median population forecast for 2100 based on information up to 2000 is 8.413 billion people. If we waited for 10 years and made the forecast for 2100 based on being above or below the median in 2010, our forecast would either be 7.652 billion or 9.328 billion. We can almost see the newspaper headlines now: "Forecasters Now Predict Almost 1 Billion More People" or "Forecasts Now Predict Almost 1 Billion Fewer People." It would seem that if we were to predict 914 million more people or 762 million fewer people in the world in 2100 than we had predicted only a decade earlier, we must have made a big mistake in 2000. Yet, this is exactly what will happen if our methodology is probabilistically correct. Clearly, our forecasts of the future will be different in 2010 than they are today. One interesting feature of probabilistic forecasting is that it can give us some idea about how much different our future forecasts are likely to be from our current ones.

It is crucial that we look not only at the effects of the passage of time on the median forecast, but also at the entire distribution of forecast population sizes. Most of the differences in the distributions based on the paths above and below the median in 2010 are in the extremes (tails) of the distributions. For example, 6.5 percent of the paths that are above the median in 2010 result in populations of less than 6 billion in 2100, compared with 22.0 percent of the paths that are below the median in 2010. The difference at the high end of the distribution is even more striking. Over 17 percent of the paths that are above the median in 2010 end the century with 12 billion people or more. In contrast, only 3.6 percent of the paths that are below the median in 2010 do so.

The tails of the distributions tell us another story as well. Even if the population path is below the median in 2010, it could still yield a population with over 12 billion people by 2100. Similarly, a population path that is above the median in 2010 could still end the century with less than 6 billion people. Being above or below the median in 2010 provides us with information about the entire distribution of outcomes, but does not rule out a population in 2100 that is in any of the population groups in *Table 3.10*.

Of course, a forecast for 2020 based on information up to 2010 will be more accurate than one based on information up to 2000. For example, our forecast for 2020 based on information up to 2000 says that 10.5 percent of the simulations lie between eight and nine billion people. After another 10 years, we would learn whether that chance is 21 percent (if we are above the median in 2010) or zero (if we are below the median in 2010).

We will learn a significant amount about future distributions of population sizes throughout the 21st century by observing whether population size is above or below the median in 2010. For example, if population size is below the median in 2010, we expect there to be a 42 percent chance that the size of the world's population in 2050 will be eight billion or lower. If population size is above the median in 2010, there is only a 7 percent chance that it will be eight billion or lower.

The fact that we can learn a great deal about population size distributions by simply observing whether or not population size is above or below the median in 2010 is reflected in our persistence measure. For 2020, this measure is 0.763 and it falls continuously to 0.271 in 2100.

Population size is so persistent because of a number of factors. First, past population size influences future population size. Paths that turn out to yield large populations in 2010 will also yield large populations in 2100, even if population growth rates after 2010 are the same. Second, some populations are large in 2010 because they have high fertility rates. These high fertility rates alter the age structure of the population, making it younger. Younger populations tend to grow more, other things being equal, a process that demographers call "population momentum." Fertility and mortality themselves have some persistence built into them, as shown in Chapter 2. The persistence of fertility and mortality means that on paths with high fertility and low mortality, which yield relatively large populations in 2010, both are likely to remain high and low, respectively, for a while. The persistence of fertility and mortality is compounded by the persistence caused by population momentum and the size effect itself.

Figure 3.9 shows the persistence index at 10-year intervals from 2020 to 2100 based on population sizes above or below the median for the world and our 13 regions. In all 14 cases, persistence falls continuously over time, but remains at a fairly high level, even in 2100. This tells us that for every region we would learn quite a bit more about its population size distribution in 2100 just through observing what actually happens by 2010.

Table 3.11 is similar to *Table 3.10*, except that it deals with population growth rates instead of population size. We divide the population paths into those that have growth rates above the median in the period 2000–2010 and those with growth

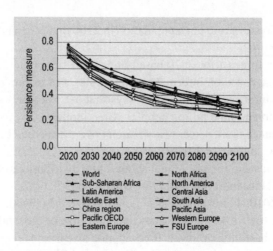

Figure 3.9. Persistence measures for what could be learned about population sizes of the world and our 13 regions from observing population size in 2010, at 10-year intervals from 2020 to 2100. *Source*: Authors' calculations.

rates below it. The two groups that we obtain in this way are exactly the same groups obtained when we divide the population paths into those with population sizes above the median in 2010 and those below it. Panel A of *Table 3.11* shows the percentages of our simulated population paths that produce average annual growth rates within the indicated ranges. For example, around 27 percent of our 2,000 population paths produce average annual world population growth rates between –0.5 and 0.0 percent per year during the decade 2090–2100.

In panel B of *Table 3.11*, we look at the distributions of growth rates separately for the paths that had growth below and above the median in 2000–2010. Panel B does not contain the RIDR, because it is not useful in cases where there are both positive and negative figures in the distribution; however, it does contain the persistence measure. The trend of the persistence measure is downward with the passage of time, as we would expect, and as is the case for population size. The persistence measure starts lower in the case of population growth and falls to practically zero.

Another way to see that population growth in 2000–2010 has little predictive value by the end of the 21st century is to look at the distributions of growth rates during 2090–2100 of those paths that were above and below the median in 2000–2010. The percentages in each group are very similar when we compare the two groups of paths, even at the extremes. For example, the proportion of paths with growth rates between 1.0 and 1.5 percent per year in 2090–2100 is 0.8 percent for those below the median in 2000–2010 and 0.9 percent for those above the median in 2000–2010.

Table 3.11. Forecast distribution of the world's population growth. Panel A = unconditional forecasts beginning in 2000; Panel B = forecasts made in 2000 and conditional on whether realized world population in 2010 was below (L) or above (H) the median population size forecast in 2000 for 2010.

Panel A: 2000 base

Distribution of average annual rates of population growth by decade

	<−1.5	−1.5 to −1.0	−1.0 to −0.5	−0.5 to 0	0 to 0.5	0.5 to 1.0	1.0 to 1.5	1.5 to 2.0	>2.0	Median
2000–2010	0.00	0.00	0.00	0.00	0.45	19.65	68.00	11.85	0.05	1.209
2010–2020	0.00	0.00	0.00	0.30	5.55	45.20	45.70	3.25	0.00	0.988
2020–2030	0.00	0.00	0.10	1.25	24.40	55.50	18.30	0.45	0.00	0.720
2030–2040	0.00	0.00	0.70	8.15	37.55	43.45	9.85	0.30	0.00	0.534
2040–2050	0.00	0.10	3.20	18.20	44.10	29.70	4.65	0.05	0.00	0.335
2050–2060	0.35	1.30	8.60	27.95	38.20	20.75	2.85	0.00	0.00	0.154
2060–2070	0.75	3.45	13.70	29.35	33.15	17.55	2.05	0.00	0.00	0.041
2070–2080	1.60	7.05	18.05	28.45	29.95	13.00	1.90	0.00	0.00	−0.086
2080–2090	4.00	10.00	21.25	26.20	22.65	14.30	1.60	0.00	0.00	−0.213
2090–2100	6.95	11.20	19.35	26.95	23.25	11.40	0.85	0.05	0.00	−0.260

Panel B: 2010 base

Distribution of average annual population growth rates conditional on being above or below the median in 2000–2010

	<−1.5	−1.5 to −1.0	−1.0 to −0.5	−0.5 to 0	0 to 0.5	0.5 to 1.0	1.0 to 1.5	1.5 to 2.0	>2.0	Median	Persistence
2010–2020/L	0.00	0.00	0.00	0.60	11.10	66.80	21.50	0.00	0.00	0.804	0.545
2010–2020/H	0.00	0.00	0.00	0.00	0.00	23.60	69.90	6.50	0.00	1.161	
2020–2030/L	0.00	0.00	0.20	2.50	37.30	53.30	6.70	0.00	0.00	0.583	0.375
2020–2030/H	0.00	0.00	0.00	0.00	11.50	57.70	29.90	0.90	0.00	0.863	
2030–2040/L	0.00	0.00	1.40	12.90	47.40	34.80	3.40	0.10	0.00	0.387	0.311
2030–2040/H	0.00	0.00	0.00	3.40	27.70	52.10	16.30	0.50	0.00	0.667	
2040–2050/L	0.00	0.20	5.40	22.90	47.20	21.00	3.20	0.10	0.00	0.231	0.195
2040–2050/H	0.00	0.00	1.00	13.50	41.00	38.40	6.10	0.00	0.00	0.442	
2050–2060/L	0.70	2.30	11.50	33.60	34.40	15.60	1.90	0.00	0.00	0.026	0.181
2050–2060/H	0.00	0.30	5.70	22.30	42.00	25.90	3.80	0.00	0.00	0.265	
2060–2070/L	1.30	4.80	16.40	32.00	29.90	14.00	1.60	0.00	0.00	−0.079	0.149
2060–2070/H	0.20	2.10	11.00	26.70	36.40	21.10	2.50	0.00	0.00	0.136	
2070–2080/L	2.00	8.70	20.00	29.30	28.60	9.90	1.50	0.00	0.00	−0.166	0.087
2070–2080/H	1.20	5.40	16.10	27.60	31.30	16.10	2.30	0.00	0.00	−0.003	
2080–2090/L	3.90	10.50	22.90	25.40	22.10	14.10	1.10	0.00	0.00	−0.244	0.039
2080–2090/H	4.10	9.50	19.60	27.00	23.20	14.50	2.10	0.00	0.00	−0.176	
2090–2100/L	7.50	10.30	19.60	28.10	22.30	11.40	0.80	0.00	0.00	−0.258	0.005
2090–2100/H	6.40	12.10	19.10	25.80	24.20	11.40	0.90	0.10	0.00	−0.265	

Source: Authors' calculations.

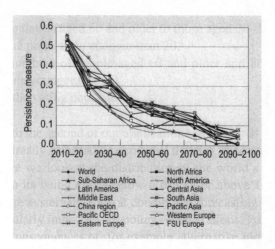

Figure 3.10. Persistence measures for what could be learned about population growth rates in the world and our 13 regions from observing population growth rates in 2000–2010, at 10-year periods from 2010–2020 to 2090–2100. *Source*: Authors' calculations.

The persistence measures for the population growth rates for the world and for our 13 regions are shown in *Figure 3.10*. The most important feature of the graph is that by 2100 the persistence measures reach a level close to zero in every region. We can learn little about what population growth will be between 2090 and 2100 from the knowledge of what it was between 2000 and 2010. The main reason that population sizes are persistent and population growth rates are not is that population size in 2100 is determined by factors that take place during the entire 21st century. Higher population growth in the early part of the century causes higher population sizes at mid-century, which translate into higher population sizes at the end of the century simply because larger populations tend to stay relatively large. In the case of population growth rates, the lingering effects of the past are much weaker.

This is a very short and simplified presentation of the basic concepts of future probabilistic forecasting with jump-off dates. It is meant to be suggestive only. Yet, even at this simple level, we can see that we learn about different population features differently. In the future, we expect to provide more detailed studies that involve demographic learning about age structures as well as population size. It also should be stressed again that this analysis only applies to what we called "passive learning," that is, learning based on the resolution of future uncertainties. "Active learning," which also improves our substantive understanding of the determinants of these trends, could be another important factor as to why we change the way we view the future. But active learning is much harder to analyze, and we leave it for future research.

3.4 Conclusions

In this chapter, we considered population aging, conditional forecasting, and passive learning. There is one fundamental lesson that runs through all of the sections. It is crucial that we think about forecasts as distributions, not just single numbers in the future. By thinking about forecasts as ranges, we can see just how uncertain forecasts of measures such as the proportions of the population aged 80 and older really are. We can see that conditional probabilistic forecasts, which look much like deterministic scenarios, are also uncertain and that their uncertainties change with the conditioning variables. In the section on future forecasting with jump-off dates, we show how a distribution of probabilistic paths can allow us not only to make forecasts, but also to predict the forecast that we would make at future times conditional on our observations between then and now.

All of these ways of measuring and presenting distributions of outcomes are vital for decision making. To decide on appropriate policies, policy makers need to know the uncertainties associated with our forecasts of age structure. Conditional forecasting helps them to understand what the potential effects of their policies could be. Finally, passive learning helps policy makers to integrate the time path of policy formulation with an understanding of what new forecasts are likely to show. They are far more likely to initiate a policy when it can be demonstrated that the phenomenon motivating them will not vanish in the next round of forecasting.

References

Lutz W (1995). Scenario Analysis in Population Projection. Working Paper WP-95-57. Laxenburg, Austria: International Institute for Applied Systems Analysis.

Lutz W & Scherbov S (2002). Can Immigration Compensate for Europe's Low Fertility? Interim Report IR-02-052. Laxenburg, Austria: International Institute for Applied Systems Analysis.

Sanderson WC, Scherbov S, O'Neill B & Lutz W (forthcoming). Conditional probabilistic population forecasting. *International Statistical Review*.

Chapter 4

Future Human Capital: Population Projections by Level of Education

Anne Goujon and Wolfgang Lutz

Chapters 1–3 look at changes in population size and age structure. These strictly demographic aspects of population change have manifold consequences for family structures, social systems, and even economic development and interactions with the natural environment. If our analysis were concerned with a specific animal population instead of the human population, the population dynamics would result in a certain population density and spatial distribution that would capture all the key elements necessary to study its interaction with the natural environment, under a certain naturally determined carrying capacity. Contrary to animal populations, the human population has the ability to learn—individually as well as collectively—and to consciously modify the way in which it interacts with the environment. This learning results in skills that can be used to alter human interactions with the environment in a way that improves human livelihood, longevity, and quality of life. It is an empirical fact that the level of these skills varies greatly among individuals within a given society, varies among different societies at a given point in time, and changes during the evolution of societies over time.

Taken in the aggregate, people's skills are an important factor of production, normally called human capital. Skills can be measured in many different ways, but, for a global comparative analysis, literacy skills and years of completed formal education are by far the most frequently used indicators. So far, educational distributions have been assessed systematically only for the past and the present. In this chapter, we present the first global-level projections of the population by age, sex, and level of education up to 2030.[1]

Education is generally assumed to have far-reaching benefits. At the individual level, better education is associated with better health, more economic opportunities, and greater autonomy, especially for women (Federici *et al.* 1993; Jejeebhoy 1995). At the aggregate level, the educational composition of the population has long been considered a key factor in economic, institutional, and social development (Benavot 1989; Bellew *et al.* 1992; Hadden and London 1996), and in the rate of technological progress (Grossman and Helpman 1991; Romer 1992). The increasing body of theoretical and empirical literature on the relationship between human capital formation and various aspects of development is not reviewed here.[2] Instead, this chapter demonstrates the feasibility of true multistate population projections for groups defined by different educational attainment. With the increasing importance of education in a knowledge-based economy, this approach has the potential to make an important contribution to the field of demography itself, but also to longer-range economic planning and the analysis of sustainable development options.

4.1 The Multistate Approach

The increasing awareness over the past decade of the paramount importance of human capital in development has stimulated several attempts to estimate and project the educational composition of the population. Most empirical studies, however, have tended to approximate educational stocks only in terms of enrolment ratios or illiteracy rates (Romer 1989; Mankiw *et al.* 1992). What is needed is a complete matrix of the composition of the population by age, sex, and level of educational attainment for different points in time. Many attempts to measure human capital stock have failed to meet this aim because of problems with data at the level of individual countries and because of the lack of appropriate demographic methodologies (Psacharopoulos and Arrigada 1986, 1992; Kyriacou 1991; Barro and Lee 1993; Nehru *et al.* 1993; Dubey and King 1994; Ahuja and Filmer 1995). Barro and Lee (2000) have produced some interesting data on educational attainment and average number of years of schooling at various levels for a large number of countries in the world. However, the data set provides estimates only for two broad age groups (15

---

[1] This chapter draws heavily on an earlier contribution by the two authors, published in *Population and Development Review* (Lutz and Goujon 2001).

[2] An extensive international bibliography is given in, for example, Brock and Cammish (1997).

and older, and 25 and older) and only for the 1960–2000 period. Ahuja and Filmer (1995) made the most progress by taking existing United Nations (UN) population projections and superimposing onto them an educational distribution estimated for two broad age groups (6–24 and 25 and older) from given sets of enrolment ratios and United Nations Educational, Scientific and Cultural Organization (UNESCO) projections. Using this approach, they project the educational composition (for four educational groups) for a significant number of developing countries. In addition to the lack of more specific information by age, this approach is also unsatisfactory because of its static nature; it does not allow the educational composition of the population to influence fertility, despite the obvious strong educational fertility differentials in most developing countries.

In this study, we apply the demographic methodology of multistate population projection to the task. This method, which is based on a multidimensional expansion of the life table (increment–decrement tables) and of the cohort-component projection method, was developed at the International Institute for Applied Systems Analysis (IIASA) during the 1970s (Rogers 1975; Keyfitz 1985). The multistate model is based on a division of the population by age and sex into any number of "states," which originally were geographic units, with the movements between the states representing migration streams. However, a "state" can also reflect any other clearly defined subgroup of the population, such as groups with different educational attainment levels, with the movements then becoming educational transition rates. Actually, the projection of human capital stocks by age and sex is an ideal example of the application of the multidimensional cohort-component model, because education tends to be acquired at younger ages and then simply moves along cohort lines. Changes in the educational composition of the total population (aged 15 and older) are typically caused by the depletion (through mortality) of less-educated cohorts and the entry of more-educated younger cohorts.

Figure 4.1 shows the specific structure of the multistate model chosen for this study. It subdivides the population into four distinct groups according to educational attainment. Each subpopulation is further stratified by age (five-year age groups) and sex, and can be represented through a separate population pyramid. The key parameters of the model are three sets of age- and sex-specific educational transition rates; that is, the age-specific proportions of young men and women who make the transition from one educational attainment category to the next higher one. Although this model can handle transitions at any age—for example, those effected by adult education campaigns—in reality, and in our model, transitions are concentrated in the age range below age 25. Another important feature that gives this model a dynamic element is the fact that it considers different fertility rates for different educational groups. Hence, even with constant status-specific fertility, a change in the relative size of the educational subpopulation results in changes in the

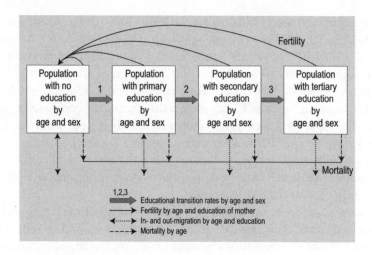

Figure 4.1. Structure of the multistate population projection model by education.

fertility rate of the total population.[3] Migration and mortality are only considered by age and sex in this application. While for international migration a hypothetical distribution by education was assumed, we did not feel in the position to do the same for mortality. As more empirical information becomes available, empirically founded educational differentials may also be assumed for these two components of change.

Social science tells us that not only fertility rates, but also school enrolment rates (flows) tend to depend on the educational composition (stocks) of the population. There is much evidence of intergenerational transmission of education. For this reason, we also run some special scenarios that take such feedbacks into account. It may be useful here to distinguish between first-order feedbacks, which refer to the compositional effects caused by educational fertility differentials, and second-order feedbacks, which represent behavioral responses to changing stocks. Although there is little reliable empirical evidence to model such responses at the macro level for different parts of the world, we describe an experimental scenario that incorporates such second-order feedbacks.[4]

It is evident that under such conditions, educational projections cannot simply be superimposed on given population projections, as has been done in previous

---

[3]This purely compositional feature significantly influences the result. Although it is not presented here, we have shown through this work that it can cause the fertility to decline further by more than 5 percent in sub-Saharan Africa, Latin America, Central Asia, the Middle East, the China region, and Pacific Asia.

[4]We thank an anonymous referee for encouraging us to present such a scenario.

studies. They require that population projections be carried out as an integral part of the exercise, since alternative education scenarios result in alternative fertility trends. The educational projections presented here are based on the assumptions of the demographic projections presented in Chapters 1–3. Contrary to the probabilistic population projections presented above, these multistate educational projections use a more conventional scenario approach, because of the greater model complexity and the significantly larger number of parameter choices involved. At some point it may also become feasible to produce probabilistic multistate projections, but for the time being we present the multistate scenarios in a way that is consistent with the above-described probabilistic population projections. The fertility, mortality, and migration assumptions in the educational projections in all 13 regions follow the median paths of the uncertainty distributions assumed and discussed for the demographic projections above. In addition, three alternative education scenarios are defined on the basis of different sets of transition rates between educational groups.[5]

Population projections by level of education are a logical next step in improving population forecasts and making them more relevant. As discussed in Lutz *et al.* (1999), adding education to age and sex as an explicitly considered demographic dimension in population forecasting also affects the demographic output parameters themselves, because a significant source of so far unobserved heterogeneity is being observed and endogenized explicitly. It may, therefore, be considered an improvement even of the purely demographic output parameters of the projection. More importantly, however, the overriding substantive importance of education means that the future educational composition of the population is of interest in its own right.

---

[5]Since fertility is assumed to be different in different educational groups, the resultant total fertility rate (TFR) of the total population will partly depend on the relative sizes of the educational groups and hence differ from one education scenario to another. To maintain consistency with the demographic projections described in Chapters 2 and 3, the "constant transition rates" scenario is taken as the standard for comparison. In other words, education-specific fertility rates are defined in such a way that the compositional changes that result from this scenario exactly give the total population TFR that is the median of the assumed uncertainty distribution for fertility in the probabilistic projections. This assumption of the fertility path thus covers the very important educational momentum effect (from past improvements in schooling) on the path of fertility decline. It does not include the aggregate fertility effects of alternatively assumed strong changes in educational transition. Up to 2030, however, the effects of alternative education scenarios on total population TFRs are only minor: in the industrialized regions there is no visible difference between the "constant" and the "American" scenarios; the strongest effect is found in sub-Saharan Africa, where the total TFR is reduced by 0.2 by 2025–2030 as a consequence of this compositional effect. Substantively, this implies that strong educational efforts in the least developed regions would result in a fertility path somewhat below the assumed median.

4.2   Data on Education

The educational projections are carried out at the level of 13 world regions.[6] For each region, the population is split into four groups according to educational attainment. The four education categories, which try to follow the international standard classification of education (ISCED) and data availability, are defined as follows:

- No education: Applies to those who have completed less than one year of formal schooling.[7]
- Primary education: Includes all those who have completed at least one year of education at the first level (primary), but who have not gone on to second-level studies.
- Secondary education: Consists of those who have moved to the second level of education, whether or not they have completed the full course, but who have not proceeded to studies at the tertiary level.
- Tertiary education: Includes those who have undertaken third-level studies, whether or not they have completed the full course.

The following procedures were applied to estimate the starting population for the year 2000 by age, sex, and education for the 13 regions. First, the population by age and sex for each region was estimated by aggregating the specific country data for the year 2000 according to the medium variant of the estimates made by the United Nations (1999);[8] next, the educational composition of the population by age and sex for 2000 was estimated based on individual country data, mostly from census and survey information. The individual countries were chosen as being representative of the region and giving a maximum coverage of the populations of the respective region. More detailed information is given in Appendix 4.1.

4.3   Regional Education Levels in 2000

The total world population for the year 2000 was slightly above 6 billion people; 4.3 billion were men and women above age 15. Of these, 18 percent of the men and 31 percent of the women were still without any formal education (see *Table A4.1*

---

[6]For a detailed listing of the countries in each region, see Appendix 2.2 in Chapter 2 of this volume.

[7]In special instances, illiteracy data are used to estimate this category. Since it may take up to four years of primary education to reach literacy, this tends to overestimate the proportion in this category. However, for several countries there is no other choice for lack of data.

[8]Since the starting year 2000 was more recent than the dates of the most recent empirical information available at the time the calculations were performed, this estimation of starting conditions includes projections for a few years, which generally followed the assumptions made in the UN medium variant for 1995–2000.

in Appendix 4.2). In 2000, there were almost as many persons without education above age 15 in the developing world as there were inhabitants of the same age in the developed world in all education categories together. The population with no education represented approximately one billion people. Of this, 88 percent was concentrated in three major regions: sub-Saharan Africa, South Asia, and the China region. Of this illiterate population, 63 percent was female. Of all the developing regions in 2000, the China region had by far the highest percentage of women among the illiterate population, with 72 percent.

At the other end of the education spectrum in 2000, 11 percent of the world's adult men and 8 percent of adult women had received some tertiary education. As in the case of no education, the share of adults with a tertiary education was very unbalanced between the more developed regions (MDRs) and the less developed regions (LDRs), as well as between men and women. North America had the highest percentage of people with a tertiary education, with 43 percent of the people above age 15 having entered third-level studies. The next region is the Pacific OECD,[9] with 24 percent, and then Europe, with less than 17 percent. In all other regions, less than 15 percent of the population had ever entered an institution for tertiary education. This figure is as low as less than 4 percent in sub-Saharan Africa, South Asia, and the China region.

Women have less tertiary education than men do. This is true for all regions of the world, regardless of their level of development. The gap between men and women is higher when rates of participation in tertiary education are lower. For instance, in sub-Saharan Africa, South Asia, and the China region, the participation of women in tertiary education is less than half that of men. In sub-Saharan Africa, less than 1 percent of women have a tertiary education. The smallest gender gap in tertiary education can be found in North America, followed by Europe. The age and education pyramid of the world (*Figure 4.2*) shows the improvements that have been made in the past half century. The shading indicates the level of educational attainment. Only 26 percent of the world's population in the 65 and older age group had a secondary or tertiary education in 2000, whereas more than 50 percent of the population in the 35–39 age group and 57 percent of those in the 20–24 age group had received some higher education.

Fertility tends to vary strongly with the level of female education in most countries, particularly in those that are in the midst of the process of demographic transition. This information can be derived from a wealth of fertility surveys (Demographic and Health Surveys [DHS], Fertility and Family Surveys [FFS], and others) that have been conducted in a large number of countries around the world. Selected DHS findings for the late 1990s are listed in *Table 4.1*. The strongest educational differentials are observed in Africa (for extreme cases in Benin and

[9]Organisation for Economic Co-operation and Development members in the Pacific region.

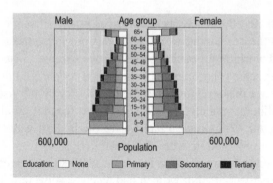

Figure 4.2. Age and education pyramid of the world in 2000. *Source*: Authors' calculations.

Togo, the DHS data show that women without formal education have well above 6 children, whereas women with some tertiary education have only 1.3 on average) and in parts of Latin America (e.g., Guatemala with 7.1 versus 1.8; Bolivia with 7.1 versus 2.2; Brazil with 5.0 versus 1.5). Asia and Europe have an intermediate position, and North America shows virtually no educational fertility differentials.

Table 4.2 lists the educational fertility differentials as estimated on the basis of available country-specific data for the 13 regions for 1995–2000.[10] Differentials by education for the 13 regions were estimated using all the information available on the level of individual countries,[11] also taking into account qualitative information for the countries without good data. The estimated relative educational differentials were then applied to the total fertility rate (TFR) and to the age-specific fertility rates for the 13 regions in the context of the multistate model described above. The future educational fertility differentials are assumed to follow an algorithm with diminishing differentials as the level of fertility falls (gradually moving from the currently observed differentials).

For educational mortality differentials, the data situation is much worse, and no attempt was made to estimate them.[12] Hence the projections do not show different mortality by education. As discussed in Lutz *et al.* (1999), such differentials only have significant effects for the size of the elderly population. They are less relevant

---

[10]The aggregate TFR for the period 1995–2000 by region was calculated from the United Nations (1999) country estimates of age-specific fertility rates weighted by number of women by age.

[11]Information was derived from the following sources: Macro-International Demographic and Health Surveys, 1988–1998; League of Arab States PAPCHILD Project, 1990s; Fertility and Family Surveys, 1990s; and several national surveys (see Appendix 4.1).

[12]Data on infant mortality by education of the mother are available from surveys, but neither this information nor the information about surviving relatives is sufficient to study.

Table 4.1. Fertility differentials by women's education level in 1995–1998 extracted from selected Demographic and Health Surveys.

Region	Total	No education (A)	Primary education	Secondary education	Tertiary education (B)	Difference, (A)–(B)
Africa						
Benin, 1996	6.0	6.6	4.8	3.0	1.3	5.3
Central African Republic, 1995	5.1	5.2	5.3	4.0	1.9	3.3
Comoros, 1996	4.7	5.3	4.8	3.6	1.8	3.5
Egypt, 1996	3.6	4.6	3.5	2.4	2.5	2.0
Kenya, 1998	4.7	5.8	5.0	3.6	3.0	2.8
Madagascar, 1997	6.0	6.8	6.5	4.4	2.0	4.8
Mali, 1996	6.7	7.1	6.5	4.2	2.3	4.8
Mozambique, 1997	5.2	5.1	5.4	3.5	1.4	3.7
Niger, 1998	7.2	7.5	6.2	5.1	2.7	4.8
Senegal, 1997	5.7	6.3	5.2	3.3	2.1	4.2
Tanzania, 1996	5.8	6.4	5.6	3.1	2.4	4.0
Chad, 1997	6.4	6.4	6.7	4.9	3.4	3.0
Togo, 1998	5.2	6.3	4.6	2.7	1.3	5.0
Uganda, 1995	6.9	7.0	7.1	5.2	2.0	5.1
Zambia, 1997	6.1	6.8	6.7	4.8	2.9	3.9
Asia						
Bangladesh, 1997	3.3	3.9	3.2	2.2	2.0	2.0
Indonesia, 1997	2.8	2.7	3.1	2.7	1.9	0.8
Nepal, 1996	4.6	5.1	3.8	2.5	2.3	2.8
Philippines, 1998	3.7	5.0	5.0	3.6	2.9	2.1
Latin America and Caribbean						
Bolivia, 1997	4.2	7.1	5.7	3.3	2.2	5.0
Brazil, 1996	2.5	5.0	3.3	2.1	1.5	3.5
Colombia, 1995	3.0	5.0	3.8	2.6	1.8	3.1
Dominican, 1996	3.2	5.0	3.7	2.6	1.9	3.1
Guatemala, 1995	5.1	7.1	5.1	2.7	1.8	5.3
Haiti, 1995	4.8	6.1	4.8	2.5	1.9	4.2
Nicaragua, 1998	3.6	5.7	4.2	2.7	1.5	4.2
Peru, 1996	3.5	6.9	5.0	3.0	2.1	4.8

Source: Selected Demographic and Health Surveys.

for the study of the working-age population. Based on the assumption that interregional migrants are usually more educated than the general population, migrants were allocated according to the following shares:

- Ten percent to the no education category.
- Forty percent to the primary education category.
- Forty percent to the secondary education category.
- Ten percent to the tertiary education category.

Table 4.2. Total fertility rates by region and by level of educational attainment for 1995–2000.

1995–2000	Total	No education	Primary	Secondary	Tertiary
North Africa	3.56	4.50	3.23	2.46	2.27
Sub-Saharan Africa	5.52	6.13	5.53	3.99	2.35
North America	1.95	1.93	1.93	1.95	1.96
Latin America	2.69	4.93	3.40	2.14	1.61
Central Asia	3.16	n.a.	1.98	3.30	2.52
Middle East	4.14	4.94	4.44	3.54	2.57
South Asia	3.38	3.80	3.34	2.54	2.18
China region	1.88	2.43	2.14	1.63	1.08
Pacific Asia	2.53	2.55	2.85	2.36	1.88
Pacific OECD[a]	1.50	1.50	1.50	1.50	1.50
Western Europe	1.64	2.24	1.71	1.64	1.52
Eastern Europe	1.44	1.62	1.64	1.44	1.15
FSU Europe[b]	1.41	1.29	1.30	1.43	1.39

[a]Organisation for Economic Co-operation and Development members in the Pacific region.
[b]European part of the former Soviet Union.
Source: Authors' calculations.

The multistate educational projections also require data on the transition of children from one level of school attainment to another. In our model, all children are born into the no education category. Transition rates between education categories for the starting period were calculated and estimated on the basis of the most recently available levels of educational attainment and enrolment rates for the 5–9, 10–14, 15–19, and 20–24 age groups. To ease the work required to estimate the transition, the first transition (from no education to primary education) occurs in the 5–9 age group. The second transition (from primary education to secondary education) occurs in the 10–14 age group, and the final transition (from secondary education to tertiary education) takes place in the 15–19 age group. Transition rates are presented in *Table 4.3*. UNESCO data on school enrolment tend to be biased upward because of an incentive structure in which school officials are usually rewarded for reporting higher numbers, so here special efforts have been made to estimate educational transition rates from the more reliable census- and survey-based information about educational attainment by age.

Future transition rates from one educational group to the next are subject to alternative scenario assumptions, as discussed in Chapter 5.

4.4 Scenarios

The results of three different scenarios are presented and discussed here:

• The "constant transition rates" (or "constant") scenario assumes that no improvements are made over time in the proportions of a young cohort that acquire

Table 4.3. Education transition rates (%) in 2000–2005 by region and sex.

Region	Transitions from					
	No education to primary education in 5–9 age group		Primary education to secondary education in 10–14 age group		Secondary education to tertiary education in 15–19 age group	
	Male	Female	Male	Female	Male	Female
North Africa	92	76	65	67	21	18
Sub-Saharan Africa	81	67	34	33	9	6
North America	100	100	97	98	52	55
Latin America	100	100	65	66	16	17
Central Asia	100	100	98	98	14	12
Middle East	92	76	65	67	16	15
South Asia	97	74	38	23	20	24
China region	99	98	73	65	6	5
Pacific Asia	97	94	53	51	22	18
Pacific OECD[a]	100	100	97	97	26	23
Western Europe	100	100	97	98	40	46
Eastern Europe	100	100	86	88	12	13
FSU Europe[b]	100	100	91	90	21	25

[a]Organisation for Economic Co-operation and Development members in the Pacific region.
[b]European part of the former Soviet Union.
Source: Authors' calculations.

different levels of education, while fertility, mortality, and migration trends follow the median demographic assumptions, as discussed above.

• The "convergence to North American transition rates by 2030" (or "American")
scenario assumes that all regions experience linear improvements in their enrolment that will bring them by 2025–2030 to the school enrolment levels of
North America today. All children will receive at least some primary education,
and up to 98 percent will receive some secondary education. The participation
in tertiary education will increase to 55 percent. The "American" scenario also
implies a closing of the gender gap at all levels of the educational scheme by
2030.

• The "ICPD" scenario reflects the quantitative goals concerning education that
were agreed at the International Conference on Population and Development
(ICPD) held in Cairo in 1994. These explicit goals are mainly related to the
spread of education in developing countries and especially refer to girls. Specifically, the Cairo Programme of Action calls for the following:

  – Elimination of the gender gap in primary and secondary education by 2005
    (operationalized as female enrolment reaching male levels by 2005–2010).
  – Complete access to primary education for all girls and boys by 2015 (oper-
    ationalized as linear interpolation to the period 2015–2020).
  – Net primary school enrolment ratio for children of both sexes of at least 90
    percent by 2010 (operationalized by 2010–2015).

Countries that have achieved the goal of universal primary education are urged
to extend education and training at secondary and higher levels. This less precise
goal was operationalized as follows. In developing countries the transition rate
from primary to secondary education reaches 75 percent by 2025–2030 for both
sexes. Transition to tertiary education increases by 5 percentage points until 2025–
2030, except for North America, where it is already above 50 percent.

Figures 4.3–4.5 give the starting conditions in 2000 and the results of the three
alternative scenarios in 2030 for sub-Saharan Africa, South Asia, and the China
region, respectively. The figures are in the form of multistate age pyramids for
women and men in five-year age groups. The improvements in schooling over the
past 20 years are clearly visible in the form of the smaller numbers without formal
education in the younger cohorts. The improvement in South Asia (*Figure 4.4*),
however, was much more pronounced for men than for women, and today this
strong gender gap in education still exists. The longer-term implications of this are
visible in the second pyramid, which gives the results of the "constant" scenario.
Past declines and anticipated future declines in total fertility mean the age structure
of South Asia is expected to age. The youngest cohorts will no longer be larger

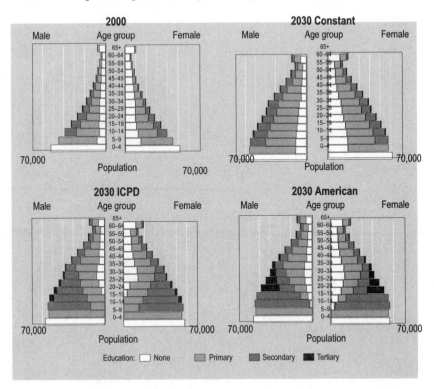

Figure 4.3. Age and education pyramids for sub-Saharan Africa in 2000 and in 2030 according to the "constant," "ICPD," and "American" scenarios. *Source*: Authors' calculations.

than the preceding ones; the mean age of the population will increase; and the population aged 65 and older will double over the next 30 years. In terms of education, the pattern reflects the gender bias in the current South Asian educational system. The "ICPD" and "American" scenarios, in contrast, show other possible futures that would significantly increase the educational attainment of the South Asian population below age 30 and narrow the educational gender gap. However, the older labor force will not be affected by 2030. This illustrates the slow speed at which recent and future investments in education affect the composition of the total population.

Some regions are likely to see stunning progress even in the "constant" scenario. Most impressive is the China region (*Figure 4.5*), where the proportion of women aged 15 and older with a secondary education will increase from 35 percent in 2000 to 60 percent in 2030, and that of men will increase from 51 to 71 percent. In North Africa and the Middle East, the proportion of women with secondary education will increase from 20 and 23 percent, respectively, in 2000 to 35 and 37 percent in 2030. These expected improvements are a direct consequence of past

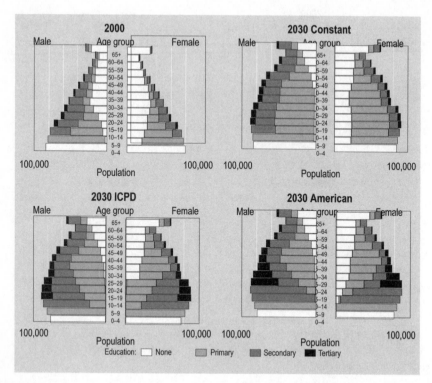

Figure 4.4. Age and education pyramids for South Asia in 2000 and in 2030 according to the "constant," "ICPD," and "American" scenarios. *Source*: Authors' calculations.

investments in female education. In sub-Saharan Africa, only minor improvements in educational attainment can be expected through this compositional effect. In a number of African countries, recent declines in school enrolment rates even imply a deterioration of the educational composition in the longer run.

At the global level, the "constant" scenario implies that in 2030 one out of five women aged 15 and older will still be without any formal education and mostly illiterate. For men this figure is only 8 percent. Under the "ICPD" scenario, which emphasizes rapid steps toward universal primary education, 7 percent of the world's male population and 14 percent of the female population aged 15 and older will still be basically uneducated in 2030. This slow improvement at the lower educational end and in the closure of the gender gap of the adult population is again because of the great inertia of the educational composition. The results of efforts become visible more quickly for secondary education in the "ICPD" scenario and for tertiary education in the "American" scenario. In 2000, 42 percent of men and 32 percent of women had some secondary education; these numbers will be, respectively, 51

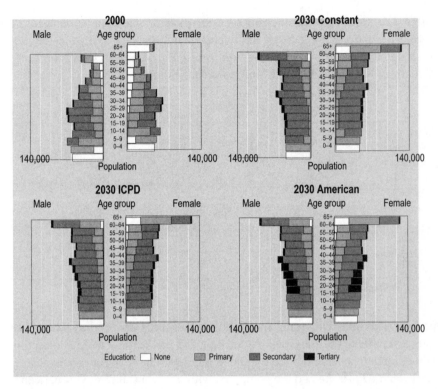

Figure 4.5. Age and education pyramids for the China region in 2000 and in 2030 according to the "constant," "ICPD," and "American" scenarios. *Source*: Authors' calculations.

and 44 percent in 2030 according to the "ICPD" scenario. Also, while currently 8 percent of all women and 11 percent of all men in the world have some tertiary education, by 2030 this will increase to only 10 and 12 percent, respectively, under the "constant" scenario, but to 17 and 20 percent, respectively, under the "American" scenario.

As discussed above, we also calculated several other scenarios, but these cannot be presented here because of space limitations. We highlight, however, the results of one special scenario that incorporates a second-order feedback, from the level of education of mothers to the enrolment ratios for girls, which goes beyond the first-order feedbacks (compositional effects) of the "constant" and "American" scenarios. Taking the "American" scenario as a basis, this special scenario assumes that the educational transition rate for secondary and tertiary education in any five-year period increases or decreases by the same rate as the proportion of women with a secondary and tertiary education in certain age groups (ages 30–39 for secondary education and 40–49 for tertiary education) changes compared with the previous

Table 4.4. Educational composition (percent) of female population aged 20–65. Special scenario with feedback from changes in proportions of educated mothers to secondary and tertiary enrolment ratios of girls, compared with "constant" and "American" scenarios for the China region and South Asia.

	2000	2030 Constant	American	American with feedback
China region				
No education	21.5	3.4	3.6	3.6
Primary	41.0	26.0	27.8	25.5
Secondary	35.3	65.5	51.5	50.9
Tertiary	2.2	5.1	17.0	20.0
South Asia				
No education	68.1	35.3	33.0	33.0
Primary	14.6	45.4	36.7	38.6
Secondary	15.3	15.7	18.6	13.5
Tertiary	1.9	3.7	11.7	14.9

Source: Authors' calculations.

period. This self-reinforcing feedback mechanism is assumed to cover both the intergenerational transmission of education and the fact that more-educated populations tend to be more productive and in turn invest more in education. The results are given in *Table 4.4* and are compared with the "constant" and "American" scenarios for the female population aged 20–65 in the China region and South Asia. Primary enrolment was not made subject to this feedback mechanism (because the "American" scenario already assumes a strong trend to universal enrolment), so the proportions with no education in 2030 are identical in both scenarios. As discussed above, this proportion is almost 10 times larger in South Asia than in the China region. For the higher educational groups, this reinforcing feedback mechanism results in a clear further improvement of the educational attainment structure in the China region, whereas in South Asia it results in an interesting bifurcation. Compared with the "American" scenario, the proportions with primary and with tertiary education increase, while the proportion with secondary education declines. This may partly reflect the bifurcation in Indian society, in which the assumed intergenerational transfer in education tends to produce a sizeable intellectual elite, on the one hand, and a large group with lower education, on the other, with the intermediate group of secondary education diminishing.

4.4.1 Regional Shifts in Human Capital

In the same way that the MDRs will have a lower and lower share of the world's population than the LDRs in the future, the human capital of the planet will be

Table 4.5. Share of the working-age population (aged 20–65) by level of educational attainment according to the "constant," "ICPD," and "American" scenarios in more developed regions (MDRs) and less developed regions (LDRs).

Education	Sex	2000		Constant		ICPD		American	
		MDRs	LDRs	MDRs	LDRs	MDRs	LDRs	MDRs	LDRs
No education	Male	1.5	23.0	0.7	8.2	0.7	7.5	0.7	7.8
	Female	2.3	39.2	0.8	20.0	0.8	16.2	0.8	18.6
Primary	Male	16.5	32.1	7.8	37.4	7.3	34.6	7.5	32.1
	Female	19.0	30.9	7.8	36.6	7.3	34.3	7.5	31.8
Secondary	Male	54.8	38.3	59.3	46.7	58.6	48.9	53.9	41.0
	Female	53.7	25.8	57.0	37.8	56.2	42.0	52.4	33.4
Tertiary	Male	27.2	6.6	32.2	7.6	33.4	9.0	38.0	19.0
	Female	25.0	4.1	34.4	5.6	35.7	7.5	39.3	16.1

Source: Authors' calculations.

concentrated increasingly in today's LDRs. Whereas 77 percent of the working-age population (aged 20–65) lived in LDRs in 2000, that figure will reach 84 percent by 2030, regardless of the scenario. The levels of educational attainment will be crucial to the development of these regions (see *Table 4.5* and *Tables A4.2* and *A4.3* in Appendix 4.2). The "constant" scenario shows what the educational structure will be if all future cohorts adopt today's enrolment rates. In this case, two major changes will occur in the educational composition of LDRs. The share without formal education will decline from one-third of the LDR's working-age population to 14 percent (8 percent for men and 20 percent for women) in 2030, and there will be a strong increase in the share of the population with a secondary education, from 38 to 47 percent in 2030 for males and from 26 to 38 percent for females. If educational improvements are implemented as in the "American" scenario, illiteracy levels will change in a way similar to that in the "constant" scenario, but more people will have a tertiary education (up to 18 percent under the "American" scenario compared with 7 percent under the "constant" scenario, up from 5 percent in the year 2000). The longer time for implementation of higher education in MDRs means that changes will not be as drastic under the two scenarios envisioned. The "constant" scenario shows a slight increase of the proportion with a higher education—secondary and tertiary together—and a proportional decrease of the proportion with a primary education. According to the "American" scenario, more than 90 percent of the population in MDRs will have at least a secondary education, compared with 80 percent in 2000, and almost 40 percent will have a tertiary education.

The changing educational composition of the population is significant not only for an individual's development and a nation's institutional and economic

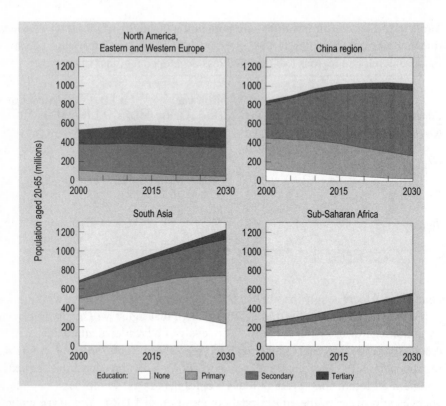

Figure 4.6. Population (in millions) aged 20–65 by level of education, according to the "ICPD" scenario in four mega-regions, 2000–2030. *Source*: Authors' calculations.

performance, but also for the relative weights, productivity, and competitiveness of major world markets. In this context, it is useful to look at absolute numbers of workers by skill level rather than at the proportions discussed above. *Figure 4.6* compares four of the economic mega-regions of the future (Europe and North America together, the China region, South Asia, and sub-Saharan Africa) in terms of trends in the size of the working-age population (aged 20–65) by educational attainment. The data presented are taken from the "ICPD" scenario. At present, the China region clearly has the largest total working-age population of these four regions, but its educated population (secondary and tertiary together) is still smaller than that of Europe and North America together. In terms of the educated working-age population, South Asia is far behind, with levels less than half those in Europe and North America, or the China region. Over the next 20 years, South Asia is expected to surpass the China region in terms of the total size of its working-age population. However, in terms of the educational composition of the population, the difference between the two regions will be stunning. While in the China region in 2030, 73 percent of the working-age population will be better educated (secondary plus tertiary), in South Asia that figure will be only 40 percent. The main reason for this divergence lies in the differences between the two regions in investment in primary and secondary education over the past two decades. Among the four major world regions, Europe and North America will continue to have the highest educational qualifications for its working-age population, but in terms of absolute numbers of educated people, this region will clearly fall behind the China region. Over the next three decades, the China region's educated working-age population is likely to increase from 390 million to 750 million, while that of Europe (without the former Soviet Union) and North America together will increase slightly from 430 million to 510 million in 2030. These significant future changes in the numbers of skilled workers are likely to have far-reaching consequences for the weights in the global economic system. In sub-Saharan Africa, low human capital associated with enormous pressure on the educational system poses significant limits to the prospects for social and economic development in the nearer term. In 2000, only 19 percent of the population in the 20–65 age group had a secondary or tertiary education. Although this percentage will almost double to 35 percent in 2030 according to the "ICPD" scenario, this shows how sub-Saharan Africa is far from converging to the other regions' levels of educational attainment.

These results also indicate that the investments in the educational system need to be increased substantially to cover the increase in levels of enrolment and the increase in population size from further population growth in developing countries. *Table 4.6* shows the absolute numbers of people aged 15–24 with some secondary and tertiary education together (higher education) from 2000 to 2030 by region, according to the three scenarios. *Figure 4.7* illustrates the data for three regions. The data show that even if all the regions keep the levels of enrolment at their present rates, the number of pupils entering an institution of higher education will increase substantially in sub-Saharan Africa, the Middle East, Central and South Asia, and the China region. The China region will be facing enormous tension in the educational system, as 53 million more students will enter higher education in 2010 than in 2000—an increase of more than 40 percent between the two periods. Similar problems will be faced in sub-Saharan Africa, where the levels of income are even lower than those in South Asia. Under the "American" scenario these changes are even more pronounced for LDRs. In contrast, *Table 4.6* shows that MDRs will face a decline in the absolute numbers of students that enter higher education as a result of the reversal of population growth.

In terms of policy priorities, this study numerically demonstrates the importance of near-term investments in education for a nation's longer-term human resources, and thus confirms an often-held qualitative view. The past decades of

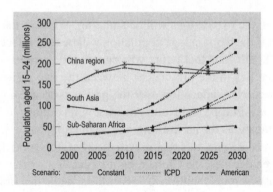

Figure 4.7. Population (in millions) in 15–24 age group with some secondary or tertiary education according to the "constant," "ICPD," and "American" scenarios in three regions, 2000–2030. *Source*: Authors' calculations.

Table 4.6. Population (millions) in 15–24 age group with some secondary or tertiary education in 2000, 2010, 2020, and 2030 according to the "constant," "ICPD," and "American" scenarios.

Regions	2000	Constant			ICPD			American		
		2010	2020	2030	2010	2020	2030	2010	2020	2030
North Africa	22.3	22.4	24.7	24.5	22.7	30.2	32.7	23.5	32.5	39.8
Sub-Saharan Africa	35.7	43.6	49.0	54.7	51.1	101.0	155.8	52.1	107.2	185.0
North America	43.1	43.8	42.3	43.9	43.9	42.9	44.9	43.8	42.4	44.1
Latin America	68.8	70.6	74.5	74.3	71.7	79.9	83.9	74.2	93.1	106.4
Central Asia	12.1	12.3	13.9	14.6	12.4	14.1	14.8	12.3	13.9	14.4
Middle East	22.0	24.6	28.8	30.6	25.4	36.0	41.0	25.8	38.0	49.6
South Asia	91.9	85.6	94.7	95.3	104.2	195.8	250.0	103.7	204.9	307.4
China region	119.9	172.6	161.9	157.7	171.1	177.0	194.0	170.6	174.8	187.0
Pacific Asia	44.2	46.5	50.4	49.6	49.0	63.9	72.6	50.7	73.8	91.5
Pacific OECD[a]	16.8	15.1	15.5	13.9	15.2	15.7	14.3	15.1	15.6	14.0
Western Europe	55.5	54.0	50.7	47.5	54.1	51.3	48.6	54.0	50.8	47.7
Eastern Europe	15.8	11.9	11.6	11.0	12.0	12.5	12.4	12.0	12.4	12.1
FSU Europe[b]	34.2	22.5	22.5	21.8	22.8	23.8	23.8	22.7	23.5	23.3

[a]Organisation for Economic Co-operation and Development members in the Pacific region.
[b]European part of the former Soviet Union.
Source: Authors' calculations.

international development have taught us that, of the countries at comparable stages of development in the 1960s, those that invested heavily in education then clearly do better today by virtually all health and development indicators. Inversely, cutting back on education and even risking a decline in enrolment rates, as has happened in many countries in the course of structural adjustment programs, is detrimental to a population's long-term future.

In the broader context of sustainable development, the educational composition of the population may also become an important factor in the ability of societies to adapt to inevitable environmental change. In the global discussion about the consequences of climate change, adaptation to such changes is becoming an increasingly important topic. However, in this discussion there seems to be a lack of useful predictors for societies' capacities for adaptation. Since education is probably the single most important determinant of empowerment versus vulnerability, at both the individual and societal levels, the kinds of educational projections presented in this chapter may also offer an analytical handle for forecasting future adaptive capacities in the context of climate change.

Appendix 4.1:
Sources of Data and Methods of Estimation

The decomposition by level of educational attainment by region was based on individual country data. These were extracted from a large variety of sources, mostly from the UNESCO *Statistical Yearbook* (1995), but also from the OECD *Education Database* (1999), EUROSTAT Data Base, Macro-International Demographic and Health Surveys (1988–1998), League of Arab States PAPCHILD Project (1990s), and several country censuses. (More detailed information on the source for each country is available on request.) The data obtained from UNESCO yearbooks on the adult population according to the highest level of education attained were collected from national population censuses or sample surveys. UNESCO presents the data available from the latest census or survey held since 1979. They are either provided by the United Nations Statistical Division or derived from national publications. Globally, the range of countries was representative of the region and was aimed at maximum coverage. The coverage was estimated at more than 95 percent of the total population in 2000 for the China region, North America, Pacific Asia, Pacific OECD, and South Asia. The coverage was between 84 and 89 percent for the regions of Central Asia, Eastern Europe, FSU Europe,[13] Latin America, and Western Europe. In the three remaining regions—Middle East, North Africa, and sub-Saharan Africa—the coverage was between 60 and 80 percent.

Some adjustments had to be made to account for differences in the data format needed for the projections. These were mostly of two sorts. First, adjusting the data to fit the 2000 base year was required in most cases, unless educational composition was available for the period 1996–2000. The age groups were moved up to reflect the aging of the population. For instance, if the population in the 20–24 age group was available for 1990 for Pakistan by education, these data were shifted to the 30–34 age group for the year 2000, and so on, for all age groups. The second adjustment that was often needed was related to data not available for all age groups. Sometimes the educational attainment of the population is available for age groups larger than the five-year age groups used for the projections. In such cases, the same educational decomposition was used for the larger age groups as for the smaller age groups. Education data were often missing for younger age groups up to 25 years of age. The missing data were then approximated by data on enrolment at different periods of times, which are usually provided by UNESCO in its yearbooks.

Sources of Input Data on Population by Education and by Education Used in Multistate Educational Projections

The education share of the population in region 1, North Africa, is estimated from the data of four countries: Egypt, Morocco, Sudan, and Tunisia. For Egypt, Morocco, and Sudan, data on levels of educational attainment were collected during the Demographic and Health Surveys (DHS) in 1995, 1992, and 1990, respectively. For Tunisia, the level of education of women aged 15–49 was taken directly from the PAPCHILD—Pan Arab Project for Child Development—(Ministère de la Santé Publique, 1996) survey of Tunisia; for older age groups as well as for the male population aged 25 and older, the distribution of population

---

[13] European part of the former Soviet Union.

by education was estimated from the UNESCO *Statistical Yearbook* (1995) data for Tunisia (1984) on educational attainment. For ages 15–25, the distribution by educational group was taken from the Global Education Database (GED).[14]

The calculation of total fertility rates (TFRs) by level of education in North Africa is based on the TFRs gathered through the DHS of Egypt (1995) and Morocco (1995), and through the PAPCHILD Project for Algeria (Ministère de la Santé et de la Population 1992), Tunisia (Ministère de la Santé Publique 1996), and Sudan (Federal Ministry of Health 1992/1993).

Levels of educational attainment of the population in region 2, sub-Saharan Africa, originate from data collected in the framework of the DHS in the following countries (the years the surveys were conducted are indicated in parentheses): Benin (1996), Burkina Faso (1992), Cameroon (1991), Central African Republic (1994), Chad (1997), Comoros (1996), Ghana (1993), Ivory Coast (1994), Kenya (1998), Madagascar (1997), Malawi (1992), Mali (1996), Mozambique (1997), Namibia (1992), Niger (1998), Nigeria (1990), Rwanda (1992), Senegal (1993), Tanzania (1996), Togo (1998), Uganda (1995), Zambia (1996), and Zimbabwe (1994).

The TFRs by women's level of education in sub-Saharan Africa were calculated based on the TFRs gathered through the DHS of the countries mentioned above.

The data on population by education for region 3, North America, are calculated from UNESCO figures for the United States of America (1994) and Canada (1991). Fertility rates by level of education are extracted from a survey on the fertility of American women (US Bureau of Census 1997) and from the Family Fertility Survey (FFS) of Canada (UNECE 1999a).

The distribution of the population by education as well as the fertility differentials by education for region 4, Latin America, are based on the DHS data for the following countries: Bolivia (1998), Brazil (1996), Colombia (1995), Dominican Republic (1996), Guatemala (1995), Haiti (1994), Nicaragua (1997), Paraguay (1990), and Peru (1996), and from the UNESCO database for Mexico (1990) (UNESCO 1995).

For region 5, Central Asia, the data were extracted from the DHS for Kazakhstan (1995) and Uzbekistan (1996), and from the UNESCO database for Tajikistan (1989). Figures on fertility differentials by level of education were only found for the countries of Kazakhstan (1995) and Uzbekistan (1996) within the results of the DHS for the two countries.

Population and education data for region 6, the Middle East, are based on the individual country data for Iran, Israel, Jordan, Lebanon, and Syria. The data from Iran were compiled from the 1996 census. Information on Israel for the year 1998 was gathered from the Statistical Abstract (Central Bureau of Statistics—Israel 1999). The data for Jordan are based on the 1990 DHS. For Lebanon, the data were extracted from the Population and Housing Survey (Ministry of Social Affairs—Lebanon 1996). Data for Syria for 1994 were compiled from Goujon (1997).

---

[14]The GED was developed by USAID's Center for Human Capacity Development to provide the Agency and its development partners with selected statistical data on international education in an easy-to-use format.

The data on fertility by level of education for the Middle East region were calculated on the basis of individual country data for Jordan (DHS 1990), Lebanon (Ministry of Social Affairs—Lebanon 1996), and Syria (Goujon 1997).

The share of the population by education for region 7, South Asia, was based on data obtained from the 1997 UNESCO *Statistical Yearbook* for four countries: Bangladesh (1981), India (1981), Nepal (1991), and Pakistan (1990). The fertility differentials by level of education for the base year were estimated from DHS data for the following countries: Bangladesh (1997), India (1993), and Nepal (1996).

Population by education figures for region 8, the China region, is based on China (Cao 2000) and Vietnam (UNESCO 1997) for 1995 and 1989, respectively. Fertility data by education were only available for China (Cao 2000).

The share of the population in region 9, Pacific Asia, by level of education is based on UNESCO (1997) data for Indonesia (1990), Korea (1995), Malaysia (1990), Myanmar (1983), Philippines (1990), and Thailand (1990). Fertility differentials by education were compiled from DHS data for Indonesia (1997) and Philippines (1998).

The population and education data for region 10, Pacific OECD, were aggregated from figures for the three countries of the region, namely, Australia, Japan, and New Zealand. The OECD education database provided the data for Australia (1996) and New Zealand (1996), and the data for Japan (1990) was extracted from the UNESCO *Statistical Yearbook* (1997).

No information could be found on fertility differentials by education in the countries of the Pacific OECD region at the time of the study. It was therefore assumed that women in all education categories had the TFR of the whole region in 2000.

Data on population disaggregated by education for region 11, Western Europe, are derived from the OECD database (1999) for the primary, secondary, and tertiary education levels for the year 1997 for Turkey and 1996 for the following countries: Austria, Belgium, Denmark, Finland, France, Germany, Greece, Ireland, Italy, Luxembourg, Netherlands, Norway, Portugal, Spain, Sweden, Switzerland, and United Kingdom. Data for the "no education" category were gathered from the UNESCO *Statistical Yearbook* (1997) for the following countries: Austria (1981), Denmark (1994), Finland (1992), France (1990), Greece (1991), Ireland (1991), Italy (1981), Portugal (1991), Spain (1991), Sweden (1995), Switzerland (1980), and Turkey (1993).

Fertility differentials by education for Western Europe were extracted from the FFS database for Austria (UNECE 1998c), Finland (UNECE 1998b), France (UNECE 1998a), Netherlands (UNECE 1997b), Spain (UNECE 1998d), Sweden (UNECE 1997a), and Switzerland (UNECE 1999b), and from the DHS of Turkey (1993).

The data on population and education for region 12, Eastern Europe, are based on country figures for Bulgaria (1992), Croatia (1991), Czech Republic (1991), Hungary (1990), Poland (1988), Romania (1992), Slovakia (1991), and Slovenia (1991) from UNESCO (1997). The figures on fertility differentials by education are based on the FFS of Hungary (UNECE 1999c) and Poland (UNECE 1997c).

The shares of the population in the four education states for region 13, FSU Europe, are based on UNESCO (1997) data for Estonia (1989), Latvia (1988), Lithuania (1989), Moldova (1989), and the Russian Federation (1994). Data on fertility differentials by education could only be found for Latvia (UNECE 1998e).

Appendix 4.2: Results of the Projections

Table A4.1. Population (in millions) aged 15 and older by education and sex in 2000 and in 2030 according to the "constant," "American," and "ICPD" scenarios.

Region	2000								2030 Constant							
	No education		Primary		Secondary		Tertiary		No education		Primary		Secondary		Tertiary	
	M[a]	F[a]	M	F	M	F	M	F	M	F	M	F	M	F	M	F
North Africa	18	31	12	9	18	11	8	5	14	34	28	21	44	35	14	9
Sub-Saharan Africa	56	90	71	59	35	21	6	2	71	128	180	157	87	69	10	5
North America	1	1	8	8	59	64	53	53	2	2	10	9	76	79	69	78
Latin America	21	27	67	69	67	67	18	16	8	11	97	103	141	147	30	32
Central Asia	0	1	1	1	14	14	3	2	0	0	0	0	26	29	5	4
Middle East	10	17	21	17	16	11	8	5	11	28	39	32	50	41	13	10
South Asia	180	284	108	74	149	65	23	9	96	279	370	329	250	113	52	27
China region	52	133	192	191	270	180	19	10	12	46	141	195	477	408	41	29
Pacific Asia	39	55	61	61	51	41	14	11	24	37	105	110	96	90	26	21
Pacific OECD[b]	0	0	12	14	33	36	16	15	0	0	5	6	40	44	19	18
Western Europe	8	14	42	53	96	94	35	29	3	6	23	29	114	112	59	62
Eastern Europe	1	2	14	20	28	25	5	4	0	0	8	10	35	36	5	6
FSU Europe[c]	1	0	20	28	53	59	15	16	0	0	8	11	61	67	16	21
World	386	656	628	606	888	690	224	179	241	570	1,014	1,013	1,498	1,272	359	322

[a] "M" stands for male and "F" for female.
[b] Organisation for Economic Co-operation and Development members in the Pacific region.
[c] European part of the former Soviet Union.
Source: Authors' calculations.

Table A4.1. Continued.

Region	2030 American								2030 ICPD							
	No education		Primary		Secondary		Tertiary		No education		Primary		Secondary		Tertiary	
	M[a]	F[a]	M	F	M	F	M	F	M	F	M	F	M	F	M	F
North Africa	13	30	21	17	44	36	22	17	12	27	26	22	45	40	16	12
Sub-Saharan Africa	60	107	132	118	115	99	41	34	52	87	150	144	130	119	16	9
North America	2	2	10	9	75	79	70	78	2	2	9	9	77	79	70	78
Latin America	8	11	78	84	136	141	54	56	8	11	91	97	144	149	34	36
Central Asia	0	0	0	0	23	25	8	8	0	0	0	0	26	29	5	5
Middle East	10	24	31	26	49	42	23	19	9	19	36	33	53	47	15	12
South Asia	93	252	269	240	296	185	111	71	91	214	309	270	295	199	73	66
China region	13	47	152	202	405	342	101	88	13	47	150	200	463	398	46	34
Pacific Asia	23	36	84	88	102	96	44	40	22	34	95	98	103	100	32	26
Pacific OECD[b]	0	0	5	6	37	41	21	21	0	0	5	6	39	43	19	19
Western Europe	3	6	22	29	112	113	62	61	3	6	22	28	110	108	64	67
Eastern Europe	0	0	7	9	32	33	9	9	0	0	7	9	35	37	5	6
FSU Europe[c]	0	0	7	10	56	64	21	25	0	0	7	10	60	67	17	22
World	224	514	819	839	1,481	1,295	588	528	212	445	908	927	1,580	1,413	412	391

[a] "M" stands for male and "F" for female.
[b] Organisation for Economic Co-operation and Development members in the Pacific region.
[c] European part of the former Soviet Union.
Source: Authors' calculations.

Table A4.2. Share of population (percent) aged 20–65 by education and sex in 2000 and in 2030 according to the "constant," "American," and "ICPD" scenarios.

| | 2000 | | | | | | | | 2030 Constant | | | | | | | |
| | No education | | Primary | | Secondary | | Tertiary | | No education | | Primary | | Secondary | | Tertiary | |
Region	M[a]	F[a]	M	F	M	F	M	F	M	F	M	F	M	F	M	F
North Africa	34	57	21	17	28	17	17	9	13	31	28	21	46	38	14	10
Sub-Saharan Africa	34	55	41	33	21	11	4	1	20	34	52	44	25	20	3	1
North America	0	0	5	4	45	46	50	50	1	1	7	6	45	42	47	50
Latin America	11	14	39	40	38	37	11	9	2	2	34	33	53	53	11	11
Central Asia	1	2	3	4	78	80	18	14	0	0	1	1	84	86	14	12
Middle East	18	34	40	34	26	21	15	11	9	23	35	29	45	39	11	9
South Asia	42	68	20	15	33	15	5	2	11	35	49	45	33	16	7	4
China region	7	21	38	41	51	35	4	2	1	3	19	26	73	65	7	5
Pacific Asia	23	33	36	36	31	23	10	7	8	12	42	43	39	37	11	9
Pacific OECD[b]	0	0	15	14	55	58	30	28	0	0	6	5	65	67	28	27
Western Europe	3	6	20	25	56	54	20	15	1	1	8	8	58	54	33	36
Eastern Europe	1	2	27	34	61	54	11	9	0	0	13	13	76	76	10	12
FSU Europe[c]	0	0	20	22	62	60	18	18	0	0	8	8	73	70	19	21
World	18	30	29	28	42	32	11	9	7	17	33	32	49	41	12	10

[a] "M" stands for male and "F" for female.
[b] Organisation for Economic Co-operation and Development members in the Pacific region.
[c] European part of the former Soviet Union.
Source: Authors' calculations.

Table A4.2. Continued.

Region	2030 American								2030 ICPD							
	No education		Primary		Secondary		Tertiary		No education		Primary		Secondary		Tertiary	
	M[a]	F[a]	M	F	M	F	M	F	M	F	M	F	M	F	M	F
North Africa	12	29	23	18	40	33	26	21	11	25	26	22	46	41	16	12
Sub-Saharan Africa	18	31	42	37	25	20	15	12	16	26	46	42	34	29	4	2
North America	1	1	7	6	44	42	48	50	1	1	6	6	45	43	47	51
Latin America	2	2	29	29	46	46	23	24	2	2	32	32	54	54	12	12
Central Asia	0	0	1	1	68	69	31	30	0	0	1	1	84	86	15	13
Middle East	8	21	30	26	38	33	24	21	8	17	33	30	48	42	12	10
South Asia	11	33	40	37	32	19	17	12	10	28	43	39	37	25	9	8
China region	1	4	21	28	59	52	19	17	1	4	21	28	71	63	7	6
Pacific Asia	8	11	35	36	36	34	21	19	8	11	39	39	41	40	12	10
Pacific OECD[b]	0	0	6	5	57	58	37	36	0	0	6	5	64	67	29	28
Western Europe	1	1	8	8	53	50	39	40	1	1	8	8	56	52	35	39
Eastern Europe	0	0	12	11	66	65	22	23	0	0	12	11	77	76	11	12
FSU Europe[c]	0	0	7	8	64	62	29	30	0	0	7	7	73	70	20	23
World	7	16	28	28	43	36	22	20	6	14	30	30	50	44	13	12

[a] "M" stands for male and "F" for female.
[b] Organisation for Economic Co-operation and Development members in the Pacific region.
[c] European part of the former Soviet Union.
Source: Authors' calculations.

Table A4.3. Population (in millions) aged 20–65 by education and sex in 2000 and in 2030 according to the "constant," "American," and "ICPD" scenarios.

Region	2000								2030 Constant							
	No education		Primary		Secondary		Tertiary		No education		Primary		Secondary		Tertiary	
	M[a]	F[a]	M	F	M	F	M	F	M	F	M	F	M	F	M	F
North Africa	14	24	9	7	12	7	7	4	10	24	22	17	36	30	11	8
Sub-Saharan Africa	43	70	51	42	27	15	5	2	55	98	146	127	71	57	8	4
North America	0	0	5	4	42	43	46	46	1	1	7	6	49	45	51	54
Latin America	15	19	53	55	51	52	15	13	4	5	74	74	116	118	24	25
Central Asia	0	0	0	1	11	11	2	2	0	0	0	0	21	22	4	3
Middle East	8	13	17	13	11	8	6	4	8	20	31	25	40	33	10	7
South Asia	151	226	72	49	117	51	17	6	68	211	308	271	207	94	43	22
China region	31	88	162	168	221	144	17	9	6	17	98	131	381	329	35	25
Pacific Asia	31	43	47	48	40	31	13	10	16	24	83	85	78	73	21	17
Pacific OECD[b]	0	0	7	7	26	27	14	13	0	0	3	2	28	28	12	11
Western Europe	5	8	28	34	78	74	28	21	1	2	11	11	79	73	45	49
Eastern Europe	0	1	10	13	22	20	4	3	0	0	5	4	27	26	4	4
FSU Europe[c]	0	0	14	16	42	44	12	13	0	0	5	6	46	47	12	14
World	299	493	474	456	699	526	188	147	170	402	792	761	1,180	975	279	244

[a] "M" stands for male and "F" for female.
[b] Organisation for Economic Co-operation and Development members in the Pacific region.
[c] European part of the former Soviet Union.
Source: Authors' calculations.

Table A4.3. Continued.

Region	2030 American								2030 ICPD							
	No education		Primary		Secondary		Tertiary		No education		Primary		Secondary		Tertiary	
	M[a]	F[a]	M	F	M	F	M	F	M	F	M	F	M	F	M	F
North Africa	9	23	18	14	32	26	20	16	9	20	21	17	37	32	12	9
Sub-Saharan Africa	50	89	119	106	71	58	41	34	46	75	127	121	95	84	11	6
North America	1	1	7	6	48	45	52	54	1	1	7	6	49	45	51	54
Latin America	4	5	63	63	100	102	51	52	4	5	71	71	117	119	26	28
Central Asia	0	0	0	0	17	18	8	8	0	0	0	0	21	22	4	3
Middle East	7	18	27	22	34	28	21	18	7	15	29	26	42	37	11	9
South Asia	66	197	248	220	203	111	108	70	65	169	272	234	233	149	55	46
China region	7	18	109	140	307	259	98	85	7	18	107	138	367	317	39	29
Pacific Asia	15	23	70	71	72	67	41	38	15	21	77	78	82	79	24	20
Pacific OECD[b]	0	0	2	2	24	24	16	15	0	0	2	2	27	28	12	12
Western Europe	1	2	11	11	72	68	53	54	1	2	10	11	77	70	48	52
Eastern Europe	0	0	4	4	23	23	8	8	0	0	4	4	27	27	4	4
FSU Europe[c]	0	0	5	5	40	41	18	20	0	0	4	5	46	47	13	15
World	162	376	682	665	1,042	869	534	473	156	326	732	714	1,220	1,055	311	288

[a] "M" stands for male and "F" for female.
[b] Organisation for Economic Co-operation and Development members in the Pacific region.
[c] European part of the former Soviet Union.
Source: Authors' calculations.

References

Ahuja V & Filmer D (1995). *Educational Attainment in Development Countries: New Estimates and Projections Disaggregated by Gender.* Mimeo. Washington, DC, USA: The World Bank.

Barro R & Lee JW (1993). International comparison of educational attainment. *Journal of Monetary Economics* **32**:363–394.

Barro R & Lee JW (2000). *International Data on Educational Attainment. Updates and Implications.* NBER Working Paper 7911. Cambridge, MA, USA: National Bureau of Economic Research.

Bellew R., Raney L & Subbarao K (1992). Educating girls. *Finance and Development* **29**:54–56.

Benavot A (1989). Education, gender, and economic development: A cross-national study. *Sociology of Education* **62**:14–32.

Brock C & Cammish N (1997). *Gender, Education and Development. A Partially Annotated and Selective Bibliography.* London, UK: Department for International Development.

Dubey A & King E (1994). *A New Cross-Country Education Stock Series Differentiated by Age and Sex.* Typescript. Washington, DC, USA: The World Bank.

Federici N, Mason KO & Sogner S (1993). *Women's Position and Demographic Change.* Oxford, UK: Clarendon Press.

Grossman GM & Helpman E (1991). *Innovation and Growth in the Global Economy.* Cambridge, MA, USA: MIT Press.

Hadden K & London B (1996). Educating girls in the third world: The demographic, basic needs, and economic benefits. *International Journal of Comparative Sociology* **37**:31–47.

Jejeebhoy SJ (1995). *Women's Education, Autonomy and Reproductive Behaviour.* Oxford, UK: Clarendon Press.

Keyfitz N (1985). *Applied Mathematical Demography*, Second Edition. New York, NY, USA: Springer Verlag.

Kyriacou GA (1991). Level and Growth Effects of Human Capital: A Cross-Country Study of the Convergence Hypothesis. Mimeo. New York, NY, USA: Department of Economics, New York University.

Lutz W & Goujon A (2001). The world's changing human capital stock: Multi-state population projections by educational attainment. *Population and Development Review* **27**:323–339.

Lutz W, Goujon A & Doblhammer-Reiter G (1999). Demographic dimensions in forecasting: Adding education to age and sex. In *Frontiers of Population Forecasting*, eds. Lutz W, Vaupel JW & Ahlburg DA, pp. 42–58. A Supplement to *Population and Development Review*, **24**, 1998. New York, NY, USA: Population Council.

Mankiw NG, Romer D & Weil DN (1992). A contribution to the empirics of economic growth. *Quarterly Journal of Economics* **107**:407–437.

Nehru V, Swanson E & Dubey A (1993). *A New Database on Human Capital Stock: Sources, Methodology and Results*. Policy Research Working Paper 1124. Washington, DC, USA: The World Bank.

OECD (1999). *Education at a Glance, Database*. CD Rom. Paris, France: Organisation for Economic Co-operation and Development

Psacharopoulos G & Arrigada AM (1986). The educational composition of the labor force: An international comparison. *International Labor Review* 125:561–574.

Psacharopoulos G & Arrigada AM (1992). The educational composition of the labor force: An international update. *Journal of Educational Planning and Administration* 6:141–159.

Rogers A (1975). *Introduction to Multiregional Mathematical Demography*. New York, NY, USA: John Wiley.

Romer PM (1989). *Human Capital and Growth: Theory and Evidence*. NBER Working Paper 3173. Cambridge, MA, USA: National Bureau of Economic Research.

Romer PM (1992). Two strategies for economic development: Using ideas and producing ideas. In *Proceedings of the World Bank Annual Conference on Development Economics*, eds Summers LH & Shah S, pp. 63–115. Washington, DC, USA: The World Bank.

UNESCO (1995). *Statistical Yearbook*. Paris, France: United Nations Educational, Scientific and Cultural Organization.

United Nations (1999). *World Population Prospects. The 1998 Revision*. New York, NY, USA: United Nations.

Bibliography for Data Sources

General

Cao, G-Y(2000). The Future Population of China: Prospects to 2045 by Place of Residence and by Level of Education. Laxenburg, Austria: International Institute for Applied Systems Analysis, IR-00-026, 44 pp.

Central Bureau of Statistics, Israel (1999). Statistical Abstract of Israel 1999. Jerusalem, Israel.

Federal Ministry of Health, Sudan (1992/93). Sudan Maternal and Child Health Survey 1992/93, Pan Arab Project for Child Development. Karthoum, Sudan, 339 pp.

Ministère de la Santé et de la Population, Algeria (1992). Enquête Algérienne sur la Santé de la mére et de l'enfant, Rapport Principal, Projet Pan Arabe pour le Développement de l'Enfance. Imprimerie Office National des Statistiques: Alger, Algeria, 256 pp.

Ministère de la Santé Publique, Tunisia (1996). L'enqute Tunisienne sur la Santé de la Mére et de l'Enfant, Rapport Principal, Projet Pan Arab pour la Promotion de l'Enfance. Imprimerie de l'Office National de la Famille et de la Population: Tunis, Tunisia, 248 pp.

Ministry of Social Affairs (1996). *Population and Housing Survey*. Republic of Lebanon, Beirut, Lebanon.

OECD (1999). Education at a Glance Database, CD-Rom. Paris, France: Organisation for Economic Co-operation and Development.

UNESCO (1995). Statistical Yearbook 1995. Paris, France: United Nations Educational, Scientific and Cultural Organization.

UNESCO (1997). Statistical Yearbook 1997. Paris, France: United Nations Educational, Scientific and Cultural Organization.

U.S. Census Bureau (1997). *Fertility of American Women*, June 1995 (update). Current Population Survey (CPS) Report. U.S. Census Bureau: Washington, D.C.

Fertility and Family Surveys

United Nations Economic Commission for Europe (1997a). Fertility and Family Surveys of the ECE Region, Standard Country Report, Sweden, Economic Studies No. 10b. UN Sales No. E.97.0.21.UNECE: Geneva, 90 pp.

United Nations Economic Commission for Europe (1997b). Fertility and Family Surveys of the ECE Region, Standard Country Report, The Netherlands, Economic Studies No. 10c. UN Sales No. E.97.0.22.UNECE: Geneva, 94 pp.

United Nations Economic Commission for Europe (1997c). Fertility and Family Surveys of the ECE Region, Standard Country Report, Poland, Economic Studies No. 10d. UN Sales No. E.97.0.28.UNECE: Geneva, 99 pp.

United Nations Economic Commission for Europe (1998a). Fertility and Family Surveys of the ECE Region, Standard Country Report, France, Economic Studies No. 10e. UN Sales No. E.97.0.27.UNECE: Geneva, 106 pp.

United Nations Economic Commission for Europe (1998b). Fertility and Family Surveys of the ECE Region, Standard Country Report, Finland, Economic Studies No. 10g. UN Sales No. E.98.0.10.UNECE: Geneva, 87 pp.

United Nations Economic Commission for Europe (1998c). Fertility and Family Surveys of the ECE Region, Standard Country Report, Austria, Economic Studies No. 10h. UN Sales No. E.98.0.24.UNECE: Geneva, 98 pp.

United Nations Economic Commission for Europe (1998d). Fertility and Family Surveys of the ECE Region, Standard Country Report, Spain, Economic Studies No. 10i. UN Sales No. E.98.II.E.26. UNECE: Geneva, 104 pp.

United Nations Economic Commission for Europe (1998e). Fertility and Family Surveys of the ECE Region, Standard Country Report, Latvia, Economic Studies No. 10f. UN Sales No. E.98.0.4. UNECE: Geneva, 110 pp.

United Nations Economic Commission for Europe (1999a). Fertility and Family Surveys of the ECE Region, Standard Country Report, Canada, Economic Studies No. 10k. UN Sales No. E.99.II.E.11. UNECE: Geneva, 82 pp.

United Nations Economic Commission for Europe (1999b). Fertility and Family Surveys of the ECE Region, Standard Country Report, Switzerland, Economic Studies No. 10m. UN Sales No. E.99.II.E.29. UNECE: Geneva, 94 pp.

United Nations Economic Commission for Europe (1999c). Fertility and Family Surveys of the ECE Region, Standard Country Report, Hungary, Economic Studies No. 10j. UN Sales No. E.99.II.E.6. UNECE: Geneva, 93 pp.

Demographic and Health Surveys

Bangladesh—Mitra, S. N.; Al-Sabir, Ahmed; Cross, Anne R.; Jamil, Kanta (1997). Bangladesh Demographic and Health Survey, 1996-1997. National Institute of Population Research and Training: Dhaka, Bangladesh; Mitra and Associates: Dhaka, Bangladesh; Macro International, Demographic and Health Surveys: Calverton, Maryland, 252 pp.

Benin—Kodjogbé Nicaise; Mboup, Gora; Tossou, Justin; de Souza, Léopoldine; Gandaho, Timothe; Guédém, Alphonse; Houedokoho, Thomas; Houndékon, Rafatou; Tohouegnon, Thomas; Zomahoun, Suzanne; Capo-Chichi, Virgile; Cossi, Andrée (1997). Rpublique du Bénin: Enquête Démographique et de Santé 1996. Institut National de la Statistique et de l'Analyse Economique: Cotonou, Benin; Macro International, Demographic and Health Surveys: Calverton, Maryland., 318 pp.

Bolivia—Instituto Nacional de Estadstica (La Paz); Macro International (1998). Bolivia: Encuesta Nacional de Demografa y Salud, 1998. La Paz, Bolivia. 278 pp.

Brazil—Sociedade Civil Bem-Estar Familiar no Brasil (Rio de Janeiro); Macro International (1997). Brasil: Pesquisa Nacional sobre Demografia e Saúde, 1996. Rio de Janeiro, Brazil, 182 pp.

Burkina Faso—Konate, Desire L.; Sinare, Tinga; Seroussi, Michka (1994). Enquête Démographique et de Santé Burkina Faso, 1993. Institut National de la Statistique et de la Dmographie: Ouagadougou, Burkina Faso; Macro International, Demographic and Health Surveys: Calverton, Maryland, 296 pp.

Cameroon—Balepa, Martin; Fotso, Medard; Barrere, Bernard (1992). Enquête Démographique et de Santé Cameroun, 1991. Direction Nationale du Deuxième Recensement Général de la Population et de l'Habitat: Yaounde, Cameroon; Macro International, Demographic and Health Surveys: Columbia, Maryland, 285 pp.

Central African Republic—Ndamobissi, Robert; Mboup, Gora; Nguélébé Edwige O (1995). Enquête Démographique et de Santé République Centrafricaine, 1994-95. Ministère de l'Economie, du Plan et de la Coopération Internationale, Division des Statistiques et des Etudes Economiques: Bangui, Central African Republic; Macro International, Demographic and Health Surveys: Calverton, Maryland, 337 pp.

Chad—Ouagadjio, Bandoumal; Nodjimadji, Kostelngar; Ngoniri, Joël N.; Ngakoutou, Ningam; Ignégongba, Keumaye; Tokindang, Joël S.; Kouo, Oumdagué Barrère, Bernard; Barrère, Monique (1998). Enquête Démographique et de Santé Tchad, 1996-1997. Bureau Central du Recensement, Direction de la Statistique, des Etudes Economiques et Démographiques: N'Djamena, Chad; Macro International, Demographic and Health Surveys: Calverton, Maryland, 366 pp.

Colombia—Ordoñez, Myriam; Ochoa, Luis H.; Ojeda, Gabriel; Rojas, Guillermo; Gmez, Luis C.; Samper, Belén (1995). Encuesta Nacional de Demografa y Salud, 1995. Asociación Pro-Bienestar de la Familia Colombiana: Bogota, Colombia; Macro International, Demographic and Health Surveys: Calverton, Maryland, 233 pp.

Comoros—Mondoha, Kassim A.; Schoemaker, Juan; Barr̄re, Monique (1997). Enquête Démographique et de la Santé Comores, 1996. Centre National de Documentation et de Recherche Scientifique: Moroni, Comoros; Macro International, Demographic and Health Surveys: Calverton, Maryland, 250 pp.

Dominican Republic—Centro de Estudios Sociales y Demogrficos (Santo Domingo); Aso-ciacin Dominicana ProBienestar de la Familia (Santo Domingo); Oficina Nacional de Planificacin (Santo Domingo; Macro International (1997). Encuesta Demogrfica y de Salud, 1996. Santo Domingo, Dominican Republic, 314 pp.

Egypt—El-Zanaty, Fatma; Hussein, Enas M.; Shawky, Gihan A.; Way, Ann A.; Kishor, Sunita (1996). Egypt Demographic and Health Survey, 1995. National Popula-tion Council: Cairo, Egypt; Macro International, Demographic and Health Surveys: Calverton, Maryland, 348 pp.

Ghana—Statistical Service (Accra); Macro International (1994). Ghana Demographic and Health Survey, 1993. Accra, Ghana, 246 pp.

Guatemala—Instituto Nacional de Estadstica (Guatemala City); Ministerio de Salud Pùblica y Asistencia Social (Guatemala City); Agency for International Develop-ment; United Nations Population Fund; Macro International (1996). Guatemala: Encuesta Nacional de Salud Materno Infantil, 1995, Guatemala City, Guatemala, 245 pp.

Haiti—Cayemittes, Michel; Rival, Antonio; Barrére, Bernard; Lerebours, Gérald; Gédéon, Michaèle A. (1995). Enquête Mortalité Morbidité et Utilisation des Services (EMMUS-II), Haiti, 1994/95. Institut Haitien de l'Enfance: Pétionville, Haiti; Macro International, Demographic and Health Surveys: Calverton, Maryland. 364 pp.

India—Ramesh, B. M.; Arnold, Fred; Roy, T. K.; Kanitkar, Tara; Govindasamy, Pavalavalli; Retherford, Robert D (1995). National Family Health Survey (MCH and family planning), India, 1992-93. International Institute for Population Sci-ences: Bombay, India. 402 pp.

Indonesia—Central Bureau of Statistics (Jakarta); National Family Planning Coordinating Board (Jakarta); Ministry of Health (Jakarta); Macro International (1995). Indonesia Demographic and Health Survey, 1994. Jakarta, Indonesia, 366 pp.

Ivory Coast—Sombo, N'Cho; Kouassi, Lucien; Koffi, Albert K.; Schoemaker, Juan; BarrŁre, Monique; BarrŁre, Bernard; Poukouta, Prosper (1995). Enquête Démographique et de Santé Côte d'Ivoire, 1994. Institut National de la Statis-tique: Abidjan, Ivory Coast; Macro International, Demographic and Health Surveys: Calverton, Maryland, 294 pp.

Jordan—Zou'bi, Abdallah A. A.; Poedjastoeti, Sri; Ayad, Mohamed (1992). Jordan Popu-lation and Family Health Survey, 1990. Department of Statistics: Amman, Jordan; Institute for Resource Development/Macro International, Demographic and Health Surveys: Columbia, Maryland, 225 pp.

Kazakhstan—Academy of Preventive Medicine of Kazakhstan (Almaty); National Institute of Nutrition (Almaty). Kazakhstan Demographic and Health Survey, 1995. Almaty, Kazakhstan, 260 pp.

Kenya—National Council for Population and Development (Nairobi); Central Bureau of Statistics (Nairobi); Macro International (1999). Kenya Demographic and Health Survey, 1998. Nairobi, Kenya, 285 pp.

Madagascar—Institut National de la Statistique. Direction de la Démographie et des Statistiques Sociales (Antananarivo); Macro International (1998). Enquête

Démographique et de Santé Madagascar, 1997. Antananarivo, Madagascar, 264 pp.

Malawi—National Statistical Office (Zomba); Macro International (1994). Malawi Demographic and Health Survey, 1992. Zomba, Malawi. 221 pp.

Mali—Coulibaly, Salif; Dicko, Fatoumata; Traoré Seydou M.; Sidibé Ousmane; Seroussi, Michka; Barrère, Bernard (1996). Enquête Démographique et de Santé Mali, 1995–1996. Ministère de la Santé de la Solidarité et de Personnes Agées, Cellule de Planification et de Statistique: Bamako, Mali; Macro International, Demographic and Health Surveys: Calverton, Maryland, 275 pp.

Morocco—Azelmat, Mustapha; Ayad, Mohamed; Housni, El Arbi (1993). Enquête Nationale sur la Population et la Santé (ENPS-II), 1992. Ministère de la Santé Publique, Service des Etudes et de l'Information Sanitaire: Rabat, Morocco; Macro International, Demographic and Health Surveys: Columbia, Maryland, 281 pp.

Morocco—Azelmat, Mustapha; Ayad, Mohamed; Housni, El Arbi (1996). Enquête de Panel sur la Population et la Santé (EPPS), 1995. Ministère de la Santé Publique, Direction de la Planification et des Ressources Financières, Service des Etudes et de l'Information Sanitaire: Rabat, Morocco; Macro International, Demographic and Health Surveys: Calverton, Maryland, 201 pp.

Mozambique—Gaspar, Manuel da C.; Cossa, Humberto A.; dos Santos, Clara R.; Manjate, Rosa M.; Shoemaker, Juan (1998).Moçambique Inquérito Demogrfico e de Saéde, 1997. Instituto Nacional de Estatstica: Maputo, Mozambique; Macro International, Demographic and Health Surveys: Calverton, Maryland, 276 pp.

Namibia—Katjiuanjo, Puumue; Titus, Stephen; Zauana, Maazuu; Boerma, J. Ties (1993). Namibia Demographic and Health Survey, 1992. Ministry of Health and Social Services: Windhoek, Namibia; Macro International, Demographic and Health Surveys: Columbia, Maryland, 221 pp.

Nepal—Pradhan, Ajit; Aryal, Ram H.; Regmi, Gokarna; Ban, Bharat; Govindasamy, Pavalavalli (1997). Nepal Family Health Survey, 1996. Ministry of Health, Department of Health Services, Family Health Division: Katmandu, Nepal; New ERA: Katmandu, Nepal; Macro International, Demographic and Health Surveys: Calverton, Maryland, 250 pp.

Niger—Attama, Sabine; Seroussi, Michka; Kourguni, Alichina I.; Koch, Harouna; Barrère, Bernard. (1999) Niger: Enquête Démographique et de Santé 1998. CARE International: Niamey, Niger; Macro International, Demographic and Health Surveys: Calverton, Maryland. 358 pp.

Nigeria—Federal Office of Statistics (Lagos); Institute for Resource Development/Macro International (1992). Nigeria Demographic and Health Survey, 1990. Lagos, Nigeria, 243 pp.

Paraguay—Centro Paraguayo de Estudios de Poblacion (Asuncion); Institute for Resource Development/Macro Systems (1991). Encuesta Nacional de Demografia y Salud, 1990. Asuncion, Paraguay, 172 pp.

Peru—Reyes Moyana, Jorge; Ochoa, Luis H.; Sandoval, Vilma; Raggers, Han; Rutstein, Shea (1997). Repéblica del Perú Encuesta Demográfica y de Salud Familiar, 1996.

Instituto Nacional de Estad`stica e Informàtica: Lima, Peru; Macro International, Demographic and Health Surveys: Calverton, Maryland, 338 pp.

Philippines—National Statistics Office (Manila); Department of Health (Manila); Macro International (1999). National Demographic and Health Survey 1998: Philippines. Manila, Philippines: 276 pp.

Rwanda—Barrere, Bernard; Schoemaker, Juan; Barrere, Monique; Habiyakare, Tite; Kabagwira, Athanasie; Ngendakumana, Mathias (1994). Enquête Démographique et de Santé Rwanda, 1992. Office National de la Population: Kigali, Rwanda; Macro International, Demographic and Health Surveys: Calverton, Maryland, 218 pp.

Senegal—Ndiaye, Salif; Diouf, Papa D.; Ayad, Mohamed (1994). Enquête Démographique et de Santé au Sénégal (EDS- II), 1992/93. Ministère de l' Economie, des Finances et du Plan, Direction de la Prévision et de la Statistique, Division des Statistiques Démographiques: Dakar, Senegal; Macro International, Demographic and Health Surveys: Calverton, Maryland, 284 pp.

Sudan—Department of Statistics (Khartoum); Institute for Resource Development/Macro International (1991). Sudan Demographic and Health Survey, 1989/1990. Khartoum, Sudan, 180 pp.

Tanzania—Bureau of Statistics (Dar es Salaam); Macro International (1997). Tanzania Demographic and Health Survey, 1996. Dar es Salaam, Tanzania, 312 pp.

Togo—Anipah, Kodjo; Mboup, Gora; Ouro-Gnao, Afi M.; Boukpessi, Bassanté Messan, Pierre A.; Salami-Odjo, Rissy (1999). Enquête Démographique et de Santé Togo, 1998. Ministère de la Planification et du Développement Economique, Direction de la Statistique: Lomé Togo; Macro International, Demographic and Health Surveys: Calverton, Maryland, 287 pp.

Turkey—Ministry of Health. General Directorate of Mother and Child Health and Family Planning (Ankara); Hacettepe University, Institute of Population Studies (Ankara); Macro International (1994). Turkish Demographic and Health Survey, 1993. Calverton, Maryland, 247 pp.

Uganda—Statistics Department (Entebbe); Macro International Demographic and Health Surveys (1996). Uganda Demographic and Health Survey, 1995. Entebbe, Uganda. 299 pp.

Uzbekistan—Ministry of Health. Institute of Obstetrics and Gynecology (Tashkent); Macro International (1997). Uzbekistan Demographic and Health Survey, 1996. Tashkent, Uzbekistan, 253 pp.

Zambia—Central Statistical Office (Lusaka); Ministry of Health (Lusaka); Macro International (1997). Zambia Demographic and Health Survey, 1996. Lusaka, Zambia, 273 pp.

Zimbabwe—Central Statistical Office (Harare); Macro International (1995). Zimbabwe Demographic and Health Survey, 1994. Macro International, Demographic and Health Surveys: Calverton, Maryland, 307 pp.

Chapter 5

Literate Life Expectancy: Charting the Progress in Human Development

Wolfgang Lutz and Anne Goujon

In Chapter 4 we describe human capital in terms of the number of people in different educational groups by age and sex. This gives a complete account of the rather complex changes in the structure of human capital over time. But the results are sometimes a bit complicated to summarize and analyze: a decrease in the proportion of women with a secondary education could result both from a deterioration of educational conditions or from more women moving on to tertiary education. Thus we must look at the full picture of all categories to arrive at the correct interpretation.

In this chapter, we present a simplified single indicator of human capital and, even more broadly, of human development that is more appropriate for direct intercountry comparisons than the multidimensional information on human capital given in Chapter 4. This indicator, called literate life expectancy (LLE), gives the average number of years a man or a woman lives in the literate state by combining the basic social development aspects of life expectancy and literacy in one number. This indicator can also be used to compare subgroups within one population, such as men and women or urban and rural residents. It is based on readily available data and (unlike most other development indicators) can even be projected into the future, based on the population and education projections described in the previous chapters.

This chapter first introduces LLE, then shows how it is calculated and how it can be interpreted. LLE is also compared with the widely used Human Development Index (HDI) introduced by the United Nations Development Programme (UNDP). Next, we present empirical data on LLE for a large number of countries, giving data on time series as well as differentials within populations. Finally, we give numerical projections of LLE to 2030 for our 13 world regions based on alternative educational scenarios.

5.1   A Clear and Meaningful Indicator of Social Development

Scientists are confronted with a strong desire for a single number that comprehensively describes a population's quality of life, can be used for comparative purposes, and has a clear meaning. Gross domestic product (GDP) per capita has been used almost exclusively for this purpose. However, it is a highly problematic indicator for a comprehensive measure of quality of life and development, as it fails to capture the distribution of income and wealth, and it does not represent other important nonmaterial aspects of well-being, such as education and health. Conscious of these shortcomings of GDP per capita, the UNDP offered a more comprehensive alternative by introducing the HDI (used since 1990). This index combines indicators of life expectancy, educational attainment, and income in one figure on a scale between 0 and 1. The HDI serves an important purpose in giving more attention to the social aspects of development, but also has some conspicuous shortcomings (see, e.g., Kelley 1991). The most problematic aspect of the HDI is that it is a highly abstract index that has no analogy in real life. Partly for this reason, GDP per capita remains highly popular because it is somehow suggestive of the average amount that people obtain as a paycheck, although it is derived very differently.

LLE was first developed at IIASA by Wolfgang Lutz in 1995 as an indicator of social development and quality of life (Lutz 1994/95); it combines the two major dimensions of survival and empowerment through literacy. It may be interpreted as the "average number of years a man or a woman lives in the literate state," based on age-specific mortality rates and age-specific proportions literate, computed using life table methods. This indicator has several advantages compared with other indicators, such as the above-mentioned HDI. Moreover, LLE is probably the only social development indicator that can be projected into the future on the basis of other already accepted forecasts and thus illustrates both the path dependence of and realistic prospects for development. It is also particularly well suited as an output and criterion variable for the type of modeling analysis presented in Chapter 6, which includes the population by age, literacy status, and mortality level. Since 1995, LLE has been applied to many settings as a descriptive indicator, ranging from the comparative analysis of Mexican provinces (Medina 1996) to the comparison of major world regions. So far, however, LLE has not been applied to projections; in this chapter, future levels of LLE under given model assumptions are calculated for the 13 world regions.

The key advantages of LLE compared with other indicators of social development are as follows:

- It has a clear interpretation in terms of the individual life cycle. LLE may be directly interpreted as the average number of years a person lives in the literate state (i.e., is able to read and write) under current mortality and literacy conditions. It is not an abstract index on a relative scale, but rather is expressed in terms of individual years of life, which is suggestive of real-life experiences (as GDP per capita is suggestive of real money).
- Unlike GDP per capita, LLE can be readily measured for men and women separately, which makes it very appropriate for gender-specific analysis. It can also be measured for other subgroups of the population, be it by urban or rural place of residence, or by province. This ability to describe within-country differentials is another great advantage over the HDI, which depends on national accounting.
- It can stand alone in its absolute value and does not require the more or less arbitrary assumption of an upper limit that changes over time (as HDI does). This is important, as it enables comparisons to be made over longer time horizons that include periods of major structural changes. In particular, no upper limit for life expectancy needs to be assumed.
- LLE can easily accommodate that not all years gained at very old ages are high-quality years of life. There is increasing concern in industrialized countries that certain parts of the additional years of life gained through increasing life expectancy are years of disability. Analogous to the concept of disability-free (or healthy) life expectancy, functional disabilities at very old ages can be reflected in lower literacy rates at those ages, a feature that makes LLE more relevant for industrialized countries. Indeed, the question of whether an elderly person is still able to read and write may be an even more useful disability indicator in terms of individual empowerment and mental quality of life than other commonly used indicators, such as the ability to climb stairs. In this chapter, however, we do not make an attempt to measure declining literacy with age. This is left to future studies.
- Finally, LLE is based entirely on clearly observable individual characteristics. In this respect, it can be seen as a benefit in terms of purity, rather than a

deficiency, that measures of increase (through concepts of national accounting) are not reflected in LLE. Finding the right level of mortality and literacy
is a largely empirical issue once an operational definition of literacy is applied.
In contrast, none of the usual measures for material wealth can be measured
directly with people. It is to a high degree dependent on the specific accounting
framework applied, whether only the formal economy is considered, whether
the depletion of natural capital is taken into account, and whether real purchasing power or distributional aspects are considered. For the HDI, the income
component is greatly "massaged" in terms of adjusting for purchasing power
and applying other nonlinear transformations that are hard to follow for the average user. It is also important to see that average life expectancy and average
literacy in themselves tend to be much less distorted by high extremes than average income is, because the possible range is much more limited. It may be
wiser not to mix these two very different kinds of indicators, one being based
on individual characteristics and the other, on an abstract economic accounting
framework and certain specific transformations.

5.2   What Does Literate Life Expectancy Represent?

Whether an indicator is useful depends not only on its properties (as described
above), but also on whether it actually measures what we want to measure. First,
it must be stressed that any single numerical indicator is necessarily reductionistic
and carries less information than a set of different indicators. However, if we are
committed to producing a single number, there is still a choice of different possible
indicators, some of which are more useful for the given purpose than others.

   LLE as a summary indicator of social development is based on two underlying
sets of indicators: age-specific mortality rates and age-specific proportions literate. There are convincing arguments for taking individual survival probabilities
and empowerment through basic education as two of the most important and least
ambiguous aspects of human quality of life. Below is an attempt to highlight some
of the underlying reasons, but its brevity means it is certainly incomplete.

   Personal survival to a mature age and the survival of immediate family and
close friends are about the most universal human aspirations that one can think of.
Individual survival is the necessary prerequisite for enjoying any kind of quality
of life. In more economic terms, increases in life expectancy at the level of society increase the expectation of returns from investments, ranging from education
to housing, consumer durables, production sites, etc. This expectation of surviving to see the benefits of investments is a basic prerequisite for modern economic
development.

However, not only does increasing life expectancy facilitate development, but its level also reflects social advancement and quality of life in a very comprehensive manner at the societal level. Life expectancy responds positively to most of the things that we consider to be important ingredients of quality of life (good diet, efficient health care, good housing, benign technologies, good social and economic infrastructure, safe working conditions, education, intellectual stimulation, etc.) and negatively to things we want to avoid (armed conflict, malnutrition, poverty, hazardous work, stress, depression, etc.). One might even go so far as to say that happiness tends to reduce adult mortality, while unhappiness increases the risk of dying; many psychosomatic studies point in that direction. Given all the problems involved in directly measuring health (not to speak of happiness), longevity is still a very useful proxy for health and possibly even indicative of comprehensive well-being. On a societal level the mortality crisis in Eastern Europe, for instance, clearly reflects a social, economic, environmental, and psychological crisis.

Basic education as an indicator of empowerment also has an individual and a societal component. On the individual level, reading and writing skills are basic prerequisites for almost every kind of professional advancement and improvement of living conditions. They are also important for securing one's basic entitlements. Not being able to read and write in most societies means being excluded from progress and carries the danger of being further disempowered. Especially for the empowerment of women in society and within their families, basic education is the key variable.

On the aggregate level of societies, it seems to make a difference whether educational budgets are spent with the aim of achieving universal literacy or whether they are allocated primarily for the higher education of small elites, while large proportions of the population remain illiterate. More generally, human capital—of which education is the most essential ingredient—seems to be by far the most important factor of economic development in the long run. A view to the historical developments of European countries over the past century shows that, without any significant natural resources or financial capital, some initially very backward countries (such as Finland) made it to the very top through early investment in general education and the achievement of nearly universal literacy as early as the beginning of the 20th century. These countries subsequently bypassed other central and southern European countries that originally had much more sophisticated cultures and significantly more physical and financial capital (Lutz 1987). In short, literacy not only shows the current level of social development, but it also characterizes a country's potential for future development.

Finally, one cannot talk about social development without mentioning equity considerations. LLE can be easily calculated for different subpopulations, which are assumed to be more homogeneous than the total, such as differentiation by sex or place of residence (urban, rural). If data are available, there is no limit to further breakdowns. Specific inequality indicators, such as the ratio of lowest and highest values of LLE among subpopulations, may be applied. Also, as mentioned above, because of the limited range of possible outcomes in survival and education, LLE is a very "democratic" measure in the sense that it is reflective of the conditions in the broad majority of the population. It cannot be distorted upward by a few extremes, as GDP per capita can be by a few super-rich individuals.

5.3 Calculations with Empirical Data

The calculation of LLE requires empirical data on age-specific mortality rates and age-specific proportions literate.[1] Age-specific mortality information is readily available in a time-series form for men and women for all countries in the world (e.g., in the United Nations [UN] assessments, although these are partly based on model life tables) and in further breakdowns for a large number of countries. On the educational side, empirical information on literacy is based on either censuses or surveys. In both cases, the information is usually collected in age-specific form, typically in five-year age groups. Hence, wherever total literacy is available, age-specific literacy also tends to be available (although it may not always be published). The United Nations Educational, Scientific and Cultural Organization

[1]On a conceptual level the two components of LLE are not isomorphic: period life expectancy—the mortality indicator used here—is based on age-specific transitions (from life to death) in one observation period; in theory, mortality can change significantly from one year to another. Age-specific literacy, on the other hand, describes the cumulative effect of past transitions (those from the illiterate state to the literate state). For this reason, literacy can only change gradually over time. Current literacy rates, especially at higher ages, are largely the heritage of past times. We know that for countries that experience rapid rises in literacy at young ages, the future literacy of these cohorts is grossly understated by the present literacy rates of the higher age groups.

If it is the future impact of current transitions to literacy that interests us, one could alternatively calculate LLE based on these age-specific transition rates instead of cumulative literacy. This can be done by applying the tools of multistate population analysis to a two-state population (illiterate and literate), simultaneously considering age-specific transition rates in both directions and age-specific mortality (see also Chapter 4). In a way, this approach is conceptually cleaner, because both components are isomorphic by constructing truly synthetic cohorts with respect to both aspects. In the case of a largely illiterate country that has recently made strong efforts to enroll all children in school, the multistate model based on the assumption of constant transition rates will show the path to a completely literate society, which can only be achieved about 70 years later.

If we wish to describe a country's current literacy and mortality conditions (without capturing possible future cohort effects in both components), we are back to combining period life expectancy with current proportions literate. As this is what we want to measure, we chose this approach, which corresponds to the methodology described in *Box 5.1.* Conceptually, under this approach literacy is not treated as an independent vital process, but rather as an attribute attached to the person-years in a life table. In that sense, we are just looking at a specific type of the years of life as implied by present conditions, namely, the literate years of life.

(UNESCO) collects age-specific proportions literate for many countries, sometimes disaggregated by place of residence. Given these data sources, some assumptions often need to be made about literacy among children and in the very high age groups. The former can be derived from information on enrolment levels and the latter, from specialized surveys on the functional reading and writing disabilities of the elderly. While the first has been done for this study, the latter will have to wait for further studies.

As described in *Box 5.1*, the calculation of LLE follows the regular life-table method used to calculate mortality-based life expectancy, with the only addition being that the number of person-years at each age is weighted by the age-specific proportion literate. This is directly analogous to the well-established method of calculating tables of working life in which the L_x column is multiplied by age-specific proportions in the labor force. LLE is always somewhat lower than regular life expectancy, because early childhood is always an illiterate state. A potential problem lies in the fact that different data sources define the literacy status of children differently. This life table method is sensitive to the different ages at which children are assumed to move from the illiterate to the literate state. For the data presented in this chapter, however, we have standardized this assumption and thus made the data directly comparable. An alternative strategy is simply to leave out childhood literacy and compare the data on LLE at age 15. LLE at age 15 can be read directly from the life table and does not suffer from the problem described above. Later in this chapter and in Chapter 6, we also give empirical data for LLE at age 15.

5.4 Trends in Literate Life Expectancy since 1970

Data available from international statistical sources allow us to reconstruct the trends in LLE for the past three decades for almost 50 developing countries and some industrialized countries. A list of data sources and estimation procedures is given in Appendix 5.1 (*Table A5.1*). Further efforts to collect data that are only nationally available (e.g., from past censuses, etc.) could certainly increase the available database for this social development indicator, both in terms of the number of countries included and in terms of the length of the historical period considered. These data sources allow us to chart the progress in human development for much longer time periods than the HDI does. Combined with the LLE projections discussed in the following section, the data presented here already cover a period of 60 years, which makes some of the secular changes in the human condition quantitatively visible.

Figures 5.1 and *5.2* contrast the trends in female and male LLE for selected countries in North Africa and sub-Saharan Africa over the past three decades. In the four countries of North Africa considered here (Algeria, Egypt, Morocco, and

Box 5.1. How to calculate literate life expectancy.

The necessary input data are the age-specific mortality rates (m_x) and the age-specific proportions literate (PL_x), see *Table 5.1*. The L_x column (total number of person-years lived in age group x in the regular life table) is then multiplied by PL_x to generate the LL_x column (literate person-years lived). The LLE at age x (Le_x^0) is then obtained by dividing the cumulative literate person-years (LT_x) by the l_x column.

Table 5.1. Example of the calculation of the literate life expectancy of rural men in Egypt, 1986.

Age (years)	Regular life table				Literate life table			
	m_x	l_x	L_x	e_x^0	PL_x	LL_x	LT_x	Le_x^0
<1	1.041	100,000	93,340	58.60	0.00	0	2,382,889	23.8
1–4	0.081	90,105	353,413	64.00	0.00	0	2,382,889	26.4
5–9	0.017	87,232	434,130	62.06	0.42	183,203	2,382,889	27.3
10–14	0.010	86,494	431,434	57.57	0.84	364,130	2,199,686	25.4
15–19	0.012	86,062	429,077	52.84	0.68	290,485	1,835,556	21.3
20–24	0.017	85,548	426,000	48.15	0.78	333,558	1,545,071	18.1
25–29	0.021	84,824	421,991	43.54	0.48	202,978	1,211,513	14.3
30–34	0.027	83,938	416,986	38.97	0.48	200,570	1,008,535	12.0
35–39	0.032	82,812	410,905	34.46	0.38	156,966	807,964	9.8
40–44	0.035	81,498	404,094	29.98	0.38	154,364	650,999	8.0
45–49	0.069	80,084	393,900	25.46	0.30	118,170	496,635	6.2
50–54	0.121	77,368	375,934	21.26	0.30	112,780	378,465	4.9
55–59	0.240	72,824	344,335	17.43	0.25	85,051	265,684	3.6
60–64	0.252	64,580	304,529	14.32	0.25	75,219	180,633	2.8
65–69	0.572	56,925	250,441	10.89	0.20	50,088	105,415	1.9
70–74	0.682	42,681	183,565	8.66	0.20	36,713	55,327	1.3
75+	1.625	30,247	186,136	6.15	0.10	18,614	18,614	0.6

Source: Lutz (1994/95).

Tunisia), LLE shows strong and almost linear improvements since the 1970s. While Tunisia has the highest absolute level of this social development indicator, both for men and women, Egyptian men show the highest rate of improvement, particularly between the late 1970s and early 1990s. For them, LLE increased by a factor of more than seven, from around 5 years in 1975–1980 to an estimated more than 38 years today. However, *Figure 5.1* also shows that sex differentials in North Africa remain strong. For all four countries, female LLE is clearly below male LLE, with both showing comparable rates of improvement. It is remarkable that even Tunisian women, the most advanced among the female populations of the four countries, have a lower LLE than Moroccan men, the least developed among the

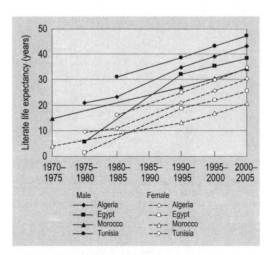

Figure 5.1. Literate life expectancy at birth for selected countries in North Africa, 1970–2005, for males and females. *Source*: Authors' calculations.

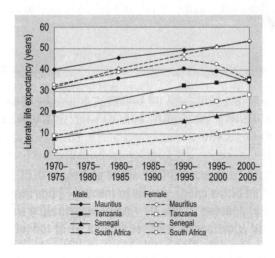

Figure 5.2. Literate life expectancy at birth for selected countries in sub-Saharan Africa, 1970–2005, for males and females. *Source*: Authors' calculations.

male populations. Only in the current period of 2000–2005 is the LLE of these two population groups estimated to be around the same level.

For sub-Saharan Africa the picture is much more diverse (*Figure 5.2*). Of the four countries included in *Figure 5.2*, Mauritius has by far the highest level of human development and the lowest sex differentials. This results from the specific history of Mauritius, with its strong investments in universal literacy of men and

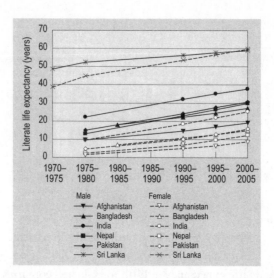

Figure 5.3. Literate life expectancy at birth for selected countries in South Asia, 1970–2005, for males and females. *Source*: Authors' calculations.

women during the 1950s and 1960s, despite extreme poverty at that time, and its subsequent economic success story (see Lutz 1994). South Africa, which was not so different from Mauritius in the 1970s, also shows some improvement up to the early 1990s, but less than Mauritius. Over the past decade South Africa, for men and women alike, shows a sharp downward trend in LLE because of AIDS mortality. This decline has nothing to do with literacy, but is entirely induced by total life expectancy, which falls to very low levels. Actually, had literacy not improved over the past decades, LLE would have fallen even below its 1970 level, as did total life expectancy. Most of the other African countries show still much lower levels of LLE. Senegal and Tanzania were chosen for this graph because Senegal has the lowest level of the 10 sub-Saharan African countries for which data are available (see *Table 5.2*) and Tanzania shows the impact of AIDS, although it does not yet outweigh the impact of improving literacy on LLE.

South Asia is the region in which LLE has been among the lowest for males and females both in the 1970s and today (*Figure 5.3*). In India in 1995–2000, the male and female LLEs were no more than 35 and 22 years, respectively; they were 25 and 13 years, respectively, in Bangladesh, and 27 years and 13 years, respectively, in Pakistan. In these countries, the gender differences are particularly large seen on a global scale. In Afghanistan, Bangladesh, Nepal, and Pakistan, LLE for men is at least twice that for women. As is shown in the following projections, this burden of generally low social development and high gender differences will not be easy to overcome, even under the most optimistic scenarios. The notable

Table 5.2. Literate life expectancy, 1970–2005.

Region	1970–1975 M[a]	F[a]	1975–1980 M	F	1980–1985 M	F	1990–1995 M	F	1995–2000 M	F	2000–2005 M	F
North Africa												
Algeria			21.0	9.4	23.3	11.1	35.1	20.9	39.3	25.7	*43.3*	*30.5*
Egypt			5.6	1.4			32.4	18.7	35.4	22.1	*38.4*	*25.6*
Morocco	14.8	4.1					27.2	13.2	30.7	16.7	*34.3*	*20.6*
Tunisia					31.2	16.0	38.8	24.9	43.3	29.8	*47.3*	*34.6*
Sub-Saharan Africa												
Cameroon	18.6	10.1					30.9	23.8	31.9	26.2	*34.1*	*29.2*
Ghana	15.5	6.4					30.9	21.6	34.0	25.3	*37.1*	*29.2*
Lesotho	21.3	34.4					31.6	45.7	30.1	41.0	*25.6*	*31.3*
Liberia	11.4	3.3					18.2	8.6	24.7	12.4	*30.8*	*16.6*
Mauritius	40.3	31.8			45.6	40.7	49.3	47.2	50.9	50.5	*53.2*	*53.7*
Reunion					57.4	60.7	47.4	56.1	49.7	58.9	*52.6*	*61.8*
Senegal	8.1	2.2					16.0	8.4	18.5	10.5	*21.0*	*12.9*
South Africa	31.2	32.7			35.9	39.0	40.5	44.9	39.3	42.7	*34.3*	*35.2*
Swaziland			21.0	20.3			33.2	33.3	31.8	31.9	*25.9*	*25.3*
Tanzania	20.1	9.0					32.7	22.5	33.9	25.2	*35.7*	*28.3*
Latin America and Caribbean												
Argentina	52.8	58.1	54.2	59.7			58.8	65.0	60.0	66.3	*61.2*	*67.6*
Bolivia	27.2	19.1					43.0	35.7	46.1	39.6	*49.2*	*43.4*
Brazil			36.4	36.1			44.2	48.0	46.2	50.9	*48.2*	*53.7*
Chile					55.1	59.8	59.8	64.2	61.1	65.8	*62.3*	*67.3*
Colombia	39.4	40.3			48.6	50.8	49.2	55.3	52.8	57.9	*55.5*	*60.2*
Costa Rica			56.0	59.3	58.4	57.9	60.7	64.2	62.1	65.8	*63.3*	*67.2*
Cuba			57.7	60.2	59.2	61.6	62.2	65.1	63.5	66.6	*64.8*	*68.0*
Dominican Rep.					38.4	38.2	44.5	45.9	46.4	48.7	*47.1*	*50.6*
Ecuador	39.1	35.9	42.2	39.6			51.5	51.3	53.5	54.0	*55.4*	*56.5*
El Salvador	28.0	24.5			32.3	32.5	41.4	41.0	45.1	44.2	*47.6*	*47.3*
Honduras	25.6	24.6			32.2	31.1	36.6	37.5	38.4	40.3	*40.0*	*42.8*
Jamaica	36.0	41.9					48.6	56.8	51.2	59.6	*53.5*	*62.0*
Martinique					56.9	63.1	62.9	69.8	64.8	71.8	*65.8*	*72.8*
Mexico	39.5	36.1			46.2	45.2	53.5	53.6	55.6	56.3	*57.4*	*58.7*
Paraguay	47.6	43.7	49.9	47.5			53.6	54.0	55.3	56.5	*57.0*	*58.7*
Peru	38.2	29.1	40.6	32.3			51.4	45.8	53.7	49.2	*55.9*	*52.5*
Middle East												
Iran	23.0	12.5					38.8	28.3	43.4	33.2	*47.4*	*38.1*
Iraq	18.8	6.7					26.9	15.7	29.4	19.3	*34.6*	*23.9*
Israel	58.0	53.7	60.7	57.6			65.1	64.3	66.8	66.7	*68.0*	*68.5*

[a] M = male; F = female.

exception in South Asia is Sri Lanka, which shows very high levels of LLE and the disappearance of the gender gap. A similar pattern is likely to appear in some of the Southern Indian states, while India as a whole shows intermediate levels of LLE.

Table 5.2. Continued.

Region	1970–1975 M^a	1970–1975 F^a	1975–1980 M	1975–1980 F	1980–1985 M	1980–1985 F	1990–1995 M	1990–1995 F	1995–2000 M	1995–2000 F	2000–2005 M	2000–2005 F
Asia												
Afghanistan			9.5	1.7			14.7	4.9	16.8	6.7	*19.1*	*8.9*
Bangladesh					17.9	6.8	22.2	10.6	24.6	12.6	*27.0*	*14.8*
Fiji			42.4	35.9			51.5	49.5	54.5	53.1	*56.9*	*56.3*
China	35.4	20.7			41.7	27.3	49.5	37.6	52.8	42.4	*55.8*	*47.2*
India			22.3	9.7			32.2	18.5	35.1	21.7	*37.9*	*25.1*
Indonesia			30.8	22.3			45.3	38.3	48.9	43.1	*52.2*	*47.8*
Malaysia	33.8	21.3			43.3	31.7	51.0	43.0	53.7	47.7	*56.3*	*52.0*
Nepal			13.0	2.3			22.8	7.0	26.2	9.4	*29.8*	*12.2*
Pakistan			15.0	4.5			24.1	10.1	27.4	12.8	*30.6*	*15.6*
Philippines	40.1	41.4	43.6	44.5			52.3	54.6	55.1	57.9	*57.3*	*60.4*
South Korea			52.3	49.4			59.2	61.8	62.0	65.3	*63.5*	*67.9*
Singapore	48.1	31.7					61.0	52.2	63.4	56.6	*65.3*	*60.6*
Sri Lanka	48.7	38.8	52.3	44.8			56.1	53.7	57.6	56.8	*59.0*	*59.6*
Thailand					51.7	47.9	55.8	54.8	56.7	58.2	*58.6*	*61.4*
Europe												
Bulgaria			59.3	59.9			59.5	65.2	59.2	65.9	*59.3*	*66.3*
Cyprus			60.6	52.4	61.8	52.5	65.5	64.5	66.8	67.5	*67.7*	*69.5*
Greece	59.6	52.3					66.0	67.4	66.8	69.7	*67.5*	*71.1*
Italy	59.2	63.1	61.3	66.1	61.5	66.6	65.5	71.1	66.7	72.4	*67.4*	*73.2*
Hungary	58.2	63.4			57.7	64.4	57.1	65.9	58.6	67.2	*60.1*	*68.2*
Malta					53.8	57.1	58.6	63.0	60.6	66.0	*62.6*	*68.2*
Poland			59.3	66.1	59.2	67.0	59.4	68.2	61.0	69.4	*62.2*	*70.4*
Portugal					52.6	52.0	58.4	60.2	60.2	63.1	*62.2*	*65.8*
Spain			60.3	61.5			65.0	70.0	66.0	71.4	*67.0*	*72.6*
Turkey	35.3	20.8					49.9	37.9	52.9	42.5	*55.7*	*46.8*

^{a}M = male; F = female.

Note: Numbers in italics represent projections; all other numbers are estimates.

Sources: Literacy data 1970–2005: UNESCO (2000); mortality data 1970–1985: US Census Bureau Web site, http://www.census.gov/ipc/www/idbnew.html; mortality data 1990–2005: United Nations (2001).

Of all developing regions, Latin America and the Caribbean show the highest levels of LLE and the most consistent upward trend. *Figure 5.4* looks unexciting, with all the trends parallel to one another and no great differentials among the countries. Also, gender differentials diminish over time, and in many countries female LLE is already higher than male LLE. This is the case in Argentina, Brazil, Chile, Colombia, Costa Rica, Cuba, the Dominican Republic, Ecuador, Honduras, Jamaica, Martinique, Mexico, and Paraguay. The reasons for this are that, under low mortality conditions, female life expectancy is several years higher than male life expectancy and there are almost no gender differentials in literacy left.

It is interesting to compare these Latin American countries with some of the economically highly successful Asian Tigers. In South Korea and Singapore, for

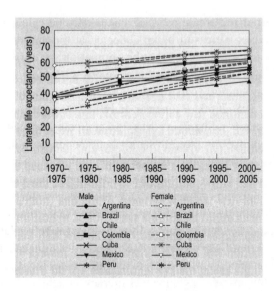

Figure 5.4. Literate life expectancy at birth for selected countries in Latin America, 1970–2005, for males and females. *Source*: Authors' calculations.

example, LLE is lower than in several Latin American countries that do much worse economically at the moment. The reason for this lies largely in the history of education. While in Singapore and Korea, strong educational efforts began only in the 1960s, many Latin American countries have a longer history of literacy. This is also reflected in the age structure of literacy. While in some of the recently developing Asian Tigers there are still some illiterate elderly men and women, this is less the case in some of the Latin American countries with higher LLEs. As is shown in Chapter 4, however, among the younger working-age population, the newly industrialized countries tend to do very well in terms of the educational composition.

The above-mentioned difference in education histories also explains some of the differences in the ranking of countries according to LLE compared with the ranking according to HDI (see *Table A5.2* in Appendix 5.1). While, generally, the ranking by LLE closely resembles that by HDI, there are some interesting exceptions. For instance, Cuba and Sri Lanka, both of which have very high literacy and high life expectancy but poor economic performance, do much better with LLE than with HDI, which also includes national income. On the other hand, countries such as Singapore and Malaysia do better under HDI than under LLE for the reasons discussed above. However, in general, for the 53 countries for which both indicators exist, the correspondence in the ranking is very close. For more than 40 countries, the ranks differ by fewer than five places.

For the industrialized countries, LLE could only be calculated for countries in which literacy rates were still being collected at the end of the 20th century, mostly because some small sections of the population were still illiterate (mostly in Southern and Eastern Europe). In those countries (*Table 5.2* lists 10 of them), LLE was already around 60 years in the 1970s and had changed by an increment of 5–10 years by 1995–2000. Women in Italy had 72.4 years of LLE at birth in 1995–2000; the corresponding figure was 71.4 in Spain and 69.4 in Poland. In all these European countries, we see the same phenomenon as in large parts of Latin America, namely, that female LLE is higher than male LLE. The only exception is Turkey, where female LLE is still almost 10 years lower than male LLE.

With respect to gender differentials, LLE provides a concise illustration of the combination of differentials in literacy and mortality that exist between males and females. In general, the gender gap in literacy is negatively related to enrolment rates; the lower the level of enrolment rates, the larger the gender gap in literacy. In the process of development, as educational attainment increases the gender gap tends to decline toward zero as universal literacy is achieved. At low levels of development, in many parts of the world, life expectancy of the male population tends to be slightly higher than that of the female population because of gender discrimination in health care, nutrition, etc.; as general health and sanitary conditions improve, the life expectancy of women tends to increase to higher levels than that of men. When a country moves from high mortality and low literacy levels to low mortality and high literacy levels, the pattern of change shows a closing gender gap in LLE, which opens again in favor of women. In South Asia, North Africa, the Middle East, and sub-Saharan Africa, female LLE is noticeably lower than male LLE, by more than 10 years in most cases, and up to 18 years in Nepal, 15 years in Pakistan, 14 years in Morocco, and 13 years in Liberia in 2000–2005. In Latin America, female LLE tends to be slightly higher than that for males across the projection period; this is the case in Southern Europe (Greece, Italy, Portugal, and Spain), with the above-mentioned exception of Turkey. In Eastern Europe, the lowest female LLE is still above the highest male LLE (as shown in *Table 5.2* for Bulgaria, Poland, and Hungary).

Subnational differentials in literate life expectancy

While estimates of mortality and literacy by sex are readily available at the national level for many countries, this is not the case for literacy and mortality rates by place of residence. Although this information might often be available from specific national data sources, it is rarely presented in international statistical yearbooks. For eight countries—Bangladesh, Belarus, Colombia, Egypt, Greece, Mexico, Romania, and Tajikistan—we found information on mortality and literacy from the *1995*

Table 5.3. Literate life expectancy for selected countries by sex and urban or rural place of residence.

	Male		Female	
	Urban	Rural	Urban	Rural
Bangladesh 1986	27.0	15.7	14.4	6.4
Belarus 1993	60.2	56.6	68.4	65.2
Colombia 1985	53.0	53.6	57.6	53.6
Egypt 1986	35.2	23.8	25.4	9.7
Greece 1991	68.9	68.4	70.8	66.5
Mexico 1990	56.7	44.9	57.2	39.6
Romania 1994	61.8	59.1	67.7	62.2
Tajikistan 1991	56.7	60.2	62.1	60.9

Source: Authors' calculations.

Demographic Yearbook (United Nations 1997) and from the *Statistical Yearbook* (UNESCO 1998),[2] respectively, and from Medina (1996).

Table 5.3 gives LLE for both sexes, for urban and rural areas separately. Although this is certainly not a representative sample of countries and one has to be very careful about the quality of this subnational data, especially with respect to differential mortality rates, we can see some general patterns. For women in all cases, the urban LLE is higher than the rural one. This is not surprising, because both literacy and mortality conditions tend to be higher in urban than in rural areas, mostly because of better availability of educational and health care facilities.

For men, the difference between urban and rural LLE is less pronounced. While the differences are clear and significant in Bangladesh and Egypt, in Colombia and Greece there is almost no difference, and in Tajikistan it is even reversed. Whatever the specific reasons for the given combinations of age-specific literacy and mortality rates in different parts of these countries, this apparent pattern makes it clear that female LLE varies more strongly by the urban–rural division than does male LLE. The reason may be because in rural areas, female literacy generally has spread more recently than in urban areas and, therefore, especially among the elderly women, there are still higher proportions of illiterates.

A recent study of Mexico calculated LLE for all 32 Mexican states for men and women separately (*Table 5.4*). For both men and women, LLE is highest in the Federal District, that is, Mexico City (with 60.4 and 62.1 years, respectively), and lowest in Chiapas (with 41.0 and 32.5 years, respectively). For the differentials within Mexico, we see essentially the same general pattern described above for

[2]The mortality data had to be adjusted downward for Romania, Belarus, and Greece to reflect data on life expectancies for the years of reference; for Bangladesh, the literacy rates for the 10–14 age group was adjusted downward to reflect the differences in the dates of observation of literacy and mortality rates.

Table 5.4. Literate life expectancy at birth for women and men of Mexico at the state level in 1990.

State	LLE of men at birth in 1990	Ranking at the national level	LLE of women at birth in 1990	Ranking at the national level
Aguascalientes	55.46	9	57.59	10
Baja California	58.31	3	61.60	2
Baja California S.	57.34	4	60.88	4
Campeche	50.37	22	48.66	21
Coahuila	57.00	5	60.21	7
Colima	52.77	14	55.72	13
Chiapas	40.96	32	32.45	32
Chihuahua	55.82	8	60.34	6
Federal District	60.39	1	62.13	1
Durango	54.33	11	58.71	9
Guanajuato	48.54	26	46.29	25
Guerrero	41.31	31	37.29	30
Hidalgo	46.75	29	42.30	29
Jalisco	53.64	13	56.16	11
State of Mexico	54.83	10	52.15	16
Michoacan	46.87	28	46.69	24
Morelos	52.54	15	51.68	17
Nayarit	51.21	20	54.98	14
Nuevo Leon	58.58	2	61.55	3
Oaxaca	42.73	30	34.79	31
Puebla	47.49	27	42.84	28
Queretaro	49.10	24	44.83	27
Quintana Roo	51.42	19	49.75	20
San Luis Potosi	49.84	23	48.52	22
Sinaloa	51.81	18	55.84	12
Sonora	56.27	6	60.52	5
Tabasco	51.86	17	48.08	23
Tamaulipas	56.13	7	58.78	8
Tlaxcala	53.72	12	49.90	19
Veracruz	48.58	25	45.01	26
Yucatán	50.79	21	49.97	18
Zacatecas	52.34	16	53.81	15

Source: Medina (1996).

a large number of countries. In the more developed states with higher levels of LLE, female LLE tends to be higher than male LLE. At the lower end we see the opposite, with female LLE significantly lower than male LLE.

This view of subnational differentials in LLE for a group of countries and Mexican states may not be representative of the global relationships. However, it may show that the concept of LLE can be applied easily to such subpopulations and may also be a useful indicator of inequalities in human development within populations, provided that the necessary empirical data are available. It should not be too difficult to derive such data from existing censuses and survey data, as well as from vital registration systems, for a large number of countries. Virtually all censuses around the world ask questions concerning education, which are cross-classified by age and sex and can also be tabulated for rather small subpopulations, even at the level of villages or census blocks. For age-specific mortality rates the data situation is a bit more difficult, since direct measurements require efficient vital registration systems. However, abundant indirect methods for mortality estimation exist that can be applied to census or survey questions about surviving children or relatives. Also, model life tables can be applied to different subpopulations, provided there is some very basic information about possible mortality differentials.

Such estimations of human development and the resultant differential empowerment of subpopulations are of particular importance in the context of sustainable development. As is discussed in Chapter 10, differential vulnerability and empowerment to cope with environmental changes are key factors for the analysis of population–development–environment interactions. As discussed above, only an indicator based on individual characteristics can serve this purpose. HDI and other indicators based on national accounting are not able to describe the differences between subpopulations.

5.5   Projections of Literate Life Expectancy to 2030

Another advantage of LLE is that it can be projected over several decades with relatively high certainty. All the components that underlie the calculation of LLE tend to change slowly and have already been projected in other contexts. Assumptions about future mortality conditions are an essential ingredient of all regular population projections and are based on a major body of literature. Reviews of this literature and its relevance for assuming certain future mortality trends, as well as their uncertainty, are given in, for example, Lutz (1996) and National Research Council (2000). The population projections discussed in Chapters 2 and 3 of this volume assume such alternative mortality paths even up to 2100. Here, we only examine projections up to 2030 and use for these 30 years the median mortality paths for the 13 world regions, as defined in Chapter 2.

Projections of literacy are less common than projections of mortality. In principle, however, it should be easier because literacy is a stock variable that changes only slowly. Typically, literacy skills are acquired in childhood, and the proportion literate within any cohort of men and women tends to be very stable after childhood. Only in rare cases of adult education programs does cohort literacy change at higher ages. Hence, if we know how many women can read and write at age 20 in 2000, we have a very good basis for projecting what proportion will be literate at age 50 in the year 2030. Here, we do not present special projections of literacy, but rather use the projections by level of education presented in Chapter 4 as the basis for projecting LLE.

For this we had to make the additional assumption that the "no education" category, defined in Chapter 4 for projections by level of education for world regions, can be used as a proxy for illiteracy. In its definition, this category includes those who have completed less than one year of formal schooling. According to this definition, this category could underestimate illiteracy, since in most developing countries four to five years of schooling are considered necessary for a child to acquire permanent literacy skills. On the other hand, literacy can be also acquired through informal channels of learning, and the number of literate persons is not necessarily limited to those who attend formal education. These two sources of error work in different directions and possibly compensate for each other. To study this empirically, in Appendix 5.1 (*Table A5.3*) we compare data on the age structure of the "no education" category in our projections in Chapter 4 with the UNESCO estimates of illiteracy rates for 2000, aggregated to recapture the world regions that we use. In general, the "no education" category is very close to the "illiterate" category in the age groups between 15 and 45 years of age. The "no education" category seems to somewhat overestimate illiteracy in South and Pacific Asia, and to underestimate it in Central Asia and the Middle East. This fit was considered good enough to use the "no education" category as a proxy for illiteracy.

In Chapter 4, we study three different scenarios in terms of future transition rates between educational groups. To summarize again, the "constant" scenario assumes that enrolment rates stay constant at the levels observed in 2000. The "ICPD" scenario reproduces the Programme of Action of the International Conference on Population and Development (ICPD) held in Cairo in 1994 concerning education. This implies full intake in primary school for boys and girls by 2015–2020 and female primary enrolment equal to male enrolment by 2005–2010. The "American" scenario is not presented here, since the assumptions in terms of literacy are very similar to those of the "ICPD" scenario.

The results of the projections are presented in *Table 5.5* for LLE at birth and in *Table 5.6* for LLE at age 15 years. As discussed above, depending on the context of analysis, one may choose either indicator. All the data given below refer to LLE at birth. In Chapter 6 we also use LLE at age 15. For this reason, the projections are presented here in terms of both indicators.

Figure 5.5 shows projected changes in female LLE at birth for six developing regions under the "ICPD" scenario. Under this scenario, the increase in female LLE will be very strong over the next 30 years. Generally, the increase will be steeper the lower female LLE is in 2000–2005. The increase is the highest in South

Table 5.5. Literate life expectancy at birth for 13 world regions, 2000–2030, according to the "constant" and "ICPD" scenarios.

Region	2000–2005		2025–2030 Constant		ICPD	
	Male	Female	Male	Female	Male	Female
North Africa	38.7	27.7	54.0	42.4	55.4	47.3
Sub-Saharan Africa	27.4	20.4	35.8	29.9	38.4	35.2
North America	69.3	75.8	74.0	80.5	74.0	80.5
Latin America	54.3	57.0	64.5	69.8	64.5	69.8
Central Asia	58.7	64.1	64.6	71.8	64.6	71.8
Middle East	48.7	38.2	61.0	51.4	62.4	56.3
South Asia	36.5	22.0	51.6	37.2	52.2	42.7
China region	56.1	48.1	65.8	67.2	65.8	67.2
Pacific Asia	46.6	43.4	58.7	58.4	59.2	59.6
Pacific OECD[a]	72.4	78.4	77.3	83.4	77.3	83.4
Western Europe	66.3	70.4	73.2	78.3	73.2	78.3
Eastern Europe	63.1	69.8	68.8	76.4	68.8	76.4
FSU Europe[b]	57.8	69.0	63.0	74.2	63.0	74.2

[a] Organisation for Economic Co-operation and Development members in the Pacific region.
[b] European part of the former Soviet Union.
Source: Authors' calculations.

Asia, where women currently can expect about 22 years of literate life. This figure will increase to more than 37 years in 2025–2030, even under the assumption of constant enrolment rates, as a result of recent efforts to improve education enrolment for girls. The "ICPD" scenario will bring female LLE up to 43 years by 2030. In Latin America, LLE will be as high as 70 years for females and 65 years for males, according to the "ICPD" scenario. The China region will also benefit from very high LLE, with 66 years for males and 67 years for females. On the other hand, as a result of low investment in education and lower survival rates at all ages (worsened by the AIDS epidemic), sub-Saharan Africa will remain behind the other regions for at least the next 30 years. The "ICPD" scenario shows that LLE will increase from 27 years to 38 years for males between 2000 and 2030, and from 20 years to 35 years for females.

Although these projections imply significant improvements in LLE everywhere, for both men and women, the bad news is that female and male LLEs in North Africa, sub-Saharan Africa, the Middle East, and South Asia are far from converging, even in 2025–2030 under the "ICPD" scenario, which supposes a rapid closing of the gender gap for those newly enrolled by 2005. This again illustrates the momentum of education. Under the "ICPD" scenario, women in South Asia in 2025–2030 have about 10 years less LLE than males (down from 14 years in 2000–2005). In all nine other regions, female LLE is higher than male LLE as a

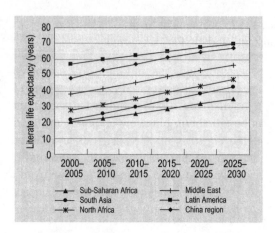

Figure 5.5. Projections of female literate life expectancy at birth for six regions, 2000–2030, according to the "ICPD" scenario. *Source*: Authors' calculations.

result of a combination of higher life expectancies for women and a closing of the gender gap in terms of literacy. In FSU Europe,[3] women can enjoy 11 more years of literate life than men can under all scenarios.

No convergence of LLE between the least developed and the more developed regions is in sight within the next 30 years. Even under the most favorable scenario ("ICPD"), the gap is more than 20 years on average between a woman born in Western Europe and a woman born in one of today's developing regions, that is, in North Africa (31 years), sub-Saharan Africa (43 years), the Middle East (22 years), and South Asia (36 years). The gap is somewhat narrower for males, but still significant.

The LLE of FSU Europe demonstrates the effect of poor quality of life for men, although literacy is universal. There, according to all scenarios, LLE will fall below that of some developing regions. Men in FSU Europe will have 63 years of LLE in 2030, according to all scenarios, which is less than the LLE of men in Latin America (64.5 years), Central Asia (64.6 years), and the China region (65.8 years) in 2030.

Table 5.6, showing the LLE at age 15, is not fundamentally different from *Table 5.5*. The ranking of countries and the trends described above remain essentially the same. However, it is interesting to see that the difference between LLE at birth and LLE at age 15 years is highest in the most advanced countries and lowest toward the end of the ranking. While, for example, male LLE under the "ICPD" scenario differs only by 0.5 years in sub-Saharan Africa, it differs by 10 years in the Pacific

---

[3]European part of the former Soviet Union.

Table 5.6. Literate life expectancy at age 15 for 13 world regions, 2000–2030, according to the "constant" and "ICPD" scenarios.

	2000–2005		2025–2030 Constant		ICPD	
Region	Male	Female	Male	Female	Male	Female
North Africa	31.9	21.5	46.7	35.9	47.3	38.5
Sub-Saharan Africa	27.8	19.3	36.5	29.7	37.9	32.8
North America	59.7	65.8	64.2	70.5	64.2	70.5
Latin America	46.5	47.8	56.1	60.2	56.1	60.2
Central Asia	52.2	55.4	57.0	62.5	57.0	62.5
Middle East	41.3	31.8	52.9	44.5	53.5	47.1
South Asia	29.0	16.1	44.0	31.2	44.2	34.2
China region	48.6	39.8	57.2	57.9	57.2	57.8
Pacific Asia	39.4	35.5	50.8	50.0	51.0	50.6
Pacific OECD[a]	62.8	68.7	67.5	73.5	67.5	73.5
Western Europe	57.7	60.7	64.1	68.5	64.1	68.5
Eastern Europe	55.0	60.1	59.8	66.6	59.8	66.6
FSU Europe[b]	52.1	59.8	56.0	64.5	56.0	64.5

[a]Organisation for Economic Co-operation and Development members in the Pacific region.
[b]European part of the former Soviet Union.
Source: Authors' calculations.

OECD region.[4] This difference mostly stems from very different probabilities of survival from birth to the age of 15. Since here we used uniform assumptions about the ages at which literacy is acquired, possible regional differentials in this factor do not influence the pattern.

5.6 Conclusions

LLE proves to be a useful and feasible new measure to describe past trends in social development in a large number of developing and developed countries and to project likely future trends over the coming decades separately for men and women. LLE, which can be interpreted directly as the average number of years a man or woman is likely to live and be able to read and write, has been increasing continuously in a large majority of countries over the past 30 years, as a result of a combination of increasing literacy and improving survival rates. The only countries in which LLE declined in the late 1990s are those affected by AIDS in sub-Saharan Africa and some East European countries. The gap between male and female LLE in developing countries is closing. The figures show that the pattern of change, as one country moves from high mortality and low literacy levels to low mortality and

---

[4]Organisation for Economic Co-operation and Development.

high literacy levels, is that of a closing gender gap in LLE, with women catching up to men and later even surpassing men because of a higher female life expectancy.

The results of the projections show that LLE will increase very strongly in most developing regions over the next 30 years. However, the momentum of education will prevent a quick closure of the gender gap for the adult population within that time period. No general convergence of LLE between developing and developed regions is in sight within the next 30 years. Even under the most favorable education scenario, the gap will remain more than 20 years of LLE, on average, between a woman born in Western Europe, North America, or Japan and a woman born in one of the developing regions. Among developing regions, the prospects are much better for Latin America, Pacific Asia, and the China region than for Africa and South Asia. This analysis clearly demonstrates that social development does not jump. Even in the case of very intensive efforts, historically rooted differences in the stage of social development cannot be overcome overnight. It requires several decades to change profoundly the educational composition of the population and effectively close the gender gap and improve health conditions in a sustainable manner.

One of the main advantages of LLE compared with other development indicators that are fully or partly derived from national accounting systems (such as GDP per capita or HDI) is that it is based on individual characteristics and hence can be calculated for men and women separately as well as for any subpopulation, and thus can describe differentials within populations. As is discussed in Chapter 10 on policies for population in sustainable development, the focus on specific vulnerable subpopulations is likely to become a major emphasis of the discussions in the years to come. Here, LLE could serve as a useful indicator that efficiently describes and projects differential vulnerability and empowerment to cope with all kinds of emerging environmental, health, and other risks.

Appendix 5.1:
Data Sources, Differences in Country Rankings, and Comparison of "No Education" and "Illiterate" Categories

Table A5.1. Assumptions and sources for calculation of literate life expectancy trends since 1970.

Category/Years	Assumptions	Sources
Literacy for age groups		
0–4	Illiterate	Authors
5–9	Half of literacy rate of age group 10–14	Authors
10–14	Equal literacy rate of age group 15–19[a]	Authors
15+		Estimates and projections by UNESCO (2000) available for 1970–2025[b]
Mortality for periods		
1970–1985		Life tables from the International Data Base of the US Census Bureau[c]
1990–2005		United Nations (2001) estimates and projections of life table survivors

[a]Clearly, literacy at younger age groups is difficult to estimate, mainly because of the differences in entrance age for primary school, as well as in the numbers of school years necessary to acquire literacy. This can range from one to two years in more developed countries, to more than four years in countries with underdeveloped education systems. To avoid making too many assumptions regarding literacy in the younger age groups, one can look at LLE starting from age 15 (when literacy has already been acquired or, if not, most likely never will be). In this chapter, both LLE at birth and at age 15 are analyzed.

[b]The approach UNESCO (1995) used in the literacy assessments in 1989, 1994, and 2000 is based on empirical findings which showed that for each country and sex, acquired literacy levels of persons older than 20 tend to remain stable over time. Further country analysis showed that literacy rates for generations over 20 years of age seem to follow a clear-cut logistic distribution, or S-curve, in most countries. The methodology consisted of fitting logistic regression models to observed literacy by generation in each country, and to projection by extending the fitted S-curve. The estimated literacy rates by generation were then applied to the corresponding age-group population estimates and projections, and aggregated to give total literacy rate estimates and projections for persons aged 15 and above for five-year intervals, and this for approximately 130 countries.

[c]The International Data Base of the US Census Bureau is a computerized data bank that contains statistical tables of demographic and socioeconomic data for 227 countries and areas of the world. It is available online at www.census.gov/ipc/www/idbnew.html.

Table A5.2. Comparison of the ranking of 53 countries according to the Human Development Index (HDI) and literate life expectancy (LLE) for both sexes (list ranks from bottom to top).

Rank	Country HDI	HDI	Country LLE	LLE	Difference in rank vs. HDI
53	Tanzania	0.421	Senegal	14.5	−1
52	Senegal	0.426	Nepal	17.8	−2
51	Bangladesh	0.440	Bangladesh	18.6	0
50	Nepal	0.463	Pakistan	20.1	−1
49	Pakistan	0.508	Morocco	23.7	−5
48	Cameroon	0.536	Iraq	24.4	−5
47	Ghana	0.544	India	28.4	−1
46	India	0.545	Egypt	28.7	−4
45	Lesotho	0.582	Cameroon	29.0	+3
44	Morocco	0.582	Tanzania	29.6	+9
43	Iraq	0.586	Ghana	29.6	+4
42	Egypt	0.616	Swaziland	31.9	−2
41	Honduras	0.641	Algeria	32.5	−3
40	Swaziland	0.644	Lesotho	35.5	+5
39	Bolivia	0.652	Tunisia	36.5	−4
38	Algeria	0.665	Iran	38.3	−6
37	El Salvador	0.674	Honduras	39.3	+4
36	Indonesia	0.681	South Africa	41.0	−2
35	Tunisia	0.695	Bolivia	42.8	+4
34	South Africa	0.695	El Salvador	44.7	+3
33	China	0.701	Indonesia	46.0	+3
32	Iran	0.715	Dominican R.	47.5	−2
31	Sri Lanka	0.721	China	47.6	+2
30	Dominican R.	0.726	Turkey	47.7	−1
29	Turkey	0.728	Brazil	48.5	−4
28	Paraguay	0.730	Mauritius	50.7	−9
27	Jamaica	0.734	Malaysia	50.7	−11
26	Peru	0.739	Peru	51.5	0
25	Brazil	0.739	Ecuador	53.7	−2
24	Philippines	0.740	Fiji	53.8	−4
23	Ecuador	0.747	Colombia	55.3	−6
22	Thailand	0.753	Jamaica	55.4	+5
21	Bulgaria	0.758	Paraguay	55.9	+7
20	Fiji	0.763	Mexico	55.9	−5
19	Mauritius	0.764	Philippines	56.5	+5
18	Cuba	0.765	Sri Lanka	57.2	+13
17	Colombia	0.768	Thailand	57.5	+5
16	Malaysia	0.768	Singapore	60.0	−13
15	Mexico	0.786	Portugal	61.7	−8
14	Hungary	0.795	Bulgaria	62.5	+7

Table A5.2. Continued.

Rank	Country HDI	HDI	Country LLE	LLE	Difference in rank vs. HDI
13	Costa Rica	0.801	Hungary	62.9	+1
12	Poland	0.802	Argentina	63.2	−1
11	Argentina	0.827	Malta	63.3	−2
10	Chile	0.844	Chile	63.4	0
9	Malta	0.850	South Korea	63.7	−1
8	South Korea	0.852	Costa Rica	63.9	+5
7	Portugal	0.858	Cuba	65.0	+11
6	Greece	0.867	Poland	65.2	+6
5	Cyprus	0.870	Israel	66.8	−1
4	Israel	0.883	Cyprus	67.2	+1
3	Singapore	0.888	Greece	68.2	+3
2	Spain	0.894	Spain	68.7	0
1	Italy	0.900	Italy	69.6	0

Sources: UNDP (1998) for HDI; Authors' calculations for LLE.

Table A5.3. Comparison of the percentage of illiterate population according to UNESCO in 2000 and IIASA percentage of population with no education in 2000 by region, age group, and sex.

Region	Sources	15–19	20–24	25–29	30–34	35–39	40–44	45–49	50–54	55–59	60–64	65+
Male population												
Western	IIASA	0.0	0.9	1.3	1.2	2.0	1.9	4.7	4.9	8.4	8.2	13.2
Europe	UNESCO	0.5	0.8	1.1	1.5	1.7	2.1	2.7	3.4	5.1	7.1	9.2
	Diff.	–0.5	0.1	0.1	–0.3	0.3	–0.2	2.0	1.5	3.3	1.1	4.0
Sub-	IIASA	20.1	21.2	25.9	29.9	33.7	40.4	44.4	54.4	58.4	66.5	73.9
Saharan	UNESCO	16.9	19.9	23.3	27.3	31.7	37.0	42.8	49.8	56.3	62.2	70.7
Africa	Diff.	3.2	1.4	2.6	2.6	2.0	3.4	1.6	4.6	2.1	4.3	3.3
South	IIASA	10.3	18.7	31.0	43.9	44.1	49.9	49.5	62.9	64.9	68.2	72.4
Asia	UNESCO	21.4	24.2	27.7	31.3	34.1	37.5	41.4	45.3	49.5	53.3	59.2
	Diff.	–11.1	–5.5	3.3	12.7	9.9	12.4	8.1	17.6	15.5	14.9	13.2
Pacific	IIASA	11.6	11.9	19.2	19.2	23.3	23.3	31.9	31.9	42.3	42.3	53.7
Asia	UNESCO	3.2	3.8	4.7	5.6	6.7	8.1	9.6	12.7	15.8	19.4	25.9
	Diff.	8.4	8.1	14.4	13.6	16.5	15.2	22.3	19.3	26.5	22.9	27.8
Pacific	IIASA	0.0	0.0	0.2	0.0	0.1	0.1	0.4	0.4	0.6	0.6	0.8
OECD[a]	UNESCO	n.a.	n.a.	n.a.	n.a.	n.a.	n.a.	n.a.	n.a.	n.a.	n.a.	n.a.
	Diff.	n.a.	n.a.	n.a.	n.a.	n.a.	n.a.	n.a.	n.a.	n.a.	n.a.	n.a.
North	IIASA	0.2	0.2	0.3	0.6	0.6	0.3	0.3	0.7	0.7	0.8	1.3
America	UNESCO	n.a.	n.a.	n.a.	n.a.	n.a.	n.a.	n.a.	n.a.	n.a.	n.a.	n.a.
	Diff.	n.a.	n.a.	n.a.	n.a.	n.a.	n.a.	n.a.	n.a.	n.a.	n.a.	n.a.
North	IIASA	14.4	16.7	23.1	27.7	31.3	38.3	48.9	56.1	64.4	67.4	78.3
Africa	UNESCO	16.1	18.8	21.7	25.8	30.0	35.0	39.4	45.2	51.4	58.5	65.9
	Diff.	–1.7	–2.1	1.4	2.0	1.3	3.3	9.5	11.0	13.0	8.9	12.4
Middle	IIASA	7.7	7.9	10.5	12.4	17.3	21.3	26.5	32.2	43.3	53.0	56.3
East	UNESCO	6.5	8.4	10.8	14.2	18.2	21.5	26.3	32.5	40.0	47.8	58.9
	Diff.	1.2	–0.5	–0.4	–1.8	–0.9	–0.2	0.2	–0.3	3.3	5.1	–2.6
Latin	IIASA	2.3	5.5	6.9	7.6	9.9	10.8	16.1	20.5	24.1	31.4	38.6
America	UNESCO	5.9	6.7	7.7	8.6	9.4	11.0	12.6	15.5	17.4	20.7	24.2
	Diff.	–3.6	–1.2	–0.8	–1.0	0.5	–0.2	3.5	5.0	6.7	10.6	14.3
FSU	IIASA	0.4	0.0	0.1	0.1	0.0	0.1	0.4	0.4	1.1	1.1	2.9
Europe[b]	UNESCO	0.2	0.2	0.2	0.2	0.2	0.2	0.2	0.2	0.3	0.5	0.7
	Diff.	0.2	–0.2	–0.1	–0.2	–0.2	–0.2	0.2	0.1	0.7	0.6	2.1
Eastern	IIASA	0.4	0.6	0.6	0.6	0.6	0.6	1.1	1.1	2.5	2.5	6.4
Europe	UNESCO	0.3	0.3	0.4	0.5	0.5	0.6	0.6	0.7	1.2	1.6	2.2
	Diff.	0.1	0.3	0.2	0.1	0.1	0.0	0.5	0.4	1.4	0.9	4.2
China	IIASA	2.1	2.6	2.5	2.4	4.1	6.5	8.6	12.8	22.0	31.0	44.8
region	UNESCO	1.0	1.4	2.2	3.4	3.4	5.5	8.1	11.2	15.8	24.6	37.7
	Diff.	1.1	1.1	0.3	–1.0	0.7	1.0	0.5	1.5	6.2	6.4	7.1
Central	IIASA	0.6	0.2	0.3	0.6	0.1	0.2	0.6	1.2	2.7	6.9	10.6
Asia	UNESCO	1.3	1.7	2.3	3.1	4.1	5.5	7.2	9.4	12.1	15.6	25.6
	Diff.	–0.6	–1.6	–2.0	–2.5	–4.0	–5.2	–6.6	–8.2	–9.4	–8.7	–15.0

[a] Organisation for Economic Co-operation and Development members in the Pacific region.
[b] European part of the former Soviet Union.

Table A5.3. Continued.

						Age group					
Region	Sources	15–19	20–24	25–29	30–34	35–39	40–44	45–49	50–54	55–59	60–64	65+
Female population												
Western	IIASA	0.0	1.6	2.6	2.7	3.4	3.9	7.3	8.4	12.3	12.4	17.0
Europe	UNESCO	2.5	3.3	4.1	5.1	6.1	8.2	10.6	12.2	14.4	17.3	18.0
	Diff.	–2.5	–1.7	–1.5	–2.4	–2.7	–4.3	–3.3	–3.8	–2.1	–4.9	–1.0
Sub-	IIASA	32.0	35.2	41.8	49.9	55.9	64.3	71.8	80.7	84.4	86.6	89.4
Saharan	UNESCO	24.0	29.5	35.8	43.2	51.3	59.2	66.3	73.5	78.5	82.5	86.8
Africa	Diff.	8.1	5.8	5.9	6.7	4.6	5.0	5.5	7.2	5.9	4.1	2.7
South	IIASA	40.0	46.9	56.3	65.4	69.9	77.4	77.2	88.4	89.6	91.4	93.9
Asia	UNESCO	37.7	42.7	48.2	53.3	58.7	64.6	70.3	74.7	78.9	82.2	86.3
	Diff.	2.3	4.2	8.1	12.1	11.2	12.8	6.9	13.7	10.7	9.1	7.7
Pacific	IIASA	13.1	16.7	26.0	26.0	32.6	32.6	46.3	46.3	56.8	56.8	69.7
Asia	UNESCO	4.8	5.9	7.7	9.4	11.7	14.4	18.5	24.5	31.3	38.4	48.2
	Diff.	8.3	10.8	18.3	16.6	20.9	18.2	27.8	21.9	25.5	18.4	21.5
Pacific	IIASA	0.0	0.0	0.2	0.0	0.1	0.1	0.1	0.1	0.1	0.1	0.8
OECD[a]	UNESCO	n.a.	n.a.	n.a.	n.a.	n.a.	n.a.	n.a.	n.a.	n.a.	n.a.	n.a.
	Diff.	n.a.	n.a.	n.a.	n.a.	n.a.	n.a.	n.a.	n.a.	n.a.	n.a.	n.a.
North	IIASA	0.2	0.2	0.3	0.2	0.2	0.5	0.5	0.5	0.5	0.6	1.2
America	UNESCO	n.a.	n.a.	n.a.	n.a.	n.a.	n.a.	n.a.	n.a.	n.a.	n.a.	n.a.
	Diff.	n.a.	n.a.	n.a.	n.a.	n.a.	n.a.	n.a.	n.a.	n.a.	n.a.	n.a.
North	IIASA	32.9	38.8	46.2	52.5	58.5	64.0	70.7	77.1	80.1	81.6	88.4
Africa	UNESCO	26.9	33.2	40.5	48.6	56.8	65.4	72.4	79.2	84.7	89.0	92.5
	Diff.	6.0	5.6	5.7	3.9	1.7	–1.5	–1.7	–2.1	–4.6	–7.4	–4.1
Middle	IIASA	19.3	16.6	22.8	27.4	34.9	42.3	50.8	55.8	66.7	70.9	80.0
East	UNESCO	14.4	18.9	25.0	31.6	39.2	46.7	55.1	63.8	72.2	77.9	81.8
	Diff.	4.9	–2.3	–2.1	–4.3	–4.2	–4.4	–4.3	–8.0	–5.5	–7.0	–1.9
Latin	IIASA	1.8	5.0	6.9	8.5	11.5	13.6	19.1	25.0	33.2	37.1	48.0
America	UNESCO	5.0	6.0	7.2	8.4	9.7	12.5	15.4	19.5	22.6	27.3	31.5
	Diff.	–3.2	–1.0	–0.3	0.1	1.8	1.1	3.7	5.5	10.6	9.8	16.5
FSU	IIASA	0.4	0.0	0.0	0.0	0.0	0.0	0.2	0.2	0.6	0.6	1.5
Europe[b]	UNESCO	0.2	0.2	0.2	0.2	0.2	0.2	0.2	0.3	0.5	0.9	1.8
	Diff.	0.2	–0.2	–0.2	–0.2	–0.2	–0.2	–0.1	–0.2	0.0	–0.4	–0.4
Eastern	IIASA	0.4	0.6	0.7	0.6	0.8	0.8	2.1	2.1	5.5	5.5	11.2
Europe	UNESCO	0.3	0.4	0.6	0.9	1.0	1.1	1.2	1.5	2.5	3.6	5.1
	Diff.	0.1	0.2	0.0	–0.2	–0.2	–0.4	0.9	0.7	2.9	1.9	6.2
China	IIASA	4.3	6.1	7.4	8.9	16.2	23.2	28.0	39.1	57.0	71.2	84.2
region	UNESCO	3.0	4.4	6.5	9.7	12.2	20.1	26.9	33.4	44.3	59.6	79.4
	Diff.	1.2	1.8	0.9	–0.8	4.1	3.1	1.1	5.6	12.7	11.6	4.8
Central	IIASA	0.4	0.7	0.4	0.3	0.6	0.8	2.1	3.0	5.7	12.9	23.0
Asia	UNESCO	3.4	4.5	5.9	7.7	9.9	12.8	16.3	20.4	25.3	30.6	44.2
	Diff.	–3.0	–3.9	–5.5	–7.4	–9.3	–12.1	–14.2	–17.4	–19.6	–17.6	–21.1

[a] Organisation for Economic Co-operation and Development members in the Pacific region.
[b] European part of the former Soviet Union.
Sources: UNESCO (2000); Goujon and Lutz (Chapter 4 in this book).

References

Kelley AC (1991). The human development index: "Handle with care." *Population and Development Review* **17**:315–324.

Lutz W (1987). *Finnish Fertility Since 1722: Lessons from an Extended Decline.* Helsinki, Finland: Finnish Population Research Institute.

Lutz W (1994). *Population–Development–Environment: Understanding Their Interactions in Mauritius.* Berlin, Germany: Springer Verlag.

Lutz W (1994/95). Literate life expectancy. *POPNET* **26**:1–5. Laxenburg, Austria: International Institute for Applied Systems Analysis.

Lutz W (1996). *The Future Population of the World. What Can We Assume Today?*, Revised Edition. London, UK: Earthscan.

Medina S (1996). *Implementing a New Indicator of Social Development in Mexico: Literate Life Expectancy (LLE).* Working Paper WP-96-103. Laxenburg, Austria: International Institute for Applied Systems Analysis.

National Research Council (2000). *Beyond Six Billion: Forecasting the World's Population*, eds. Bongaarts J & Bulatao RA, Panel on Population Projections, Committee on Population, Commission on Behavioral and Social Sciences and Education. Washington DC, USA: National Academy Press.

UNDP (1998). *1998 Human Development Report.* New York, NY, USA: United Nations Development Programme.

UNESCO (1995). *Methodology Used in the 1994 Estimation and Projection of Adult Illiteracy.* Statistical Issues STE-18. Paris, France: United Nations Educational, Scientific and Cultural Organization, Division of Statistics.

UNESCO (1998). *Statistical Yearbook.* Paris, France: United Nations Educational, Scientific and Cultural Organization.

UNESCO (2000). Estimation and Projection of Adult Illiteracy. Computer file. Paris, France: United Nations Educational, Scientific and Cultural Organization.

United Nations (1997). *Demographic Yearbook 1995.* New York, NY, USA: United Nations, Department of Economic and Social Information and Policy Analysis, Statistics Division.

United Nations (2001). World Population Prospects: The 2000 Revision. File 4: Life Table Survivors, lx, for Both Sexes Combined, by Age, Major Area, Region and Country, 1990–2050. Electronic file. New York, NY, USA: United Nations, Population Division, Department of Economic and Social Affairs.

Chapter 6

Population–Environment–Development–Agriculture Interactions in Africa: A Case Study on Ethiopia

Wolfgang Lutz, Sergei Scherbov, Paulina K. Makinwa-Adebusoye, and Georges Reniers

6.1 Background

Over the past two decades, Africa has experienced a severe crisis manifested in, among other things, the constant decline of its economic growth rate. Since 1994, the economic situation of the continent has improved steadily, but economic growth is still below the level necessary to have a significant impact on poverty. Although the proportion who live in extreme poverty in Africa may have declined by a few percentage points in the past couple of years, high population growth rates mean that the absolute number of poor continues to increase on a daily basis. Additionally, Africa's economic performance seems to be highly dependent on the international economic environment and weather conditions, two exogenously determined factors that do not embody any guarantee of future growth (UNECA 1999). Two basic pressures account for the continued deterioration in the quality of life in Africa. First, the population growth rate exceeds those of economic growth and food production in most African countries. Additionally, the rapid deterioration of the environment prevents the desired increase in agricultural productivity. Today, over three-fourths of sub-Saharan African countries produce less food per capita than they did in the 1980s. Daily calorie availability is well below the recommended minimum, and as much as 30–40 percent of the population is undernourished. Malnutrition affects even more people now than it did in the 1980s.

Inspired by the notion of sustainable development, there is an increasing realization of the need to go beyond the traditional sectoral approach in national development planning. It has been demonstrated that, at least in the medium to long term, a country's economic performance and the food security of its citizens are closely related to its demographic and educational trends, as well as to the health of the natural environment. Since these issues are closely interconnected in the real world, they should also be viewed together in national politics and development planning. The scientific understanding of their mutual interdependencies is, however, not yet sufficiently reflected in the political institutions of individual countries. There is tremendous inertia in such systems, partly because of the traditional training of experts, which is often characterized by the compartmentalization of disciplines, and partly because the impact of developments in one sector is often invisible in another sector in the short term.

Hence, convincing policy makers and country experts of the negative synergy that arises from the interconnections of population growth, environmental deterioration, and declining agricultural production is a major objective of the Sustainable Development Division (SDD) of the United Nations Economic Commission for Africa (UNECA). With that goal in mind, the SDD began to develop a computer simulation model intended to illustrate the interactions between population changes (P), the environment (E), socioeconomic development (D), and agriculture (A), the PEDA model. In this chapter, we present a theoretical introduction to the PEDA model as well as an illustration of its application to Ethiopia.

6.1.1   PEDA in brief

PEDA is an interactive computer simulation model designed to demonstrate the medium- to long-term impacts of alternative national policies on the food security status of the population (Lutz and Scherbov 2000). Through the manipulation of scenario variables, the model enables the user to project the proportions of the population that will be food secure and food insecure for a chosen point in time. As food security is directly dependent on trends in the fields of population, agriculture, environment, and socioeconomic development, the model demonstrates the relationships between these domains as well. The current version of the PEDA model includes the results of the first experiments to introduce an HIV/AIDS component and to illustrate its impact on the other variables in the model. As such, the

---

Box 6.1. Policy questions.

- What is the impact of increased educational enrolment over the next 5 years on food security over the next 20 years?
- How does a decrease in fertility rates influence agricultural production and land degradation in a country?
- What is the impact of different HIV/AIDS scenarios on agricultural outputs?
- How would the food security status of the elderly female rural population be affected by increased fertilizer use versus better education for the young?

PEDA model is able to give answers to a wide range of policy questions regarding the nexus interactions (*Box 6.1*).

As a model with a focus on a specific chain of interactions, the mission attributed to PEDA at its conception was one of advocacy from an integrated view: illustrate the negative development spiral that results from high population growth, environmental degradation, and decreasing per capita agricultural production. The goal is to demonstrate the magnitude of the existing interactions and to suggest alternative policy strategies to break this vicious circle in African countries. Since its conception and after several rounds of evaluation and review, the different components of the model have grown and have been refined to support ambitions that may exceed the original function.

6.1.2 Theoretical inspiration for PEDA

A theoretical construction, often labeled the "vicious circle model," has become an influential paradigm in the discussion surrounding population, poverty, food security, and sustainable development. It essentially assumes that high fertility, poverty, low education, and low status of women are bound up in a web of interactions with environmental degradation and declining food production in such a way that stress from one of the sources can trap some rural societies, especially those that live in marginal areas, in a vicious circle of increasingly destructive responses. One illustration of this mechanism is the parable of firewood (Nerlove 1991). In many countries the collection of firewood takes a lot of time, and more children can help to collect more firewood. However, this leads to the depletion of firewood near the villages and to the desire for more children to help collect firewood from greater distances, which thereby deprives the children of educational opportunities. Das-gupta (1993) presents this argument in a more generalized form. The condition of poverty and illiteracy in the households concerned prevents substitution of alterna-tive fuel sources or alternative livelihoods. A gender dimension is added through a worsening of the status of women and girls because of the increasing amount of time and effort that they must devote to daily household tasks (Agarwal 1994; Sen 1994). The result is faster population growth, further degradation of the re-newable resource base, increasing food insecurity, stagnating educational levels, and yet further erosion of the status of women. From a theoretical point of view, this vicious circle model is a useful contribution toward a unifying framework that causally links fertility, poverty, low female status, environmental degradation, and agricultural efficiency (O'Neill *et al.* 2001).

In terms of its empirical relevance, the vicious circle assumption is more con-troversial. The economic reasoning of this model largely operates at the household level, so empirical studies on the issue have been confined mostly to that level and have reached mixed results. At the macro level of different population seg-ments, this model could be very relevant—particularly in the African context—even though some of the assumptions of the stricter version are empirically un-confirmed and contentious. The assumption that environmental degradation may actually lead to increases in fertility is especially difficult to defend at a time when fertility rates are falling rapidly all over Africa within a context of degrading envi-ronmental resources. This does not necessarily imply that the assumed effects are entirely absent, but it does seem to imply that if they operate, they are overlain by the powerful and dominating processes of the demographic transition. Hence, it may be reasonable to assume alternatively that food insecurity is associated with a slower decline in fertility, although under certain conditions and in the short run famines may well induce declining fertility. Whatever the position on this issue, the PEDA model as outlined below is flexible enough to represent alternative as-sumptions through alternative parameter choices and scenarios.

The PEDA model was used recently to illustrate the differences between full models of this sort based on empirical data and highly stylized, reduced-form mod-els that address the same sort of nonlinear interdependencies between population, human capital, agricultural production, and the natural environment. For this pur-pose, an empirical application of the full model for Mali was compared with a reduced-form model centered on the food distribution function as given by the Lorenz curve. This comparison, published in Lutz *et al.* (2002), concludes that strongly reduced, stylized models can serve the important aims of both gaining more insight into a specific form of nonlinear dynamics and aiding the numerical sensitivity analysis, but they cannot replace a full empirical model. In the following sections, we apply the full model to the specific conditions of Ethiopia, a country

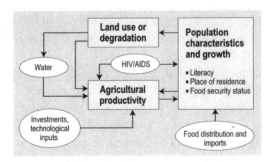

Figure 6.1. Structure of the PEDA model.

that faces very serious, real-world challenges as a consequence of the interactions between differential growth of different segments of the population, food production, food distribution, land degradation, and water scarcity.

6.2   The Structure of the PEDA Model

As illustrated in *Figure 6.1*, the PEDA model consists of three sub-modules or segments:

- a population module;
- a natural resources module (land and water); and
- an agricultural production module with a food distribution function.

The vicious circle in PEDA operates through the negative impact of a fast-growing, food-insecure segment of the population on the natural resources stock. This adversely affects agricultural production, which in turn induces more food insecurity. This negative chain of interactions is, however, not part of the model structure itself. As is highlighted below, the user can easily change the assumptions of the relationships between population growth, the natural resources stock, and agricultural production.

In the population segment of PEDA, multistate population projections are carried out to determine the size of the population by urban or rural place of residence, literacy status, and food security status. The food production and availability in PEDA is influenced by a set of endogenous and exogenous variables. An important resource for agricultural production is land. Although the user can omit this effect, the model by default assumes a negative impact of population growth on land. Agricultural production is influenced further by the size and qualification level of the labor force, the availability of water, and efforts in fertilizer and machinery use.

The contribution of water to agricultural outputs is dependent on climatic conditions, but also on the status of land degradation and efforts in irrigation and water management (building of reservoirs).

In addition to the produced food, the model allows for both post-harvest losses and food imports and exports to estimate the net food availability. In the final step, the available food is distributed over the population following a nonlinear food distribution function to determine the proportion of the population that is food insecure. PEDA also has an HIV/AIDS component to account for its demographic impact through excess mortality and for its negative impact on agricultural production through the reduction of the labor force because of illnesses related to HIV/AIDS.

The different segments in the PEDA model touched upon above are treated in more detail below. An even more elaborate treatment of the different aspects and features of the PEDA model can be found in the *PEDA Technical Manual* (UNECA, forthcoming).

6.2.1   Vicious versus virtuous circle dynamics

Although the PEDA model is flexible with regard to the underlying theoretical assumptions, by default it is set to be compliant with the main principles of the vicious circle at the macro level described earlier. In other words, the growth of the (illiterate and food-insecure) population in rural areas contributes to the degradation of land and thus lowers agricultural production and further increases the number of food-insecure people. If not broken, this vicious circle leads to ever-increasing land degradation and increases in the food-insecure population. The model does not assume increasing fertility as an automatic response to food insecurity, which is the most problematic part of some vicious circle models. Rather, the food-secure and food-insecure fractions of the population are assumed to have different fertility levels (subject to exogenously defined trends), and hence the aggregate fertility level only responds to changes in food insecurity through the changing weights of the groups in the calculation of the overall fertility.

The vicious circle can be broken through several possible interventions in the fields of food production, food distribution, education, environmental protection, and population dynamics, which thus allows for more Boserupian visions on the nexus of population, the environment, and agricultural production. The power of the PEDA model is that these assumed positive or negative interactions form part of the scenarios that can be set by the user and are not hardwired into the model. Hence PEDA does not prescribe a certain view of the world.

More optimistic projections can, for example, be carried out by defining scenarios that assume no negative (or even a positive) effect of increasing population densities on the natural resources stock, or increasing technological inputs in agriculture (e.g., fertilizer, machinery, or irrigation), and so on.

6.2.2 The population segment

PEDA is different from most macroeconomic models in that it uses a population-based approach. The population-based approach views human beings with their specific characteristics (such as age, sex, education, health, food-security status, urban or rural place of residence, etc.) as agents of social, economic, cultural, and environmental change. However, the population is also at risk of suffering from the negative repercussions of these changes, as well as benefiting from positive implications. In this sense, human beings are seen as a driving force of these changes and the first to be affected by the consequences of these changes. Economics, if it comes into the picture (e.g., through the importance of markets in distributing goods), plays only an intermediate role; economic indicators are not seen as the primary objective of the modeling exercise. In this sense, the population-based approach differs from much of development economics literature.

The population-based approach does not assume that population growth or other demographic changes are necessarily the most important factors in shaping our future. Instead, the phenomena that we want to model are studied in terms of different characteristics that can be attached directly to and (at least theoretically) measured with individual members of the population. Characteristics such as age, sex, literacy, urban or rural place of residence, and even nutritional status can be assessed at the individual level. The sum over these individual characteristics makes up the distribution of the total population. In using these individual characteristics, PEDA differentiates itself from models that rely on other frequently used economic indicators such as gross national product (GNP) per capita. Although GNP is indicative of the average amount of money that an individual has in his or her pocket, it cannot be measured directly at the individual level. It results from aggregated indicators of national accounting with various conceptual and measurement problems. Although many of the powerful quantitative economic tools (such as general equilibrium models) cannot be applied within this framework, other very powerful but less well-known tools of demographic analysis and projection can be used. The tools of multistate population analysis allow for the projection of the population by several characteristics (such as age, sex, education, and place of residence) at the same time. Multistate projections group all individuals of a given population into different subpopulations, which are then simultaneously projected into the future, while at each time interval, people can also move from one subpopulation to another.

In PEDA, the population is broken down into eight sub-groups according to urban or rural place of residence, level of education, and food-security status. Place of residence and food-security status are core elements of the vicious circle, as mentioned earlier. Significant educational–fertility differentials give a strong rationale to the explicit consideration of education in the model (see Lutz *et al.* 1999), but there are also good reasons to assume a positive effect of literacy on agricultural production.

Each of these eight sub-groups is further subdivided by age (in single-year age groups) and sex (i.e., each of the eight groups has its own age pyramid). During each one-year simulation step, a person moves up the age pyramid by one year within the same sub-group, or moves to another sub-group while aging by one year (or dies). It is also possible for some people to make multiple transitions within one time step (e.g., from rural–food insecure–illiterate to urban–food secure–illiterate). For education and rural–urban migration, the model is hierarchical (i.e., people can only move in one direction, from lower to higher education and from rural areas to urban areas). Movement between food security states can happen in both directions, depending on the food conditions in the relevant year and the food distribution function.

The PEDA population module is in itself a useful piece of software for multi-state population projections. As part of the initialization process, the user can set, for each of the eight states, age- and sex-specific fertility, mortality, and educational transition rates. As scenario variables, dynamic future paths can be defined for fertility and mortality. The model automatically adjusts age-specific fertility and mortality patterns according to the levels of the total fertility rate and life expectancy chosen for each year. The methods of multistate population projections are well described in the literature (e.g., Rogers 1975; Keyfitz 1979; Scherbov and Grechucha 1988). Here, it is sufficient to mention that the multistate population projection model is a generalization of the one-dimensional cohort-component model of population projections that takes into account transitions that occur between different states.

Education and rural–urban migration are defined in terms of the proportion of male and female cohorts that become literate and move from rural to urban areas. While education is concentrated in childhood, rural–urban migration tends to follow a typical pattern, with the highest migration intensities in young adulthood. The standard internal migration schedule used here (Rogers and Castro 1981) reflects this pattern. The model also uses sex- and age-specific educational transition rates like those described in Chapter 4.

The PEDA model also accounts for the demographic and developmental consequences of the HIV/AIDS pandemic. We discuss how we deal with the disease in the model and what its predicted effects are in more detail below.

6.2.3   Land and water

Land (arable land and pasture) is a key environmental resource for agricultural production. Like many of the variables that affect agricultural production, land is treated as an index variable set to 1.0 in the starting year. This value describes

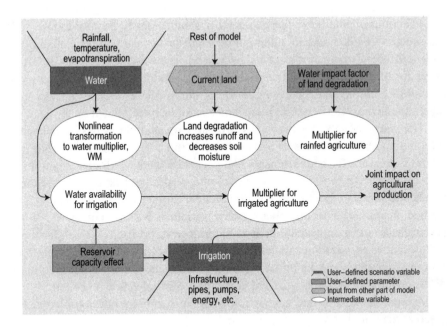

Figure 6.2. Water module.

both the quantity and quality of land. In a more general manner, one can label the land variable as "the natural resources stock." The change in the stock of natural resources is the result of a combination of indigenous growth or regeneration and a reduction through population-induced environmental degradation. It is also assumed that the pace of resource recovery diminishes as the saturation level is approached. The population-induced depletion of the natural resource depends on the change in overall population density and on the change in size of the rural illiterate, food-insecure segment of the population. An exact, formal description of the dynamics of the land variable is given in Appendix 6.1.

For its key role in food security and sustainable human development, water also deserves particular attention in models that deal with the nexus issues. In the PEDA model, water is treated in a separate module (see *Figure 6.2*), with an eventual multiplier effect on agricultural outputs. The water module contains two externally defined scenario variables (water and irrigation) that can be changed dynamically, and two user-defined parameters:

- the reservoir capacity effect (RCE); and
- a parameter that specifies the impact of land degradation on water availability (subsequently labeled as the water impact factor, WIF).

The value of the latter two parameters should ideally be determined during the process of initialization, although different values can still be defined by an advanced user as part of the scenario settings. The water segment in PEDA also relies on the input from other variables in the model, such as the quantity and quality of land, and calculates a number of intermediate variables. This input is determined completely endogenously and cannot be manipulated by the user.

The water module essentially has two parts, one that refers to rain-fed agriculture and another that refers to irrigated agriculture. The scenario variable water, $W(t)$, is relevant for both segments and covers the general climatic conditions in year t, particularly with respect to rainfall and evapotranspiration. It therefore can be used to simulate both short-term or cyclical droughts and longer-term climate change. Unlike most of the other scenario variables, water is not set to 1.0 in the starting year; its initial value is defined in terms of its position on a nonlinear curve that describes the relationship between water availability and agricultural production. This definition of the initial value depends on the specific climate conditions of the country in the initial year and is part of the initialization procedure.

A more detailed formal description of the segments for both rain-fed and irrigated agriculture is given in Appendix 6.1.

6.2.4   Agricultural production segment

The total agricultural production in one year, measured in total calories produced (in index form), is calculated through a Cobb–Douglas-type agricultural production function. Many agricultural production functions exist, but most of them do not consider the labor force and its skills as a production factor. Instead, they largely focus on physical and financial inputs. The production function chosen for the PEDA model is a notable exception. Based on pooled data sets of time series for most countries of the world, Hayami and Ruttan (1971) estimated a large number of Cobb–Douglas-type production functions with different combinations of input factors for different groups of countries. The equation that seemed most appropriate for PEDA Africa is the principal components regression for developing countries, including educational variables. The estimated elasticities are given as default values in PEDA. If more recent estimates or ones that are more appropriate for the country under consideration are available, the elasticities are changed accordingly. In a thorough initialization for a new country, the inclusion of other variables should even be considered. In this respect, much depends on the mix of crops under production and the share of livestock in the total outputs.

The total production is a function of the labor and land inputs, and investments in fertilizer use, mechanization, etc. In PEDA, some of these inputs are endogenously determined by the other segments in the model and others are treated in terms of externally defined scenario variables.

The population by age and sex in the eight defined categories affects total agricultural production in two different ways. First, the population projections produce an estimate of the size of the rural labor force. In addition to their technical training (an externally defined scenario variable), their productivity is affected by the proportion literate within each category (determined endogenously). The values for all these variables directly enter the agricultural production function, as discussed below.

The other chain of causation is a reflection of the vicious circle reasoning: the factor land is degraded as a function of the relative increase in the rural illiterate, food-insecure segment of the population and of the population density in general, as discussed above. Other main factors that influence the agricultural output of a country, such as mechanization and fertilizer use, need to be specified in externally defined scenario variables. The specific numerical values of the production function used, as well as the way in which imports and/or exports and loss during harvest, transport, and storage are dealt with, are given in Appendix 6.1.

Abundant theoretical and empirical evidence indicates that inequality in food distribution is at least as important to food insecurity as is the total production of food. The work of Amartya Sen (1981) in particular demonstrated that some of the worst famines occurred under conditions in which there would have been enough food for everybody had the distribution been appropriate. For this reason it is evident that a model that focuses on food security but does not pay attention to the distributional aspects is incomplete, if not misleading. The main problem with considering such distributions, however, lies in the fact that hardly any empirical data exist on distributive mechanisms in the African countries of today, and that theoretical distributions are hardly appropriate because the conditions tend to vary significantly from one country to another. PEDA opts for another solution to approximate the inequality in the access to food through household income distribution functions that exist for a number of African countries on the basis of household expenditure surveys (World Bank 1997, Section 15). Hence, PEDA relies on the assumption that inequalities in access to food follow a distribution similar to that for inequalities in access to income in urban and rural areas separately.

In each one-year step of the projections, food is allocated to rural and urban areas according to population size and using an urban bias factor, and within each of these areas the food distribution function determines the new sizes of the food-secure and food-insecure subpopulations. *Figure 6.3* gives an example of such a food distribution function. It is a Lorenz curve with the cumulated proportion of the population on one axis and the cumulated calories available for distribution on the other. If the Lorenz curve coincides with a 45° diagonal, the slope of the curve is equal to 1.0 and everyone in the economy has access to the mean available calories

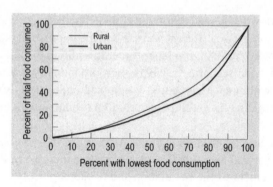

Figure 6.3. Food distribution function for urban and rural areas.

(i.e., a 45° diagonal describes a situation of perfect equality). The convexity of the curve, therefore, measures the degree of inequality.

The curves given in *Figure 6.3* indicate that, in this case, the most privileged 10 percent of the urban population (those between 90 and 100 percent on the x-axis) consume 30 percent of the available food. Moving down the curve, about half the urban population consumes more than 75 percent of the food. The borderline between the food-secure and the food-insecure population is established by applying an externally defined minimum calorie requirement per person. The iterations are carried out in steps of 1 percent of the population. The borderline for the proportion of the population that is considered to be food insecure is established at the point where the food allocation of the percentile falls below the minimum food requirement specified. Over time, the proportions of food insecure may change as a consequence of changes in the population size and food availability, or possible changes in the assumed food distribution function. In this application, however, the food distribution function is assumed to remain constant over the whole projection period.

6.2.5 HIV and AIDS in PEDA

As a model to demonstrate the interactions between population, education, environment, and food security, PEDA was not initially designed to explicitly cover the possible sustainable development and food security consequences of HIV/AIDS. However, since this pandemic has become such a challenge to many African countries, and because it is not meaningful to talk about a future development path without explicitly considering HIV/AIDS, this section discusses how HIV/AIDS is incorporated in PEDA. As there is still relatively little empirical knowledge on the trends and consequences of the pandemic, especially on its effect on the different sectors on the economy, the model is necessarily experimental in its conception and treatment of HIV/AIDS.

The most obvious impact of HIV/AIDS on the nexus is through excess mortality, and thus indirectly through a reduction of the labor force. As the age pattern of AIDS mortality differs from that observed in a population without AIDS, it was decided to include this effect using a user-specified scenario variable. In that scenario variable, the user needs to specify AIDS-related morbidity rates. The morbidity rates are translated into age-specific mortality rates, which are incorporated in the age-specific mortality pattern of each of the eight different sub-groups in the population. The additional age-specific mortality pattern caused by AIDS has been estimated on the basis of a model for Botswana (see Chapter 7 of this volume). AIDS mortality has a typical shape, with very high rates in early adulthood and, through vertical transmission, also in early childhood. The specified age-specific excess mortality caused by AIDS is scaled up or down depending on the morbidity level set by the user in the HIV/AIDS scenario variable and incorporated with the mortality from other causes.

In this application, identical AIDS morbidity schedules were applied to the eight sub-groups. However, the user can make different assumptions as to the expected reduction in the level of life expectancy and thus account for different potential impacts of HIV/AIDS in rural and urban areas, among literates and illiterates, etc.

HIV/AIDS not only induces increased mortality with its impact on the population structure, but it also seriously affects agricultural production through different mechanisms. Most of these effects are not endogenized in PEDA and need to be dealt with in the form of consistent user-defined scenarios. One can choose the various model parameters and scenario variables in such a way that they describe consistent "stories" or scenarios of possible future trends.

AIDS mortality and morbidity reduce educational enrolment and technical education through AIDS orphanhood, fewer qualified teachers (who may die), and AIDS-induced financial and economic constraints. These likely negative consequences of AIDS on the incomes of affected households may also reduce investments in fertilizer, irrigation, and mechanical inputs in agriculture. The only endogenized feedback from the AIDS morbidity rates on agricultural production is the reduction in productivity of the labor force. By default the model assumes a linear decline in the productivity of the labor force at the rate of the morbidity level. Put more simply, people who are sick (i.e., symptomatic with HIV/AIDS) are subtracted from the labor force. The rationale is that the capacity of sick people to work is greatly reduced and that some healthy people will have to look after their sick relatives instead of working, which thus reduces their productivity in agriculture.

Taken together, these different effects may have a drastic impact on agricultural outputs and the development of a country, but at the moment hardly any systematic empirical evidence exists on these issues. Hence, the assumptions are necessarily highly speculative at this point.

6.3   PEDA Projections for Ethiopia

To date, the PEDA model has been initialized for nine African countries. The initialization for Ethiopia goes furthest in terms of customization to country-specific conditions. When considering the outcomes of these PEDA projections, it must be recognized that this customization is not exhaustive. To estimate agricultural outputs, for example, the model mainly relies on a generic agricultural production function for Africa. Consequently, the projection results are to be seen as indicative and could still be improved upon. Aspects of the current application of PEDA for Ethiopia that are open to revision include the definition of the food distribution function, the elasticities of the agricultural production function, the water saturation curve, and the parameters of the land module.

Before discussing the projection results for Ethiopia, we first give a descriptive overview of the situation in the country with regard to the nexus issues and the policy responses.

6.3.1   The Ethiopian population–environment–agriculture nexus: Beyond the threshold of a sustainable livelihood?

Over the past couple of decades, Ethiopia has been the subject of many headlines that report recurrent war and famine. Although the latter is often caused by factors that cannot be modeled by PEDA, the model is able to illustrate the fragile equilibrium between population growth, environmental stress, and performance of the agricultural sector that serves as the context within which these tragedies take place. In such situations, it is often only slight disturbances, caused by a period of reduced rainfall, isolation through conflicts, or a malfunctioning distribution system, that lead to acute food-security problems. In the case of Ethiopia, occasionally these have escalated to catastrophic proportions.

To speak of an equilibrium when describing the population–environment–agriculture nexus in Ethiopia is, however, optimistic. The country is facing structural problems in all three sectors, and they often reinforce one another. The scope of the problem is captured in the fact that about 50–60 percent of the population is considered to be chronically food insecure (Befekadu and Berhanu 2000, p. 176). Over half of Ethiopian children under the age of five are stunted, and more than one in four is stunted severely. Further, 11 percent are wasted moderately and 1 percent are wasted severely (CSA and Macro International 2000, p. 17).

Like many African countries, Ethiopia's population is growing fast. It is only since the early 1990s that fertility started to decline from rates above 7.5 children per woman at the national level. Combined with slight improvements in the control of mortality since the 1960s, this is responsible for population growth rates of up to 3 percent annually. Around 85 percent of the estimated 65 million inhabitants live in rural areas, mostly concentrated in the northern and central highlands (CSA 1999).

According to the official national medium-variant population projections, the population will more than double by the year 2030, which implies an average growth rate of around 2.4 percent (CSA 1999, p. 343). Even under this "favorable" scenario, which assumes a decline in fertility to 3.32 by 2030, population growth will continue to exert serious pressure on the environment and will remain an enormous challenge to agriculture.

Although these data are usually difficult to obtain, the fragmentary information presented below suggests that environmental degradation, whether through deforestation, soil erosion, or the depletion of soil nutrients, will be one of the major constraints to finding a sustainable livelihood for most of those who live in rural areas. Over the past century, the land covered by forests has decreased from approximately 40 to 3 percent.[1] In the early 1990s, the annual rate of deforestation was estimated at 88,000 hectares (ha) per year, while the rate at which this loss is being replaced through afforestation is estimated to be 6,000 ha per year (TGE-OPM 1993, p. 7). The causes are related to the expansion of settlements and agriculture, and the use of fuelwood as a primary source of energy. One estimate regarding soil erosion states that by 2010, 17 percent of the highlands will not be suitable for sustained farming (Befekadu and Berhanu 2000, p. 180). In addition to the cropping pattern and techniques, the nature of the terrain and the intensity of rainfall in peak periods are two important factors that contribute to soil erosion. About one-third of the highlands has a slope that exceeds 30 percent, which makes it susceptible to soil erosion once the vegetation is removed. In addition, land degradation is exacerbated by centuries of crop production without fertilizer use or any other investment in land conservation. Crop residues are used to feed cattle, and animal manure is used for fuel instead of put back into the land. Not surprisingly, these practices have resulted in a net outflow of vital nutrients and a reduction of the soil's capacity for moisture retention (Befekadu and Berhanu 2000, p. 180).

---

[1]Other sources are somewhat more optimistic, reporting that in 1995 around 6.9 percent of the 1.11 million square kilometers of land area was covered by forests and woodland (UNDP 1998, p. 69).

The situation described above is particularly worrying, since agriculture is, and will long remain, the mainstay of the Ethiopian economy. The share of agriculture in the country's gross domestic product (GDP) is around 51 percent (Befekadu and Berhanu 2000, p. 155); it provides employment for 85 percent of the population, generates up to 90 percent of the export earnings, and is also the main supplier of raw materials for the manufacturing sector (Dejene 2000, p. 13). Regardless of its prominent position in the Ethiopian economy, the prospects for the performance of the agricultural sector are not bright at all. In addition to the environmental problems, farmers face numerous constraints related to diminishing farm sizes, low tenure security, imperfect agricultural markets (partly through a lack of infrastructure), and the weak agricultural research base and extension system (Befekadu and Berhanu 2000, pp. 177–195). Many of these constraints act together, and so condemn farmers to subsistence agriculture and consequently limited investments in the land and exacerbated land degradation.

Agricultural land in Ethiopia is managed at the communal level, and farmers do not have the right of private ownership. Throughout history, agricultural land has been redistributed frequently, often with a reduction in farm sizes. The need to accommodate an increasing population has required many local authorities, particularly in the northern highlands, to distribute grazing land for farming, and thereby seriously reduce the already insufficient animal fodder (Befekadu and Berhanu 2000, p. 199).

The average farm size at the national level is 1 ha per household, but 62 percent of the households cultivate less than this. On these small plots, subsistence and survival agriculture is the primary concern. All income, from both farm and nonfarm activities, is invested in food. There simply is no surplus for investment in land conservation or agricultural intensification (Befekadu and Berhanu 2000, pp. 178–179). In the mid-1990s, only 4.6 percent of the arable land was irrigated (UNDP 1998, p. 69), less than 2 percent of the farmers were reported to use improved seeds (Befekadu and Berhanu 2000, p. 184), and fertilizer use was about 7 kilograms (kg) of nutrients per hectare of arable land, compared with an average of 9 kg for sub-Saharan Africa and 65 kg for the world (Dejene 2000, p. 14). These limited technological inputs make agricultural production very susceptible to fluctuations in rainfall.

In addition to all other constraints, many farmers have little incentive to produce an agricultural surplus, since markets to sell their goods are inaccessible. Around three-quarters of the farms are more than half a day's walk from an all-weather road. Farmers' produce must be carried long distances by pack animals or by humans to locations at which buyers are found (Befekadu and Berhanu 2000, p. 189).

Disturbed by recurrent conflict and war over the past decades, per capita agricultural production declined at a dramatic rate of 1.15 percent per year on average between 1970 and 2000. Over the past decade, per capita food production declined at a somewhat slower pace of 0.64 percent per year (FAO/WFP 2001, p. 3). Considered in isolation, these figures support a Malthusian disaster scenario. However, improved economic management, currency and trade liberalization, and grain and agricultural input liberalization are considered to be important factors that have contributed to an average economic growth rate of 6.5 percent, while inflation was kept under 4 percent between 1993 and 1998. A period of favorable rainfall in the mid-1990s added to this impressive growth in GDP, but once again war, a multi-year drought, and the increased burden of HIV/AIDS virtually stalled economic growth toward the end of the 1990s (FAO/WFP 2001, p. 3). UNECA is more optimistic about Ethiopia's more recent economic performance. They put the real GDP growth for the 2001–2002 period at around 6.6 percent (UNECA 2002).

The fast economic growth rates observed in the mid-1990s and early 2000s indicate that a scenario of declining per capita production along with increasing poverty and food insecurity is not inevitable, but, as illustrated by the PEDA simulations (see discussion below), preventing such a scenario requires a concerted and sustained effort in multiple sectors of the society and economy.

6.3.2 The policy response

The Ethiopian government is aware of the challenges posed by the negative interactions between demographic, environmental, and agricultural variables. In 1993, just after the downfall of the military socialist regime, it recognized that

> demographic and developmental factors reinforce each other. High fertility and rapid population growth exert negative influences on economic and social development and low levels of economic and social development provide the climate favoring high fertility and hence rapid population growth. Because of an unholy combination of these forces, Ethiopia finds herself in a vicious cycle of failure and defeatism. (TGE-OPM 1993, pp. 24–25)

To tackle these problems, the government committed itself to holistic planning and even established a multidisciplinary office within the Office of the Prime Minister and a National Population Council to be composed of members from various ministries. Among the general objectives of the National Population Policy are the following (TGE-OPM 1993, pp. 24–25):

- To close the gap between high population growth (total fertility rate of 4.0 by 2015) and low economic productivity through planned reduction of population growth and increased economic returns.

- To reduce the rate of rural–urban migration.
- To maintain and improve the carrying capacity of the environment.
- To raise the economic and social status of women and other vulnerable groups.

The current agricultural development strategy of the government is known as agricultural development led industrialization (ADLI). This strategy gives high priority to smallholder farmers in terms of provision of incentive packages and technologies for increased agricultural productivity (Dejene 2000, p. 13). As a result, fertilizer use has increased in the past couple of years, but because of high prices (caused by the removal of subsidies in 1997) and a poor distribution and credit system, 40 percent of the fertilizer made available remained unsold in 1996–1997 (Befekadu and Berhanu 2000, p. 192). Fertilizer use well below the planned quantity remains a constraint to agricultural intensification up to the present time (FAO/WFP 2001, p. 8).

In 1997, the Ethiopian government approved an environmental policy that is cross-sectoral and integrative, that supports decentralized initiatives, and that proposes a legislative framework and a monitoring and evaluation system (Dejene 2000, p. 23–24). The Ethiopian government is thus clearly aware of the vicious circle of increasing poverty, environmental degradation, and decreasing agricultural outputs. It has developed policies to break this circle and even made institutional reforms to support these policies. However, relatively few quantitative objectives have been formulated, and evidence of the performance of the agricultural sector and economy does not give a clear indication that the implementation of these policies will be sufficient to reverse the current negative development trend.

6.3.3   PEDA applied to Ethiopia

In preparing the baseline data for Ethiopia and a baseline scenario for making projections, we relied as far as possible on observed data and on time series that were extended into the future.[2] However, some data are simply not available or are very difficult to obtain. In these cases, we have made estimates, usually on the optimistic side.

The Baseline Data and the Baseline Scenario for PEDA Ethiopia

The total population by single years of age and by sex, and the age-specific fertility and mortality schedules for each of the eight states were prepared following the procedures illustrated in the *PEDA Technical Manual* (UNECA, forthcoming). The data are from the 1994 Population and Housing Census (CSA 1999). Since disaggregated information on fertility and mortality for each of the eight states is

---

[2]The PEDA model for Ethiopia was initialized in 2001 and only uses data available at that time.

not always available, some estimation procedures had to be followed. In making these estimates, it was always verified that the disaggregated values were consistent with the observed or reported aggregated figures.

The food distribution functions for urban and rural areas were prepared following the procedures outlined in the *PEDA Technical Manual*, using household expenditure data published by the World Bank (1997). At the time of the initialization of PEDA for Ethiopia, no household expenditure data were available. Therefore, we used data for Uganda as a proxy. Together with the food availability in a country, the food distribution curves are important in determining the proportion of the population that is food insecure. In this case, the estimate of the share of the population that is food insecure for the initial year of the projections is around 65 percent, and thus is somewhat higher than the figures often cited for Ethiopia.

A comprehensive listing of the specific model specifications and parameter settings for this application to Ethiopia is given in Appendix 6.1. Here we only discuss the data and assumptions made for the eight sub-groups of the population and its education, as well as the treatment of HIV/AIDS in this model. We then move directly to a discussion of the results of alternative scenarios.

Sub-Group Parameters

Total fertility rates (TFRs) and life expectancy values for each of the eight states were estimated following the procedures described in the *PEDA Technical Manual* (UNECA, forthcoming). This is done in such a way that the nested values are consistent with the aggregated values reported in the census monograph (CSA 1999). Under the baseline scenario, we make assumptions similar to those made by the Central Statistical Authority for their medium variant population projections (CSA 1999). These include a steep decline in fertility and an important increase in life expectancy (see *Table 6.2* for more details).

According to the 1994 census (CSA 1999, p. 85), only 23.3 percent of the population was considered literate.[3] As is illustrated in *Table 6.1*, the discrepancies between males and females, and especially between urban and rural areas, are considerable. Under the baseline scenario (*Table 6.2*), we assume not only that enrolment rates will increase rapidly, but also that the gender gap will be reduced significantly. In urban areas, we assume that 95 percent of all children will make the transition from the illiterate to literate status. In rural areas, we assume that 60 percent of the boys and 55 percent of the girls will enter school and become literate. Since education is treated statically in the PEDA model, these transition rates are applied from the first year of the projection period. Again, these are very optimistic scenario assumptions, as the gross enrolment rates increased by only 25

---

[3]This figure is much lower than the 35 percent reported by UNESCO for 1995 (UNESCO Web site).

Table 6.1. A description of the fertility, mortality, and literacy conditions in Ethiopia in 1995.

State (St)	TFR[b]	$e_0{}^a$ Males	Females	Percentage literate Males	Females
St1: Urban, literate, food secure	4.28	60.4	64.7	–	–
St2: Urban, literate, food insecure	4.28	55.8	59.8	–	–
St3: Urban, illiterate, food secure	4.83	53.5	57.5	77.4	60.6
St4: Urban, illiterate, food insecure	4.83	49.4	53.8	77.4	60.6
St5: Rural, literate, food secure	5.97	56.6	59.5	–	–
St6: Rural, literate, food insecure	6.86	52.4	55.1	–	–
St7: Rural, illiterate, food secure	6.73	50.3	53.0	21.8	8.6
St8: Rural, illiterate, food insecure	7.74	46.6	49.0	21.8	8.6
Aggregate	6.74	50.0	51.6	–	–

[a] Life expectancy at birth.
[b] Total fertility rate.

Table 6.2. Fertility, mortality, and literacy assumptions for Ethiopia under the baseline scenario (by 2030).

State (St)	TFR[b]	$e_0{}^a$ Males	Females	Educational transition rates Males	Females
St1: Urban, literate, food secure	2.28	79.9	84.8	–	–
St2: Urban, literate, food insecure	2.28	73.7	78.4	–	–
St3: Urban, illiterate, food secure	2.58	70.8	75.4	95.0	95.0
St4: Urban, illiterate, food insecure	2.58	65.3	69.7	95.0	95.0
St5: Rural, literate, food secure	3.18	74.8	78.0	–	–
St6: Rural, literate, food insecure	3.66	69.3	72.2	–	–
St7: Rural, illiterate, food secure	3.59	66.5	69.4	60.0	55.0
St8: Rural, illiterate, food insecure	4.13	61.6	64.2	60.0	55.0
Aggregate	3.51	65.0	68.0	–	–

[a] Life expectancy at birth.
[b] Total fertility rate.

and 20 percentage points for boys and girls, respectively, between 1970 and 1996 (UNESCO Web site).

HIV/AIDS

The first cases of AIDS in Ethiopia were reported in the mid-1980s. By 1989, the adult HIV prevalence rate (ages 15 and older) was estimated at around 1 percent. In the 1990s, prevalence rates grew rapidly, reaching 3.2 percent in 1993 and 7.4 percent in 1997. Large discrepancies still exist between rural and urban areas. In the former, the adult prevalence rate was believed to be around 4.5 percent in 1997,

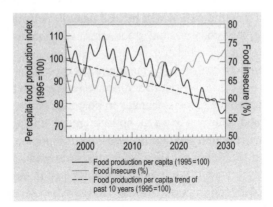

Figure 6.4. Evolution of the per capita food production and the percentage of food insecure under the baseline scenario.

and for urban areas, around 17 percent (Ministry of Health 1998, p. 5). Conservative official estimates are that prevalence rates will increase to 9 percent by 2006 and will stabilize at that level (Ministry of Health 1998, p. 16).

Reporting on the prevalence between the ages of 15 and 49,[4] the Joint United Nations Programme on HIV/AIDS (UNAIDS) estimate for the end of 1997 was 9.3 percent (UNAIDS 1998, p. 3). By the end of 1999, that figure had increased to 10.6 percent. This means that around three million adults and children are living with HIV/AIDS in Ethiopia. Around 280,000 people are believed to have died from AIDS-related illnesses in 1999 alone (UNAIDS 2000, p. 3).

6.3.4 Simulation results for the baseline scenario

In the assumptions for the baseline scenario, we chose rather optimistic values. The moment has now come to verify whether the projection results are equally optimistic. The answer is ambivalent. As mentioned earlier in this chapter, per capita food production in Ethiopia declined in the 1990s on average by 0.64 percent per year. For illustrative purposes, this linear trend is extended in *Figure 6.4* throughout the projection period. Our projections to 2030 present a slightly more positive image (they do not consider the year-by-year variations in per capita production caused by fluctuations in rainfall). Nevertheless, the overall tendency of per capita agricultural production continues to decline at an alarming rate. Even under the optimistic conditions elaborated upon above, the per capita agricultural production

---

[4]This is the new standardized definition of adult HIV prevalence adopted by UNAIDS. The values are usually higher than those for the 15 and older definition. Based on the data reported for 1997 by the Ministry of Health (old definition) and UNAIDS (new definition), we assume that the prevalence rates of the population aged 15–49 is 1.5 percent higher than that of the population aged 15 and older.

by the end of the projection period will be less than 80 percent of what it was in 1995. In that sense, the prospects under our optimistic baseline scenario are still very poor.

Similarly, the proportion that is food insecure is expected to increase by almost 10 percent over the projection period. In addition to food production and population growth, this output variable reflects changes in post-harvest losses and changes in the net import of food. Our positive assumptions are not able to resolve the food-security problem in the country either. It seems that the population–environment–agriculture nexus in Ethiopia has fallen below the threshold of sustainability. To give one more example: under the conditions summarized in the baseline scenario, it is estimated that the food imports will have to increase by more than 7 percent annually to stabilize the proportion of food-insecure people in the country. This figure is almost three times higher than the current population growth rate.

Underlying the negative tendency in per capita food production is the degradation of the natural resources stock. PEDA assumes that a fast-growing population contributes to increasing land degradation, and land is one of the most important production factors. In particular, the rural illiterate and food-insecure segment of the population is expected to deplete natural resources in their quest for survival. In our projections, the total population is expected to double by 2030, and despite all our assumptions regarding improvements in the literacy rates, decreasing fertility, and increased inputs in agriculture, the rural food-insecure segment of the population is expected to grow the fastest (more than doubling by 2030). As a result, the land stock is estimated to maintain only 86 percent of its productive capacity by the year 2030 (see *Table 6.4*).

6.3.5 Other scenarios: HIV/AIDS, drought, and migration

Let us now turn to a less optimistic scenario, one in which HIV/AIDS plays a more prominent role. To ease our task, we assume that HIV prevalence rates are similar in rural and urban areas. To correct for the overestimation of the prevalence in rural areas, we use a relatively conservative estimate of the evolution of the pandemic in Ethiopia. We assume that AIDS morbidity levels rapidly increased in the second half of the 1990s to reach 2 percent by the year 2000 (this stands for an adult HIV prevalence rate of around 10 percent). We then assume that morbidity levels stay at around 2.15 percent for the next decade and then start to decline gradually. Life expectancy assumptions are modified to be around 10 years lower by the year 2030 compared with a situation without AIDS.

Although a number of studies point to the socioeconomic impact of HIV/AIDS (see, e.g., Bollinger *et al.* 1999; Stover and Bollinger 1999), none of them has quantified the nationwide impact of HIV/AIDS on the different sectors of the economy and human development. Most of the reported effects result in the reduction of the labor force through excess mortality and morbidity, and in a reduction of the household income. The latter is often an outcome of the reduction of the labor force itself and of the costs for medical treatment and funeral services. These two effects have many spin-offs. A reduction in the labor force has to be compensated by other family members (often children who are withdrawn from school) or it leads to reduced labor inputs in agriculture. A reduction of the household income induces farmers to economize on the technological inputs in agriculture and land preservation, and even on the education of their children. Other often-mentioned side effects of the HIV/AIDS pandemic are cutbacks in qualified personnel, such as teachers, and a reduction of the transfer of skills from one generation to another. The arguments summarized here justify the scenario assumptions presented in *Table 6.3*, though their values remain relatively arbitrary because of a lack of more precise empirical information.

For illustrative purposes, we define two other alternative scenarios in addition to the HIV/AIDS scenario. One scenario assumes two three-year periods of reduced rainfall, and the second incorporates a higher rate of rural–urban migration. For these two scenarios, all the other assumptions are similar to those of the baseline scenario (see *Table 6.3*).

As would be expected, the prospects under the HIV/AIDS scenario are even worse than under the baseline scenario. In addition to the important human impact, per capita food production drops to less than three-fourths its value in 1995. As a result, the share of the food-insecure segment will increase to more than 75 percent of the population by 2030 (*Table 6.4*). If our assumptions on the effect of the AIDS pandemic are correct, it will have a major effect on both the food-security situation in the country and on a number of other variables related to human development. Although mostly a direct result of our scenario assumptions, both life expectancy and literate life expectancy[5] of the population are expected to be much lower than under the baseline scenario.

The results of the projections for the other two scenarios are also worth mentioning. Apart from the acute food-security problems that arise during periods of reduced rainfall, drought has a long-term negative effect on the population–environment–agriculture nexus, which extends the period of the drought itself. This is illustrated in the value of the natural resources stock, $R(t)$, at the end of the projection period, which is lower than under the baseline scenario, and in the higher proportion of the population that is food insecure (see *Table 6.4*). The migration scenario, on the other hand, has perhaps unexpected positive results. Its gains are visible both in terms of the food-security status of the population and in terms of

---

[5]The number of years a person is expected to live in a literate state from the age of 15 onward. See Chapter 4 of this volume for more details on this output variable.

Table 6.3. A comparison of assumptions for the baseline, HIV/AIDS, drought, and migration scenarios.

Indicator	Scenario			
	Baseline	HIV/AIDS	Drought	Migration
HIV/AIDS morbidity	Constant at 1.1%	Peak at 2.18% in 2010	*	*
Life expectancy	See *Table 6.2*	Reduction of 10 years by 2030 compared with the scenario without HIV/AIDS	*	*
Urban literacy transition rates	95% for males 95% for females	90% for males 85% for females	*	*
Rural literacy transition rates	60% for males 55% for females	40% for males 35% for females	*	*
Increase in the technical eduction of the labor force	1.5% annually	0.9% annually	*	*
Reduction in post-harvest losses	1% annually	0.75% annually	*	*
Increase in fertilizer use	5% annually	4% annually	*	*
Increase in machinery use	0.5% annually	0.4% annually	*	*
Increase in irrigation	1% annually	0.75% annually	*	*
Land regeneration parameter (a)	0.0175	0.015	*	*
Water	Values based on rainfall time series for the period 1992–1999	*	Two three-year periods of reduced rainfall (value 0.7 for the water scenario variable)	*
Rural–urban migration	6% of each rural cohort migrates	*	*	25% of each rural cohort migrates

*Same assumptions as under the baseline scenario.

Table 6.4. Projection results for the baseline and alternative scenarios.

Indicator	Year	Scenario			
		Baseline	HIV/AIDS	Drought	Migration
Total population (millions)	2030	132.80	119.90	133.00	130.30
	2050	195.30	164.70	195.70	186.80
Food insecure (%)	2030	73.30	76.20	75.20	72.50
	2050	92.80	98.00	98.00	83.30
Life expectancy (years)	2030	66.50	56.00	66.40	67.00
	2050	65.80	55.00	65.60	67.10
TFR[a]	2030	3.50	3.60	3.50	3.30
	2050	3.60	3.70	3.60	3.30
LLE[b] (aged 15+)	2030	19.90	13.60	19.90	20.70
	2050	23.40	14.50	23.30	25.60
Land, $R(t)$	2030	0.86	0.84	0.85	0.90
	2050	0.49	0.51	0.48	0.61

[a]Total fertility rate.
[b]Literate life expectancy.

the human development component. Increased migration facilitates a fertility decline and increases in life expectancy and literate life expectancy, and also relieves the pressure on the natural resources stock. As suggested by PEDA, rural–urban migration should thus be considered as part of a policy strategy to tackle the food-security problem in the country. Currently, the government of Ethiopia considers internal migration to be a problem rather than part of the solution to their development concerns (see discussion above). Increased rural–urban migration, of course, adds to the challenge of creating jobs for the migrants and, with already high urban unemployment rates, the solution is not self-evident.

6.3.6 What needs to be done to break the vicious circle?

None of the scenarios presented so far is able to break the vicious circle of high population growth, increasing environmental degradation, and decreasing per capita agricultural outputs. Therefore, to gain an idea of the magnitude of the efforts that are required to break the negative development cycle in the case of Ethiopia, we have defined three other scenarios.

All three scenarios depart from the assumptions of the baseline scenario. The first entails increased technological inputs in agriculture. It assumes an annual increase in fertilizer use of 6 percent, in machinery use of 1 percent, and in irrigation and technical education of 2 percent each. This means that by 2030, fertilizer use will be more than 7.5 times higher than in the initial year, that irrigation and technical education will double, and that machinery use will be 1.5 times higher. The second scenario assumes almost universal education (95 percent) in both urban and

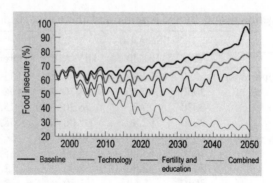

Figure 6.5. Evolution of the percentage of food insecure under the baseline, technology, fertility and education, and combined scenarios.

rural areas and a steeper fertility decline to reach a TFR of 2.4 by the year 2030. The third scenario combines these efforts in terms of the inputs in agriculture, education, and fertility reduction.

The projection results, presented in *Figure 6.5* in terms of the share of the population that is food insecure, are clear. Only concerted efforts in the different sectors are likely to break the negative development vicious circle. Increased efforts in agricultural intensification or education and fertility alone may be able to improve the situation in the short run, but the proportions of food insecure tend to increase again after 20 to 30 years.

Although the scenario assumptions of the combined scenario presented here may not be feasible or realistic (e.g., they do not include the potential negative consequences of HIV/AIDS), the PEDA projections clearly illustrate that a solution to the food-security problem in Ethiopia is unlikely to be found in one sector alone. The exact constellation of policies to solve the food-security problem may be different and may include migration, intensified industrialization, and higher food imports. However, the important message that underlies the projection results is that a single sector solution is unlikely to be sustainable in the long term, although the effect in the short run may be clearly positive.

Another lesson to be drawn from the PEDA projections is that time plays a crucial role: the faster policies are implemented, the lower the efforts needed to break the vicious circle. To give but one example, in the technology scenario above, fertilizer use is assumed to increase at 6 percent per year to reach a level of fertilizer use that is more than 7.5 times higher by 2030 than in 1995. The same per capita agricultural outputs would be reached by 2030 if the fertilizer use were increased to only 5 times the level of 1995, but under the condition that this increase be implemented within the first five years of the projection period (after which the fertilizer use remains constant).

6.4   Conclusions

Ethiopia's recent past has been marked by political turmoil and a succession of famines. Its future, if different, will depend crucially on the proper management of the population–environment–agriculture nexus. With the majority of the population already living on the edge of survival, the challenges are enormous. Breaking the vicious circle of rapid population growth, environmental degradation, and decreasing per capita agricultural production will require fast and concerted efforts in many sectors of society and the economy, not only in those that directly affect agriculture.

The Ethiopian government is aware of the issues at stake and has developed policies and new institutions to tackle the development problems it is facing. Almost 10 years after their formulation, the time has come for an evaluation and possible adjustment of the policies where necessary. Tools like PEDA could be useful to support the formulation of alternative policies and also to assess and anticipate the effects of the proposed policy mix. To use the PEDA model effectively in such a manner, a number of challenges to both scientists and policy makers remain. To render policies open to evaluation, they should be accompanied by quantitative objectives, which requires much political courage. On the other hand, it is the responsibility of the scientist to further elaborate and specify the intricate interactions between demographic, socioeconomic, environmental, and agricultural variables to feed into models like PEDA and to make them better reflect country-specific situations.

Acknowledgment

We are grateful to Israel Sembajwe, Han Chol, and the other staff members of the Sustainable Development Division at UNECA for their contributions to the development of the model and for their comments on earlier versions of this chapter.

Appendix 6.1:
Model and Parameter Specifications

Land

The change in the stock of natural resources $R(t)$ is the result of a combination of indigenous growth or regeneration $g(R(t))$ and a reduction through population-induced environmental degradation $D(t)$:

$$R(t) = g(R(t)) - D(t) , \tag{6.1}$$

where $R(t)$ for the initial year is equal to 1 and indigenous growth or regeneration is defined as

$$g(R(t)) = a(\overline{R} - R(t)) . \tag{6.2}$$

Parameter a reflects the speed at which the resources recover. However, it is assumed that the pace of resource recovery diminishes as the saturation level $\overline{R}$ is approached. The saturation level is the stationary solution for R if the resources are not degraded. The saturation level has to be chosen in accordance with the specific conditions in the country of application and remains constant over the whole projection period.

The model allows the user to assume that the rural illiterate food-insecure segment of the population, in particular, depletes natural resources in their quest for survival. As this is often used as an assumption in natural resources modeling, this impact diminishes as the stock of resources decreases. In mathematical form this is given by

$$P_I(t) \frac{R(t)}{R(t) + \eta} , \tag{6.3}$$

where $P_I(t)$ stands for the relative change in the number of rural illiterate food-insecure in the population compared with the starting conditions, and η is a constant factor that has a default value of 4.

The scale of environmental degradation is also a function of the change in the overall population density. Mathematically, this is expressed as

$$\frac{P(t)}{\overline{R}} , \tag{6.4}$$

where $P(t)$ stands for the relative change in the total population compared with the initial year. The denominator reflects the upper limit of the natural resource stock and has a constant value that is country specific and reflects the relative status of the resource stock in the year for which the initial data are prepared.

The complete mathematical expression for environmental degradation $D(t)$ is thus

$$D(t) = \gamma \frac{P(t)}{\overline{R}} P_I(t) \frac{R(t)}{R(t) + \eta} \,. \tag{6.5}$$

The only parameter not yet described in this function is γ. This parameter, called the land degradation impact factor in PEDA, influences the intensity of the effects described above. The value of γ can be adjusted in the PEDA user interface. Although the value of γ is subject to country-specific conditions, by default it is set to equal 0.02. Setting the value of γ to 0.00 implies that increasing population densities has no negative effect on the natural resources stock. For experimental purposes, the user could also set a negative value for γ, which means that increasing population densities has a positive effect on the natural resources stock, but in that case the natural resources upper limit $\overline{R}$ may be exceeded easily.

The expression of land degradation used here implies that if resources are degraded completely (i.e., $R(t) = 0$), the value of $D(t)$ will automatically be zero, as there is nothing to be depleted. Similarly, if the stock of rural illiterate food-insecure population is zero, environmental degradation will also be zero.

Rain-fed agriculture

To calculate the impact of the scenario variable "water" on rain-fed agriculture, a nonlinear transformation into a water multiplier $WM(t)$ is introduced, because an increase of one unit of water does not always have an equal impact on agricultural production. The assumed relationship is derived from the hydrological and agricultural literature, and the specific shape of this nonlinear relationship greatly depends on local conditions and the kind of crops and/or livestock under consideration. For in-depth applications of PEDA, the definition of this curve requires serious attention. For the current version of PEDA, a hypothetical curve was assumed. Its general features are that in cases of serious drought nothing can grow; but after this point, small increases in water availability can produce great returns. With further increases in water availability, the curve flattens and eventually reaches a saturation level, starting from which more water adversely affects agricultural outputs. Beyond this point, flooding starts to be harmful to production and may ultimately destroy all production.

The assumed nonlinear relationship of water on agricultural outputs only holds if other relevant determinants of soil moisture remain constant over time. Unfortunately, land degradation and land erosion tend to increase the runoff of rainfall

and therefore decrease the moisture that will be stored in the soil, and thus negatively affect agricultural productivity. Since land degradation is modeled explicitly
in other parts of PEDA, the impact of land degradation can be directly taken into
account. To do this in quantitative terms, another user-defined input parameter was
introduced, the water impact factor WIF of land degradation. WIF is defined in
the form of an elasticity applied to current land (defined as $R(t)$). This results in
an effective water multiplier EWM for rain-fed agriculture:

$$EWM(t) = WM(t) * R(t)^{WIF} . \tag{6.6}$$

Values greater than 1.0 for WIF increase the effect of the status of the land or
resources in the calculation of the EWM; values smaller than 1.0 decrease its
elasticity.

Irrigated agriculture

For irrigated agriculture, the dynamics by which water availability and irrigation
efforts have a joint effect on agricultural outputs are even more complex. The
functional relationships defined here are a great simplification, but should still be
able to capture the most important dynamics. The formula given below creates
an intermediate variable, effective irrigation EIR, which enters the agricultural
production function as a multiplier. To determine the value of EIR, PEDA makes
a distinction between the situation in which water availability is already at or above
the saturation level of 1.0 and when it is still below. If the water supply is above
the saturation level, efforts in irrigation do not make any difference to agricultural
production. If, on the other hand, the water supply is below the saturation level, the
positive effect of irrigation efforts further depends on the level of the water supply
and RCE. The reservoir capacity parameter stands for the potential to stock water
for later use in irrigated agriculture.

In the mathematical expression, $W(t)$ stands for the value of the scenario variable water at time t and $IR(t)$, for the value of the irrigation variable. In the
production function, Frt is the elasticity of fertilizer applied to irrigation, because
of the lack of better data on the effect of irrigation on agricultural production:

$$EIR(t) = \begin{cases} 1; \text{ if } W(t) \geq 1 \\ \left[RCE * \frac{IR(t)}{IR(0)} * \frac{W(t)}{W(0)} \right]^{Frt}; \text{ if } W(t) < 1 . \end{cases} \tag{6.7}$$

The second line of the above formula may require some explanation, since it is an
approximation of several more complex mechanisms. The main reasoning is that,
even under high irrigation efforts, water must be available to have any effect, and
even a high reservoir capacity does not help if it does not rain for a long time.

Ideally, we should calculate the cumulative water-storage effects over time. A simple approximation is obtained by multiplying by a ratio of current water over initial water in cases where the current water availability is still below the saturation level. This also implies that if there are no extra irrigation efforts, but simply more water, positive returns are also generated in terms of agricultural outputs. This can be interpreted as an additional direct effect of water on production that is weighted by improvements in irrigation and reservoir capacity.

Both effective irrigation $EIR(t)$ and the effective water multiplier $EWM(t)$ are added to the agricultural production function as additional multipliers. In this setup, the two water-related variables and current land enter the agricultural production function twice, but in two different forms and after transformations as outlined above. The water variable enters both through rain-fed and irrigated agriculture, as discussed. Land degradation, as captured by current land, enters as a regular production factor with a given elasticity and through the impact of land degradation on increasing runoff and therefore decreasing soil moisture. Depending on the other settings of the model and the specific parameter choice, this indirect effect of land degradation through declining soil moisture may be even more relevant than the direct effect through the production function.

Agricultural production

All these inputs to agricultural production are considered on a relative scale; their values are set to 1.0 in the starting year and change over time as a result of effects that emanate from the other segments in the model or as defined in the scenario settings for the exogenous variables. If, for example, we assume an increase in fertilizer use of 20 percent by 2005, this means that the value of that scenario variable is set to increase to 1.2 by that year.

In sum, total agricultural production in terms of total calories produced is calculated in the following multiplicative manner, in which the final two factors are the water multipliers discussed earlier:

$$\mathrm{Pr}\, odIndex = LF(t)^{0.534} * R(t)^{0.088} * FER(t)^{0.162} * MECH(t)^{0.072}$$
$$* LITLF(t)^{0.276} * TE(t)^{0.158} * EIR(t) * EWM(t). \quad (6.8)$$

Food availability and distribution

Not all the food produced in a country is consumed by its citizens. A fraction is lost during harvest, transportation, and storage, and a part of it may be intended for use as seeds in the next cropping season or for export. Imports may complement the food produced locally. Mathematically, the net food available FA can be expressed in the following manner:

$$FA_t = FP_t * (1 - LT_t) + imports_{t_0} * FIE_t. \tag{6.9}$$

In this expression, the net food production is equal to the gross production FP times the proportion that remains after deduction of the post-harvest losses and seedlings LT. The post-harvest losses are expressed as a proportion of the total production and can be manipulated in a dynamic scenario variable.

The net food imports are added to the net food production to obtain the net food availability. For the initial year of the projection period, an absolute value of imports has to be specified by the user ($imports$) in terms of the daily supply of kilocalories per capita. This is usually done as part of the initialization process. FIE is a dynamic scenario variable that has the default value of 1 for the initial year and allows the user to account for fluctuations in the volume of imports.

After the correction for post-harvest losses and net imports, the estimated amount of available food is distributed over the population in two steps. First, an "urban bias factor" (external scenario variable) determines which fraction of the available food is consumed by the rural and urban populations. As with the other scenario variables, this is done on a relative scale—1.0 reflects a condition of equality between rural and urban areas in the access to food. A value of 1.1 means that urban areas receive 10 percent more food than would have been attributed if food had been distributed in proportion to the size of the population who live in urban areas.

In addition to the urban bias factor, the PEDA model also accounts for inequality in the access to food within urban and rural areas. The distribution of food is often unequal because some people simply have more purchasing power than do others or have privileged access to food by other means. The result is that some people remain food insecure even though the total amount of food that reaches the population is theoretically sufficient to provide the necessary minimum diet for everybody. As access to food is usually more unequal in urban than in rural areas, PEDA works with two food distribution functions, one for rural and one for urban areas.

General settings and model parameters

These parameters apply to the country as a whole and deal with the start and end of the projection period, food production, and imports in the initial year, the parameters of the land module, and the rural–urban migration parameter. Their values for the PEDA Ethiopia projections are specified in *Table A6.1*.

Table A6.1. General settings and model parameters.

Parameter	Value	Comments
Initial year	1995	
End of the projection period	2030	To present the long-term dynamics, the projections are sometimes extended to 2050. The fertility and life expectancy assumptions (see text) are, in these cases, assumed to remain constant after 2030.
Production (and imports) of kilocalories per capita (kcal/capita) in the initial year	1,756.8	This figure refers to the net daily per capita production in the initial year. In addition to the production, the model also accounts for the net imports to calculate the net food availability in the initial year.
		On the ANDI Web site, 1,830 is reported as the average (net) supply of kcal/capita for the 1995–1997 period. Although other sources report lower figures for the daily per capita supply in 1995 (e.g., 1,750 in UNDP [1998, p. 68] and 1,727 in the FAOSTAT database), we have chosen to use the most optimistic figure.
		Between 1980 and 1998, food imports accounted, on average, for 11.8 percent of the gross available food, with extremes as low as 4.8 percent and as high as 18.3 percent (Dejene 2000, p. 17). Depending on the sources used, data on the food imports (including food aid) vary greatly. Dejene (2000, p. 17) reports the share of net food imports for the year 1994–1995 as 14 percent. In the FAO food balance sheets, (net) food imports in 1995 accounted for only 4 percent of the total available food for consumption (FAOSTAT Web site). Given our philosophy to present an optimistic baseline scenario for the food-security situation, we assume that only 4 percent of the total food supply in 1995 was imported. The 4 percent of net food imports stood for around 620,000 tons of food. The World Food Programme (WFP) reports that, for 1995, 652,000 tons of food were delivered to Ethiopia as food-aid alone (WFP Web site). Our estimates of food deficits and imports are therefore likely to be on the conservative side.
Assumed minimum consumption of daily kcal/capita to be food secure	1,700	Values with respect to the minimum and desirable daily per capita energy intake for Ethiopia vary between 1,700 and 2,100 kcal. The former was used as a threshold below which relief aid was distributed. The nationally recommended minimum is 2,100 kcal (Dejene 2000, p. 15).
Land degradation impact factor	0.03	Since no reliable empirical information is available with respect to the impact of population pressure on land resources, estimates of the respective parameters were made that would result in an expansion of the productivity of land resources of 1.9 percent by 2005. Again, this is a rather optimistic scenario, since the possibilities for land expansion under rain-fed agriculture are not very high and new land brought under cultivation may be offset or even outstripped by land degradation (Befekadu and Berhanu 2000, p. 146). The values of the parameters of the land module in the baseline scenario for PEDA Ethiopia are $\gamma = 0.03$, $\eta = 4$, and $a = 0.0175$.
Proportion of cohort moving to cities	0.06	In the census of 1994, 4 percent of the population reported that they had moved from rural to urban areas over their lifetime (CSA 1999, p. 196). In the case of PEDA Ethiopia, we have chosen a slightly higher figure for the baseline scenario. Given the lower fertility rates in urban areas, this scenario would, more or less, result in a status quo of the proportion who live in rural and urban areas.

HIV/AIDS

For several technical reasons, PEDA works with HIV/AIDS morbidity rates. As the symptomatic period (1–3 years) is much shorter than the incubation period (5–10 years), morbidity rates tend to be less than one-third of the adult (aged 15–49) prevalence rates. Given an estimate of a prevalence rate of 5.5 percent for the population aged 15–49 in 1995, we would have a morbidity rate of 1.1 if we consider the morbidity rate to be one-fifth of the prevalence rate. This value is used as an input to reflect the conditions in the initial year of the projections.

In the baseline scenario, this HIV/AIDS morbidity level is assumed to remain constant. As only relative increases in the HIV/AIDS morbidity levels from one year to another are used to calculate a reduction in the productivity of the labor force, the impact of HIV/AIDS in the baseline scenario is assumed to remain constant at the 1995 level as well. The purely demographic impact of HIV/AIDS through excess mortality is mainly manipulated by setting the life expectancy levels (see UNECA [forthcoming], for more details on the treatment of HIV/AIDS in PEDA). It must be stressed that these are unrealistically optimistic baseline scenario assumptions.

Other scenario variables that affect food production and supply

For the initial year, the net food imports were determined to be 4 percent of the domestically produced food, or 620,000 tons (see discussion above). Under the baseline scenario we assume that food imports increase by 2 percent per year, to reach a level of approximately 1,240,000 tons annually by the year 2030.

The agricultural production function in PEDA calculates the gross agricultural production. To determine the net food supply to the population, assumptions need to be made about post-harvest losses and net imports. The post-harvest losses, which include deduction of the produce used as seeds for the next season, are estimated at 15 percent of the production (Dejene 2000, p. 17). Although these losses may be even higher in years of good yields, because the on-farm storage capacity is limited and crop protection chemicals are not available (FAO/WFP 1996, p. 2), the baseline scenario assumes a slight reduction of post-harvest losses of 1 percent per year.

For the initial-year data, the user has to determine how favorable the water conditions were for agriculture in that year (i.e., the position on the water saturation curve). To do so, we relied on rainfall time series during the two main cropping seasons (*belg* and *meher*) for the period 1992–1999 (Tucker 2000) and on food production assessments in the same period. FAO/WFP (1996) reports that the 1996 harvest (1996–1997) is considered to be an exceptionally good year, with "a bumper crop." The value of the water scenario variable for the year 1996 is thus set to equal to 1 (i.e., the figure that describes optimal water conditions for agricultural production). Once the optimal value of rainfall for agriculture is determined, the water scenario values can be determined accordingly. For the baseline scenario, the observed rainfall pattern during the cropping seasons is used for the period 1995–1999. From the year 2000 onward, the observed rainfall pattern for 1992–1999 is repeated. Since that period was characterized by relatively favorable rainfall conditions, the baseline water scenario settings are, again, of an optimistic nature.

The share of irrigated agriculture in Ethiopia is very low. According to UNDP (1998), only 4.5 percent of the arable land (or 23,000 square kilometers) is irrigated. In the FAOSTAT database, no significant increase in irrigated land has been recorded since 1993. Under the baseline scenario, we nevertheless assume an annual increase in irrigated land of 1 percent.

Following efforts of the current government to expand the National Extension Program, fertilizer use in the mid-1990s increased rapidly at times, but its application fluctuates considerably. From one year to another, fertilizer use increased by 5 percent in 1996 (FAO/WFP 1996), decreased by 20 percent in 1997 (FAO/WFP 1997), increased by 27 percent in 1998 (FAO/WFP 1998), and increased by 2.6 percent in 1999 (FAO/WFP 2000). The important reduction in fertilizer use in 1997 was caused by the removal of subsidies and credit restrictions. It is thus difficult to forecast how future fertilizer use will evolve. In the baseline scenario, we assume a steady increase in fertilizer use of 5 percent per year. If only 7 kg of nutrients per hectare of arable land were used in 1995, the increase would thus be to almost 40 kg by 2030.

Few data are available on machinery use in Ethiopian agriculture. The small plot size, abundance of manual labor, and the relatively high cost of machinery mean its use is virtually nonexistent outside commercial or state farms. According to the FAOSTAT database, only 3,000 tractors were in use in the early 1990s, a figure that has not changed. In the baseline scenario, we assume that machinery use will increase by 0.5 percent per year.

In addition to the literacy of the labor force, the agricultural production function also takes the technical education of the workforce into account. This covers a variety of skills directly related to agricultural production techniques and may be improved through governmental extension services and the activities of nongovernmental organizations. It is, however, difficult to obtain empirical data on this issue. A project in the 1980s, known as the Peasant Agricultural Development Program, which included a training and visit approach, is not considered a success. A new system of agricultural extension, known as the Participatory Demonstration and Training Extension System, was launched by the current government in 1994–1995. The system includes a training component and the application of a package including fertilizer, improved seeds, and pesticides. The objective for the 1997–1998 season was to reach 2.9 million participants. Although the government has given the program high priority, it is not very clear whether the objectives have been reached. Problems faced in the implementation of the program are related to the increasing prices of these packages after removal of the subsidies in 1997, the limited financial capacity of farmers, decreasing farm sizes, and the required moisture level for the seeds and fertilizers to generate an improved production. Thus, fertilizers increase the risk of failure under high rainfall variability, which is the case in most parts of the country (Befekadu and Berhanu 2000, pp. 185–186).

The baseline scenario assumes that the level of technical education of the agricultural labor force increases at an annual rate of 1.5 percent. In the baseline scenario, we do not assume any urban or rural bias. Food is distributed in proportion to the quantity of people who live in rural and urban areas.

Other adjustments made to the default settings of PEDA for application to Ethiopia

Other adjustments made to the default settings of the PEDA model in its application to Ethiopia are the reduction in the elasticity of the size of the labor force in the agricultural production function and the manipulation of the water saturation curve.

Depending on the amount and timing of the rainfall, agricultural production in Ethiopia can easily go up or down by 20–30 percent. The default water saturation curve was not able to capture the responsiveness of the agricultural outputs to the fluctuations in the rainfall pattern. The water saturation curve was therefore changed to make the agricultural production much more a linear function of the quantity of rainfall. Note that a different shape to the water saturation curve may strongly influence the year-to-year fluctuations in agricultural outputs, but it does not influence the medium- to long-term pattern dynamics that much.

The agricultural production function used by default in PEDA attributes a relatively large elasticity of the growth of the rural labor force on agricultural outputs. Such an agricultural production function is suitable to describe a situation in which a growing population can move into previously unused land to increase production. However, the potential for cropland expansion is very limited in Ethiopia, and a growing workforce would not necessarily result in increased production. We therefore reduced the elasticity of labor in the agricultural production function from 0.534 to 0.2, and thereby give the general educational level of the population more weight than the size of the workforce itself.

References

Agarwal B (1994). The gender and environment debate: Lessons from India. In *Population and the Environment: Rethinking the Debate*, eds. Arizpe L, Stone MP & Major DC, pp. 97–124. Boulder, CO, USA: Westview Press.

Befekadu D & Berhanu N (2000). *Annual Report on the Ethiopian Economy, Vol. I, 1999–2000*. Addis Ababa, Ethiopia: The Ethiopian Economic Association.

Bollinger L, Stover J & Seyoum E (1999). The Economic Impact of AIDS in Ethiopia. Working Paper. Washington, DC, USA: The Futures Group International (www.tfgi.com/ecimaids.asp).

CSA (1999). *The 1994 Population and Housing Census of Ethiopia. Results at the Country Level, Volume II, Analytical Report*. Addis Ababa, Ethiopia: Federal Democratic Republic of Ethiopia, Office of Population and Housing Census Commission, Central Statistical Authority.

CSA & Macro International (2000). Ethiopia Demographic and Health Survey 2000. Preliminary Report. Addis Ababa, Ethiopia: Central Statistical Authority and Macro International.

Dasgupta PS (1993). *An Inquiry into Well-Being and Destitution*. Oxford, UK: Oxford University Press.

Dejene A (2000). *Report on Food Security, Environment and Population in the Context of a Policy Framework for Sustainable Development. Case Study of Ethiopia*. ECA/EA-SRDC/2000/6(ii)/NCS(1). Kigali, Ethiopia: UNECA, SRDC-EA.

FAO/WFP (1996). *Global Information and Early Warning System on Food and Agriculture*. Special Report. Rome, Italy: FAO/WFP Crop and Food Supply Assessment Mission to Ethiopia (www.fao.org/waicent/faoinfo/economic/giews/english/alertes/sptoc.htm).

FAO/WFP (1997). *Global Information and Early Warning System on Food and Agriculture*. Special Report. Rome, Italy: FAO/WFP Crop and Food Supply Assessment Mission to Ethiopia (www.fao.org/waicent/faoinfo/economic/giews/english/alertes/sptoc.htm).

FAO/WFP (1998). *Global Information and Early Warning System on Food and Agriculture*. Special Report. Rome, Italy: FAO/WFP Crop and Food Supply Assessment Mission to Ethiopia (www.fao.org/waicent/faoinfo/economic/giews/english/alertes/sptoc.htm).

FAO/WFP (2000). *Global Information and Early Warning System on Food and Agriculture*. Special Report. Rome, Italy: FAO/WFP Crop and Food Supply Assessment Mission to Ethiopia (www.fao.org/waicent/faoinfo/economic/giews/english/alertes/sptoc.htm).

FAO/WFP (2001). *Global Information and Early Warning System on Food and Agriculture*. Special Report. Rome, Italy: FAO/WFP Crop and Food Supply Assessment Mission to Ethiopia (www.fao.org/waicent/faoinfo/economic/giews/english/alertes/sptoc.htm).

Hayami Y & Ruttan V (1971). *Agricultural Development: An International Perspective*. Baltimore, MD, USA: Johns Hopkins University Press.

Keyfitz N (1979). Multidimensionality in population analysis. In *Sociological Methodology 1980*, ed. Schuessler KF, pp. 191–218. San Francisco, CA, USA: Jossey-Bass.

Lutz W & Scherbov S (2000). Quantifying vicious circle dynamics: The PEDA model for population, environment, development and agriculture in African countries. In *Optimization, Dynamics and Economic Analysis. Essays in Honor of Gustav Feichtinger*, eds. Dockner EJ, Hartl RF, Luptacik M & Sorge G, pp. 311–322. Heidelberg, Germany: Physica-Verlag.

Lutz W, Goujon A & Doblhammer-Reiter G (1999). Demographic dimensions in forecasting: Adding education to age and sex. In *Frontiers of Population Forecasting*, eds. Lutz W, Vaupel JW & Ahlburg DA, pp. 42–58. A Supplement to *Population and Development Review*, **24**, 1998. New York, NY, USA: Population Council.

Lutz W, Scherbov S, Prskawetz A, Dworak M & Feichtinger G (2002). Population, natural resources, and food security: Lessons from comparing full and reduced-form models. In *Population and Environment. Methods of Analysis*, eds. Lutz W, Prskawetz A & Sanderson WC, pp. 199–224. A Supplement to *Population and Development Review*, **28**, 2002. New York, NY, USA: The Population Council.

Ministry of Health (1998). *AIDS in Ethiopia. Background, Projections, Impacts, Interventions*. Addis Ababa, Ethiopia: Ministry of Health, Epidemiology and AIDS Department.

Nerlove M (1991). Population and the environment: A parable of firewood and other tales. *American Journal of Agricultural Economics* **73**:1334–1347.

O'Neill BC, MacKellar FL & Lutz W (2001). *Population and Climate Change*. Cambridge, UK: Cambridge University Press.

Rogers A (1975). *Introduction to Multiregional Mathematical Demography*. New York, NY, USA: John Wiley.

Rogers A & Castro L (1981). *Model Migration Schedules*. Research Report RR-81-30. Laxenburg, Austria: International Institute for Applied Systems Analysis.

Scherbov S & Grechucha V (1988). "DIAL"—A System for Modeling Multidimensional Demographic Processes. Working Paper WP-88-36. Laxenburg, Austria: International Institute for Applied Systems Analysis.

Sen A (1981). *Poverty and Famines: An Essay on Entitlement and Deprivation*. Oxford, UK: Clarendon Press.

Sen G (1994). Women, poverty, and population: Issues for the concerned environmentalist. In *Population and the Environment: Rethinking the Debate*, eds. Arizpe L, Stone MP & Major DC, pp. 67–86. Boulder, CO, USA: Westview Press.

Stover J & Bollinger L (1999). The Economic Impact of AIDS (in Africa). Working Paper. Washington, DC, USA: The Futures Group International (www.tfgi.com/ecimaids.asp).

TGE-OPM (1993). *National Population Policy of Ethiopia*. Addis Ababa, Ethiopia: Transitional Government of Ethiopia, Office of the Prime Minister.

Tucker MR (2000). *Food Security and Food Aid Contract: Strengthen the Capability of the National Meteorological Services Agency in Ethiopia to Provide Meteorological*

Services to Agriculture and Food Production. Final Report. Addis Ababa, Ethiopia: European Commission.

UNAIDS (1998). *Ethiopia. Epidemiological Fact Sheet on HIV/AIDS and Sexually Transmitted Diseases*. Geneva, Switzerland: UNAIDS/WHO.

UNAIDS (2000). *Ethiopia. Epidemiological Fact Sheet on HIV/AIDS and Sexually Transmitted Infections, 2000 Update*. Geneva, Switzerland: UNAIDS/WHO.

UNDP (1998). *Human Development Report. Ethiopia 1998*. Addis Ababa, Ethiopia: United Nations Development Programme.

UNECA (1999). *Economic Report on Africa*. Addis Ababa, Ethiopia: United Nations Economic Commission for Africa.

UNECA (2002). *Economic Report on Africa. Tracking Performance and Progress*. Addis Ababa, Ethiopia: United Nations Economic Commission for Africa.

UNECA (forthcoming). *The Population–Environment–Development–Agriculture Model. Technical Manual*. Addis Ababa: United Nations Economic Commission for Africa.

World Bank (1997). *African Development Indicators*. Washington DC, USA: The World Bank.

Web sites

ANDI: Africa Nutrition Database Initiative Web site (World Bank, FAO, UNICEF, and WHO): www.africa-nutrition.net/

FAOSTAT: FAO Statistical Databases Web site: apps.fao.org/

UNESCO: UNESCO Institute for Statistics Web site: unescostat.unesco. org/

WFP: World Food Programme Web site: www.wfp.org/

Chapter 7

Interactions between Education and HIV: Demographic Examples from Botswana

Warren C. Sanderson

7.1 Introduction

Understanding the past course of the HIV/AIDS pandemic in sub-Saharan Africa and how it is likely to evolve from here would be a difficult task even with good data, but the data that we must use as the foundation of any analysis are sparse and often of poor quality. Nevertheless, it is important to try to learn from the past and to forecast the future, because some decisions that need to be made today depend on what we expect the future to be. For example, in water-scarce regions, decisions on whether or not to start building expensive water infrastructure depend, in part, on the likely future population size. Similarly, if we wanted to try to understand the effects of the epidemic on economic growth, we would need to assess, among other things, the likely number of deaths of more-educated and less-educated workers.

Even good information on the past, though, would not be sufficient to provide us with a reasonable indication of what is likely to happen in the future. Even without any policy innovations or changes in behavior, the evolution of the epidemic is still impossible to understand without an appropriate mathematical model. The normal dynamics of the epidemic are just too complex. Two developments, however, make forecasting even more difficult. First, government policies in sub-Saharan Africa are changing. New programs that provide antiretroviral medications and education about risky sexual behavior are becoming ever more common. Second, in many sub-Saharan African countries, the educational composition of the population has been changing and is expected to continue to change in the future, and educational attainment interacts with these new government programs.

This chapter describes the scarce empirical information about the relationship between the level of education and HIV prevalence, and applies a model that allows the study of different possible interactions between the two. The educational structure of the population so far has received insufficient attention as a key factor in the spread of the epidemic, and almost no data have been collected. The model-based analysis presented here may help to strengthen the rationale for giving more attention to education and for collecting more empirical information on this key driver of the dynamics of the epidemic.

Recent tidbits of evidence suggest that when HIV/AIDS first became seeded in sub-Saharan African heterosexual communities, prevalence rates were higher among the more-educated population. In addition, it appears that, as the danger of HIV/AIDS became clearer, the more educated may have begun to change their behavior more rapidly, attenuating or eliminating the positive education–prevalence relationship. For a number of reasons, it is also likely that education will be associated with the extent and success of medication use. Medication programs are more likely to be set in urban areas, where a greater proportion of the more-educated people live. Proportionally, more doctors work in urban areas, which makes it easier for people who live there to obtain checkups and have their medications altered as they become less effective. The more educated are also more likely to be active in gathering information on testing and counseling programs. Education, therefore, plays a pivotal role in understanding how behavioral change and medication use are likely to vary over time.

In a world with data commensurate with the seriousness of the epidemic, it would be much easier to incorporate education in terms of its effects on the riskiness of sexual behavior and on the extent of medication use. We do not live in such a world. Our knowledge base on this subject is miniscule. Instead of proceeding by analyzing data, we can only make progress indirectly. We have to create models of how education could influence the spread of HIV and then look at what those models predict for things about which we do have information. If the model forecasts and observations match, then we have a framework that could be consistent with the dynamics of the epidemic and therefore one that could be useful for understanding and forecasting.

In a world with spotty information, it is very easy to make mistaken inferences from the tidbits of data we do have. For example, a deceleration in the spread of the epidemic can be interpreted mistakenly as a sign that a government program is working, when really it is not. Decelerations are often seen in models of HIV/AIDS, even in the absence of effective government policies. We can only assess which programs work and which do not on the basis of a model that produces predictions about what would happen in specific cases. For example, it seems plausible that more-educated people would change their behavior more strongly when informed about the dangers of HIV/AIDS, but the empirical proof of this matter is not so straightforward. If HIV prevalence were initially higher among the more educated, even with invariant behavior we could observe a convergence in the prevalence rates by education over time. Higher death rates in the subgroup of the more educated with the riskiest sexual behavior would leave behind only those with relatively low-risk behavior, which could cause prevalence among the more educated to fall. It is also possible that increases in prevalence in the normal progression of the HIV epidemic could mask decreases caused by behavioral change.

In this chapter, we incorporate the interrelationships between educational attainment, behavioral change, and medication use into a model of the evolution of the HIV epidemic in Botswana. Botswana is especially interesting in this context for a number of reasons. First, Botswana has the highest rate of HIV prevalence in the world. In 2001, over 50 percent of women 20–29 years of age were already HIV-positive. Second, Botswana is a stable democracy that has had governments famous for formulating and implementing successful social and economic policies. Now that around one-third of the population of voting age is HIV-positive,[1] the government of Botswana has introduced Africa's first national antiretroviral medication program that aims to provide medication to all its citizens who need it. In addition, it has begun a nationwide program of education about HIV that focuses on informing people about the importance of reducing the riskiness of their sexual behavior. This means that the interrelationships between government policies and education that we discuss in this chapter are potentially realistic ones. If appropriate data become available, we will be able to test the results presented here against observations.

The third reason that Botswana is especially interesting is that it is experiencing an educational revolution. The government of Botswana has made increasing investments in human capital. Ironically, these were just beginning to bear fruit at the same time that the HIV epidemic started to spread rapidly. The large past and expected future changes in the educational composition of the population should make it easier to observe the changes that education causes. The fourth reason is that the model has already been calibrated and tested on Botswana data. It starts

---

[1]The one-third figure is a result of our model and is based on HIV prevalence rates that have been corrected for known biases, including those introduced by educational differences in fertility. For more details about these biases, see Appendix 7.2.

in 1993 and is constructed to match age-specific national prevalence data for 1993 and 1997. It predicts the population of Botswana in 2001 quite accurately. The model was used previously to forecast a number of aspects of Botswana's future, and including these in our discussion below provides additional depth.

There are two main disadvantages of using Botswana here. First, because of its economic success and the stability of its democratic political system, Botswana is an atypical African country. It could be dangerous to apply lessons derived from Botswana uncritically to other countries in which the economic and political circumstances differ. Second, as in almost all sub-Saharan African countries, there are no historical data on the relationship between HIV prevalence and education in Botswana. The model produces statements of the "if-then" type. They show what would happen in certain hypothesized situations. If the past relationship between education and HIV prevalence is stipulated and if future programs cause particular education-specific changes in the riskiness of behavior and in medication use, then we can generate a detailed forecast of population size, age structure, educational structure, and many other important demographic features of the country.

This use of scenarios in simulations of the future has a long history and is well established in the literature. One of its strengths is that it allows us to explore the quantitative nature of a number of uncertainties. Some uncertainties involve the nature of anti-HIV programs and how they will affect different education groups. By performing simulations on Botswana, we can begin to see how different resolutions of these uncertainties would affect outcomes of interest. A second strength arises in the comparisons of scenarios. This allows us to pose and answer questions about how much difference alternative policies make. A third is that we can distinguish between data patterns that are plausible and those that are not. If we find implausible changes in data, we know immediately to be cautious about our interpretations. Unlikely patterns in our observations may indicate that the data are biased and need to be corrected before we can make use of them.

There is, of course, a significant limitation to this approach. It allows us to understand certain aspects of the HIV epidemic in quantitative terms, including the effects of various sorts of policy regimes. Still, we cannot, by any stretch of the imagination, forecast exactly what Botswana's future will be. The uncertainties involved are much too great.

We begin our inquiry, in the second section, with a very brief look at the evidence on education and HIV prevalence elsewhere in sub-Saharan Africa. An overview of the methodology of the model is presented in the third section. The fourth section contains our new results with respect to education and HIV in Botswana. Specifically, we use the model to compute forecasts of Botswana's total population, the proportion of the working-age population with secondary schooling or more, and the prevalence rates of young women under various scenarios that involve education-specific behavioral changes and medication utilization rates. The model used here was developed as part of a larger project that studied population–development–environment interactions in Botswana, Namibia, and Mozambique.[2] In the fifth section, we review some of our conclusions from previous work and show how they pertain to our understanding of the connections between education and HIV in Botswana. In particular, we discuss Botswana's economic growth, the affordability of medication programs, the limited effectiveness of medication programs in increasing life expectancy, and the effects of the expected urbanization and economic growth on the need for further investments in water infrastructure. Concluding remarks are given in the final section. A more detailed presentation of important elements of the model's structure can be found in Appendix 7.1. A discussion of how the data used were corrected for biases and how education-specific figures were computed appears in Appendix 7.2.

Before leaving this introduction, it is important to emphasize once more that little is known about education and HIV prevalence in Africa. There are fragmentary data and educated impressions. At best, this study can provide some idea of the relative magnitudes and possible patterns of evolution in important HIV-related quantities. In an era when AIDS deaths number in the millions and when much concern is expressed about HIV/AIDS, it is barely short of a crime against humanity that so little is known about the people in Africa who suffer from the disease. Hopefully, the analysis presented here can be used to demonstrate the need for more data on AIDS and education.

7.2 Some Tidbits of Evidence

Three types of data are considered here:

- Observations on HIV prevalence.
- Self-reported survey data on changes in behavior.
- Educated impressions.

Table 7.1 shows the evidence reported in Fylkesnes *et al.* (2001). It presents HIV prevalence in Zambia by years in school, age, and place of prenatal care checkup for 1994 and 1998. The data were obtained anonymously from women who sought prenatal care. The biases inherent in these data are discussed below. The data are clear. In 1994, holding age and location of the prenatal care fixed, women

---

[2]The project was the fourth in a series of studies of the interactions between population, development, and the environment. Details about the project, including its methodology and findings, can be accessed at www.iiasa.ac.at/Research/POP/pde/index.html?sb=16. Information about the other three studies can be found in Lutz *et al.* (2002).

Table 7.1. Trends in HIV prevalence among women who attended a prenatal clinic in Zambia, 1994 and 1998, by age, years in school, and location of clinic (in percent).

Site/Age group	Year	Years in school				
		0–4	5–6	7	8–9	10+
Lusaka						
15–19	1994	19.6 (46)	25.3 (79)	21.1 (133)	24.8 (129)	
	1998	9.1 (77)	18.5 (81)	16.9 (177)	13.5 (215)	
20–24	1994	23.4 (64)	29.9 (97)	29.3 (191)	32.2 (92)	40.2 (92)
	1998	30.9 (94)	29.5 (112)	28.4 (222)	27.2 (180)	27.5 (171)
25–29	1994	6.9 (29)	31.7 (41)	33.7 (95)	29.6 (71)	51.2 (86)
	1998	24.7 (81)	32.1 (53)	46.3 (149)	40.0 (105)	29.8 (131)
Other urban[a]						
15–19	1994	12.5 (40)	19.0 (79)	20.4 (147)	21.8(197)	
	1998	19.2 (63)	13.4 (112)	15.9 (232)	16.8 (351)	
20–24	1994	21.6 (74)	18.4 (87)	27.7 (238)	41.5 (217)	40.3 (139)
	1998	29.0 (107)	28.8 (163)	28.8 (347)	31.7 (334)	30.3 (218)
25–29	1994	27.5 (40)	27.5 (51)	27.4 (135)	40.0 (115)	52.4 (105)
	1998	26.4 (91)	29.5 (88)	33.7 (196)	40.6 (192)	41.6 (113)
Rural[b]						
15–19	1994	6.7 (255)	6.9 (144)	9.8 (123)	12.0 (83)	
	1998	4.7 (274)	5.8 (171)	7.2 (152)	5.4 (111)	
20–24	1994	10.7 (290)	8.9 (192)	14.2 (176)	19.2 (125)	40.0 (20)
	1998	9.0 (301)	9.0 (210)	13.2 (227)	17.0 (141)	21.7 (46)
25–29	1994	9.1 (187)	12.6 (103)	18.3 (120)	29.3 (41)	35.5 (31)
	1998	12.4 (194)	10.5 (133)	15.7 (140)	19.2 (78)	12.9 (29)

[a]Ndola, Livingstone, Solwezi, Kabwe, and Mansa.
[b]Kashikishi, Minga, Isoka, Kasaba, Ibenga, and Mukinge (Macha excluded because no information on education was collected in 1994).
Note: Figures in parentheses are numbers of observations.
Source: Fylkesnes *et al.* (2001, Table 2, p. 911).

with higher education had higher HIV prevalence. In 1998, that pattern vanishes in some instances and is much weaker in others. One example is enough to illustrate this. Data from prenatal care sites in the urban areas outside of Lusaka show that in 1994, 21.6 percent of women with 0–4 years of schooling were HIV-positive, while 40.3 percent of those with 10 or more years of education were infected. In other words, the prevalence rate was almost twice as high among those in the highest education group compared with those with the least education. By 1998 that pattern had changed. The prevalence rate increased for those with 0–4 years of education (going from 21.6 percent to 29.0 percent) and decreased for those with 10 or more

Table 7.2. Prevalence rates in Fort Portal, Uganda, cross-classified by age, education, and time period.

Age group	Education	1991–1994	1995–1997
15–24	Illiterate	23.8 (19.3–28.4)	19.8 (15.6–24.0)
	Primary education	24.5 (20.9–28.0)	18.5 (15.0–21.9)
	Secondary education	27.2 (20.2–34.1)	14.8 (8.9–20.7)
25–49	Illiterate	14.7 (10.9–18.5)	19.2 (14.1–24.2)
	Primary education	18.9 (14.5–23.4)	16.7 (11.8–21.6)
	Secondary education	35.1 (22.3–47.9)	27.6 (15.7–39.4)

Note: 95 percent confidence intervals are given in parentheses.
Source: Kilian *et al.* (1999).

years of education (going from 40.3 percent to 30.3 percent). In 1998, prevalence rates were almost independent of education.

It is unwise to make too much of any single comparison in *Table 7.1*. For example, the prevalence rate in 1994 among 20–24 year olds who sought care in Lusaka and had 10 or more years of education was 40.2 percent. In 1998, the rate for 25–29 year olds with the same level of education was 29.8 percent. It is highly unlikely that HIV deaths alone could have caused such a large decrease. We discuss anomalies in *Table 7.1* in more detail below. Nevertheless, at least in Zambia, it appears that HIV initially spread more quickly among more-educated women, and that subsequent variations in the speed of behavioral change rapidly reduced the prevalence differentials.

Our second and third fragments of information come from Uganda. In the early 1990s the government there instituted an effective program aimed at behavioral change, the results of which are evident in *Table 7.2*. Prevalence fell over time in all cases except for illiterate women aged 25–49. *Table 7.2* has the same striking features as *Table 7.1*, with higher initial prevalence among the more educated followed by a much more rapid decrease.

Survey data also show that the more-educated people have changed their sexual behavior to a greater extent than the less educated. *Table 7.3* presents the responses people gave in the 1995 Uganda Demographic and Health Survey (DHS) to a question that asked how they changed their behavior to avoid contracting HIV. Among females with no education, 42.6 percent said that they made no behavioral changes. Only 24.2 percent of women with a secondary education or more said that they made no changes in their behavior.

Finally, a recent working paper from the International Labour Organization (ILO) Program on HIV/AIDS and the World of Work provides an educated impression:

Table 7.3. Percentage of people who have heard of HIV/AIDS and have had intercourse, by specific changes in behavior to avoid HIV/AIDS, Demographic and Health Survey, Uganda, 1995.

Gender/ Education	No change	Stopped sex	Began using condom	Restricted to one partner	Fewer partners	Avoid sex with prostitutes	Number of obs.
Females							
No education	42.6	6.1	0.1	48.6	2.9		2,016
Primary	33.9	6.9	2.1	54.1	3.9		3,537
Secondary or above	24.2	10.6	7.6	57.7	4.5		766
Males							
No education	18.0	14.6	3.4	51.7	18.4	13.6	206
Primary	11.4	8.6	7.2	57.0	28.2	12.9	1,104
Secondary or above	6.6	12.0	23.2	50.9	35.0	12.8	428

Proximate Source: de Walque (2002, Table 8).

> While evidence on the social class gradient of infection is very partial and mostly absent for most countries in sub-Saharan Africa, there [are] some data that support the argument that HIV infection in the past decade or so did positively correlate with income, educational level and occupational status. (Cohen 2002, p. 5)

The citations in Cohen (2002) are different from those above, and so the paper can be read as being consistent with the empirical data that have been presented.

All told, the evidence about the relationship between education and HIV prevalence in sub-Saharan Africa is fragmentary, but suggestive enough to be worth pursuing. We cannot add anything to the evidentiary base here, but we can examine the kinds of patterns we would expect to see in data under various assumptions about the relationship between education and HIV/AIDS prevalence in the hope that some of these can improve our understanding of what has happened and what is likely to occur in the future. To do this, we must first have an analytic model of the spread of HIV that incorporates education. It is to this task that we now turn.

7.3 Overview of the Methodology

To assess the role of education in the evolution of the HIV/AIDS pandemic requires a model. We introduce one here that is designed specifically for this purpose. Models differ according to the questions they are designed to address and the modeling philosophies they use. This model focuses on the analysis of populations with high HIV prevalence rates. It includes education and considers its effects on changes in HIV-relevant behavior and on medication programs. Our modeling philosophy is to stay as close as possible to the available data and to the accepted demographic methodology.

At the core of the model is a standard population forecasting framework that requires the population to be disaggregated by age and sex. To this we add disaggregation by education and by a set of variables required to deal with HIV/AIDS. Below, we discuss the population states and look at the flows from one state to another. In Appendix 7.1, we look in detail at the most crucial part of the model, the relationship between prevalence rates and incidence rates. The incidence rate is the fraction of the HIV-negative people with risky sexual practices who are newly infected in a given year. The prevalence rate is the fraction of the population who are HIV-positive at any moment in time. The higher the HIV prevalence rate, the more people there are who spread the infection. The more people who spread the infection, the more people there are who will become infected. The more people who are infected, the more people they can infect and so on. In Appendix 7.1, we discuss how that relationship is modified because of the use of antiretroviral medication and because of behavior change. In the final section of Appendix 7.1, we discuss the other transition rates between states in the model. Unfortunately, observed data on HIV prevalences are biased. In Appendix 7.2, we discuss those biases in detail and show how they can be corrected. The relationship between education and HIV prevalence is a crucial part of the correction procedure.

7.3.1   Population states

The model is based on a population disaggregated by

- 100 single years of age;
- two genders;
- three types of education (primary or less, secondary, and more than secondary);
- two types of sexual behavior (risky and not risky);
- four HIV statuses (HIV-negative, HIV-positive asymptomatic and unmedicated, HIV-positive asymptomatic and medicated, and AIDS [symptomatic]);
- 15 single years since infection (for those HIV-positive asymptomatic and unmedicated); and
- two sexual activity states (initiated sexual activity or not).

An earlier version of the model, as well as a detailed description of its use in studying population, development, and environment interactions in Botswana, Mozambique, and Namibia is given in IIASA (2001). The model can be downloaded and run from there. The model has also been used in Hellmuth and Sanderson (2001) and Sanderson (2001a, 2001b, 2002a, 2002b).

In working with populations with high HIV prevalance, it is important to make forecasts in steps of one year using a population disaggregated by a single year of age. In the HIV epidemics in sub-Saharan Africa, the situation has changed with amazing rapidity. Educational distributions can also change rapidly. Interventions can occur at different times. A behavioral change program can begin in one year, and a medication program, in another.

There are four HIV statuses in the model. We need all four in order to study the effects of medication programs. Among those who are asymptomatic and unmedicated, we keep track of the duration of their infection to determine the probabilities that they will become symptomatic in each year. For simplicity and because of a lack of information, we do not keep track of the duration of medication use among those who are asymptomatic and medicated. We implicitly make a distinction between the initial rate of discontinuation and subsequent rates when we specify the nature of the medication programs.

In the Botswana example, the initial distribution of women into those who are HIV-negative and those who are HIV-positive is made using adjusted Sentinel Surveillance prevalence rates.[3] There are no usable data for men, so their distribution is based on the data for women adjusted for the facts that in widespread HIV epidemics, prevalence rates are typically lower for men than for women and that teenage girls have considerably higher rates than teenage boys.

For a number of reasons, some people are not at risk for contracting HIV. We have chosen a base rate of 10 percent for all groups of the population. The model allows different choices for different education groups and allows that value to change over time at different rates, depending on education. Finally, we divide young people into those who have and those who have not initiated sexual activity by a given age. There are two reasons for doing this. First, the age at the first sexual contact can differ by education. Second, observed prevalence rates for young people significantly overstate their true rates. The same risky behavior produces both pregnancies and HIV infections. The Sentinel Surveillance data on HIV prevalence are based on observations of pregnant women. Young women who initiate sexual activity early are at greater risk of both pregnancy and HIV than young women in general. The use of Sentinel Surveillance data for young women, without adjustment, could result in incorrect inferences and policy recommendations.

7.3.2 Population flows

The pattern of flows through the states of the model is shown in *Figure 7.1*. For clarity, the effects of normal mortality and educational differentials are omitted from *Figure 7.1* and this discussion, but are, of course, part of the model. The

---

[3] The nature of these data and their biases are discussed in the appendices.

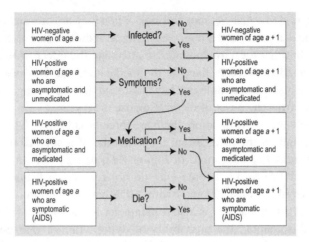

Figure 7.1. The pattern of flows through the states of the model.

boxes on the left- and right-hand sides of the diagram represent the number of women in each state at the beginning of age a and $a + 1$, respectively. The center part of the diagram shows most of the transitions possible in the model.

A woman at her ath birthday who is HIV-negative and susceptible may on her next $(a + 1)$ birthday be either HIV-negative or HIV-positive. The proportion of the initially HIV-negative women who become HIV-positive between the two birthdays is the age-specific incidence (or new infection) rate. The determination of HIV incidence rates is the heart of the model and is discussed in more detail in the next subsection. When a woman becomes HIV-positive, she enters the state of being HIV-positive, asymptomatic, and unmedicated. Once in this state, we keep track of the number of years since infection. This is important because HIV has a long latency period. People typically remain infected for around a decade with no symptoms. The probability of making a transition out of the asymptomatic and unmedicated state into another state depends on the woman's duration in the unmedicated state.

A woman who makes a transition out of the asymptomatic and unmedicated state can go either into the symptomatic (i.e., AIDS) state or into the medicated state. The model assumes that women start to take medication at the first sign of symptoms. This is very close to what is happening in Botswana today, and there are a number of reasons to expect that future programs in other countries will be organized along the same basic lines. First, in an environment of scarce resources, we would expect that the people most in need would have the highest claim on the medications and the attention of physicians. Second, the medications have serious side effects. Many people may not be able to discipline themselves to follow a regime that makes them feel sick, when they are otherwise feeling fine. HIV/AIDS medication is not a cure. Experience indicates that it can extend life considerably, but that the virus mutates to attenuate the effect of the medication. The average number of years lived in the medicated state is a parameter of the model. In the Botswana example, we have assumed that the average symptom-free life expectancy from the onset of medication use is 10 years.

Once people are on medication, there are three possibilities. They may remain symptom free and on the medication, they may die of a non-AIDS related cause (such normal mortality is ignored in *Figure 7.1*), or they may come down with AIDS, as may HIV-positive people who do not receive medication. The AIDS state is considered terminal. Women with AIDS have a high probability of dying each year, and this probability is also a parameter in the model. In the Botswana examples in this chapter, the probability of dying within a year once a woman becomes symptomatic is one-half, which implies a life expectancy with symptoms of two years.

Details about the transition rates shown in *Figure 7.1* are presented in Appendix 7.1. Information about how incidence rates by education were estimated for the mid-1990s appears in Appendix 7.2. All the projections in the following section start from those estimated rates.

7.4   Examples from Botswana

There are no usable data on the relationship between HIV prevalence and education in Botswana, so what we can show here are not forecasts, but the investigation of the consequences of various scenarios. Our goal is to learn about the sensitivity of the evolution of the epidemic to changes in behavior associated with education. Observed patterns can then, possibly, provide hints as to the association between behavioral changes and education.

7.4.1   The scenarios

For the purpose of this exploratory analysis, we ran the model with six scenarios. The model distinguishes three education groups:

- those with a primary education or less;
- those with at least some secondary education; and
- those with at least some post-secondary education.

In the base scenario, it is assumed that women with a post-secondary education have age-specific prevalence rates during the 1993–1997 period that are 67 percent higher than women with a primary education or less. Women with a secondary education are assumed to have prevalence rates that are 33 percent higher than those with a primary education or less.[4] The resultant prevalence rates by age are used to estimate the incidence rates in the 1993–1997 period. The riskiness of sexual behavior is always viewed in terms of the relationship between prevalence rates and incidence rates. Behavior is riskier if, holding prevalence constant, the incidence rate is higher.

In the base scenario, the age-specific relationships between the estimated prevalence rates and incidence rates are held fixed for the remainder of the projection at their levels estimated for the 1993–1997 period.[5] The base scenario, then, reflects part of the story of the relationship between education and behavior. It assumes more-educated women have higher HIV prevalence early in the epidemic and that their behavior does not change over time. Their relatively risky behavior is permanent.

The fragmentary empirical data that we present above suggest that the more-educated women change their behavior more rapidly when they learn about how HIV is transmitted. The next three scenarios explore this. In the scenario entitled "convergence," the levels of riskiness of the sexual behavior[6] of the two higher education groups stay at their initial values from 1993 through 2001 and then converge over the next five years to the level of riskiness of the lowest education group. After 2006, the extent of the riskiness for all three education groups remains fixed at the initial (low) level estimated for the lowest education group. In other words, if prevalence rates in the three education groups were the same after 2006, their incidence rates would be the same as well. In this scenario, behavioral change is fastest for the group with the highest education, slower for the group with a secondary education, and nonexistent for the lowest education group. All the scenarios, except the base case, assume that government policies are phased in over time. This is consistent with what is happening in Botswana now and what is likely to happen elsewhere in Africa in the future.

It is interesting to think about the possibility that more-educated women will ultimately engage in sexual behavior that is even less risky than the behavior exhibited by less-educated women. We explore this in the scenario entitled "crossover." The assumptions in this scenario are the same as those in the "convergence" scenario, with an additional period of change between 2006 and 2011. Between 2006 and 2011, the riskiness of sexual behavior decreases, so that after 2011, for the same

---

[4]Given the notation in Appendix 7.1, $p(2, 1995) = 1.33$ and $p(3, 1995) = 1.67$. The values of κ derived from these assumptions are assumed to remain constant in the base scenario.

[5]More information about the prevalence–incidence relationship can be found in Appendix 7.1.

[6]In terms of the notation in Appendix 7.1, the riskiness of sexual behavior is reflected in the set of age- and education-specific values of κ. When the κs remain constant, the riskiness of sexual behavior remains constant, even though incidence rates will change as the prevalence rates change.

prevalence rate, women with more than a secondary education have only 50 percent of the incidence rate of women with the lowest education. Women with a secondary education have only 66 percent of the incidence rate of less-educated women with the same prevalence rate.

We call the last of the three comparative scenarios "differential." Between 2001 and 2006, a period of rapid behavioral change occurs. Women with the most education change their behavior the most. Their incidence rates fall by 60 percent from what they were in 2001 (again holding prevalence constant). Women with an intermediate level of education have rates that fall by an intermediate amount, 40 percent from their 2001 levels. Women with the least education have only a 20 percent decrease. After 2006, behavior is assumed to stabilize in all three education groups.

Education not only plays a role in behavioral change, but it also influences the use and effectiveness of medication. Space restrictions limit us to only two medication scenarios here. In the first, "medication1," we combine the "convergence" scenario with the assumption that initiation of antiretroviral medication use increases linearly, from 0 percent in 2001 to 40 percent in 2006, among those who first begin to experience AIDS symptoms. After 2006, the proportion remains fixed at 40 percent. In the "medication2" scenario, also based on the "convergence" scenario, we assume that the utilization of medication differs by level of education. Women with the least education have usage rates of 20 percent in 2006. Women with a secondary education have utilization rates that increase to 40 percent. Among women with more than a secondary education, the rates increase to 60 percent by 2006. After 2006, all utilization rates remain constant.

Education is also likely to be associated with dosage compliance and therefore associated with the effectiveness of medication use. We do not consider this here, although it potentially could be quite important.

7.4.2   The results

Figure 7.2 shows the total population of Botswana under four scenarios: base, "convergence," "crossover," and "differential." The population of Botswana in 2001 was around 1.67 million. In all the scenarios, the population of the country remains roughly constant for around the next 15 years and then begins to decline. In the base scenario, Botswana's population in 2051 is 1.04 million.[7] In the "convergence" scenario, the behavior of the more-educated women begins to change rapidly after 2001 and ultimately becomes as risky as that of women with a primary education

---

[7]The year 2051 was chosen as the end point in the graphs to allow us to view the situation in Botswana in the long run. The graphs represent working through particular assumptions and are not forecasts. Hopefully, well before 2051 there will be a vaccine against HIV and a cure for those who are already infected.

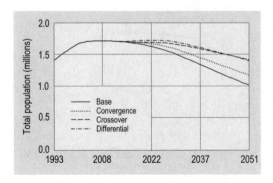

Figure 7.2. The total population of Botswana under four scenarios, 1993–2051.

or less. In that scenario, Botswana's population in 2051 would be just 1.19 million. Simply reducing the riskiness of the behavior of the two more-educated groups to that of the least-educated group clearly does not keep the population from declining substantially.

The "crossover" and "differential" scenarios assume more behavioral change. In the "crossover" scenario after 2011, incidence rates for the most-educated group are half those in the least-educated group (holding prevalence constant). For women with a secondary education, they are two-thirds as large. Here, the behavior of the more-educated women in the early 1990s was much riskier than that of the less-educated women, but by 2011 it has crossed over and become much less risky. The result is that in the "crossover" scenario the population declines to 1.43 million people in 2051. The "differential" scenario envisages substantial behavioral changes in all three education groups in the period from 2001 to 2006. The riskiness of behavior falls by 20 percent for the least educated, by 40 percent for the intermediate group, and by 60 percent for those with the most education. The upshot for the "differential" scenario is that Botswana's population in 2051 is 1.41 million people.

The population of Botswana projected under the two medication scenarios is shown in *Figure 7.3*. Both of these build upon the "convergence" scenario. Using "medication1," in which 40 percent of those who need it receive medication, the population of Botswana is 1.41 million in 2051. The implication of the "medication2" scenario, in which the utilization of medication increases with education, but the average usage rate is about the same as in "medication1," is that Botswana's 2051 population will be 1.37 million.

Two conclusions are clear. First, more behavior change and/or medication use than we have assumed in our scenarios is needed to keep Botswana's population from shrinking in the long run. Second, combining medication programs with the "convergence" scenario results in about the same population in 2051 as going

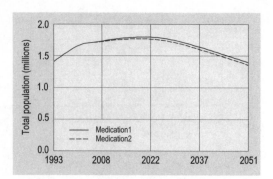

Figure 7.3. Botswana's population under the two medication scenarios.

beyond the "convergence" scenario with the additional behavioral change assumed in the "crossover" or "differential" scenarios.

HIV/AIDS affects not only the total population, but its educational composition as well. We take a step toward understanding the educational composition effect and its possible impact on the economy by considering the proportion of the working-age population with at least a secondary education.[8] We exclude people who are symptomatic and therefore in the terminal phase of their illness. These people are often too sick to work. *Figure 7.4* shows the proportion of the working-age population with at least a secondary education. Past policies have produced a significant and ongoing increase in this proportion. Regardless of which scenario we consider, the proportion increases dramatically in the next 50 years, even in the face of the HIV epidemic. Our projection shows that the proportion of the (asymptomatic) working-age population with a secondary education or more is around 34 percent in 2001.[9] It reaches 50 percent about 20 years later.

The "convergence" and "medication1" scenarios assume that the riskiness of behavior is the same for all education groups after 2005. The proportion of the the working-age population is virtually the same in both scenarios in 2051, around 71 percent. In the "crossover" and "medication2" scenarios, behavior is quite different across the education groups, but nevertheless the proportions of the working-age population with a secondary education or more in 2051 do not differ much, reaching 76 percent for the "crossover" scenario and 72 percent for the "medication2" scenario.

---

[8] We define the working-age population here as people between the ages of 20 and 64. Small changes in the age boundaries have no effect on qualitative conclusions.

[9] This figure is based on our projection that is based on data from the 1991 census. The model has not been calibrated to match detailed information from the 2001 census, because that information was not available at the time this chapter was written.

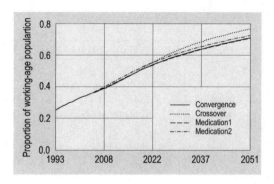

Figure 7.4. Projections of the proportion of asymptomatic (non-AIDS) working-age population (20–64 years old) who have a secondary education or more, Botswana 1993–2051, using four scenarios.

The differences in behavior by education have such a small effect on the projected proportions of the population with at least a secondary education because secondary education is already so widespread in Botswana. In countries where secondary education is less common, such behavioral differences will matter more. In Botswana, at least, the argument that a large medication program is needed to maintain the country's stock of human capital needs to be qualified. Population declines in all the scenarios considered here, but the proportion of more-educated people among those of working age is greatest in the "crossover" scenario, in which antiretroviral medications are not used.

Table 7.4 shows how HIV prevalence evolves from 1996 to 2031 in the six scenarios for women in the three education categories. This table contains information similar to the observations presented in *Tables 7.1* and *7.2*. Although *Table 7.4* is large, three important features stand out. First, holding the level of education constant, high prevalence among 20–24 year olds does not lead to low prevalence among 25–29 year olds five years later, although in *Table 7.1* we present data from Zambia that do show this. The prevalence rate among 20–24 year olds with 10 or more years of education in Lusaka in 1994 was 40.2 percent (based on 92 observations), while four years later the rate for 25–29 year olds was 29.8 percent (based on 131 observations). Although the four-year interval is not exactly what we need, such a decline does not seem to be consistent with the information in *Table 7.4*. The same phenomenon appears for women who sought care in rural areas, though this is based on far fewer observations.

The inconsistency of the model and the observations calls for further investigation. There are four possibilities:

Table 7.4. Hypothetical HIV prevalence rates, Botswana, 1996–2031, under six scenarios.

Scenario	1996	2001	2006	2011	2016	2021	2026	2031
Base								
Primary education								
20–24	0.36	0.47	0.48	0.48	0.48	0.48	0.49	0.49
25–29	0.36	0.55	0.60	0.60	0.60	0.60	0.60	0.61
Secondary education								
20–24	0.48	0.58	0.58	0.58	0.59	0.59	0.59	0.60
25–29	0.49	0.70	0.73	0.73	0.73	0.73	0.73	0.73
Tertiary education								
20–24	0.61	0.69	0.70	0.70	0.70	0.71	0.71	0.71
25–29	0.64	0.82	0.82	0.82	0.82	0.82	0.82	0.82
Convergence								
Primary education								
20–24	0.36	0.47	0.48	0.48	0.48	0.48	0.49	0.49
25–29	0.36	0.55	0.60	0.60	0.60	0.60	0.60	0.61
Secondary education								
20–24	0.48	0.58	0.54	0.47	0.46	0.46	0.46	0.46
25–29	0.49	0.70	0.71	0.64	0.60	0.59	0.59	0.59
Tertiary education								
20–24	0.61	0.69	0.63	0.49	0.45	0.46	0.46	0.46
25–29	0.64	0.82	0.80	0.69	0.60	0.59	0.59	0.59
Crossover								
Primary education								
20–24	0.36	0.47	0.48	0.48	0.48	0.48	0.49	0.49
25–29	0.36	0.55	0.60	0.60	0.60	0.60	0.60	0.61
Secondary education								
20–24	0.48	0.58	0.54	0.43	0.32	0.29	0.29	0.29
25–29	0.49	0.70	0.71	0.62	0.50	0.42	0.40	0.40
Tertiary education								
20–24	0.61	0.69	0.63	0.43	0.25	0.20	0.20	0.20
25–29	0.64	0.82	0.80	0.66	0.45	0.32	0.30	0.29
Differential								
Primary education								
20–24	0.36	0.47	0.46	0.40	0.37	0.38	0.38	0.38
25–29	0.36	0.55	0.58	0.55	0.51	0.50	0.50	0.50
Secondary education								
20–24	0.48	0.58	0.53	0.39	0.35	0.35	0.35	0.35
25–29	0.49	0.70	0.70	0.61	0.52	0.50	0.50	0.50
Tertiary education								
20–24	0.61	0.69	0.60	0.36	0.29	0.29	0.29	0.29
25–29	0.64	0.82	0.80	0.66	0.51	0.48	0.48	0.48

Table 7.4. Continued.

Scenario	1996	2001	2006	2011	2016	2021	2026	2031
Medicine1								
Primary education								
25–29	0.36	0.55	0.60	0.62	0.63	0.62	0.63	0.63
30–34	0.30	0.49	0.55	0.61	0.63	0.63	0.63	0.63
Secondary education								
25–29	0.49	0.70	0.71	0.67	0.62	0.61	0.61	0.62
30–34	0.40	0.65	0.68	0.68	0.65	0.63	0.62	0.62
Tertiary education								
25–29	0.64	0.82	0.80	0.71	0.63	0.61	0.61	0.61
30–34	0.52	0.78	0.75	0.73	0.67	0.63	0.62	0.62
Medicine2								
Primary education								
25–29	0.36	0.55	0.60	0.61	0.62	0.61	0.62	0.62
30–34	0.30	0.49	0.55	0.58	0.59	0.59	0.59	0.59
Secondary education								
25–29	0.49	0.70	0.71	0.67	0.62	0.61	0.61	0.62
30–34	0.40	0.65	0.68	0.68	0.65	0.63	0.62	0.62
Tertiary education								
25–29	0.64	0.82	0.81	0.72	0.64	0.62	0.62	0.62
30–34	0.52	0.78	0.76	0.76	0.71	0.66	0.65	0.65

Source: Author's calculations.

- The problems could result from sampling variability.
- The observed four-year interval instead of the desired five-year interval can affect the results.
- It is possible that the model has some failings that account for the inconsistency, or that a model for Zambia would be very different from one for Botswana.
- The data in *Table 7.1* could be biased in some way.

It seems doubtful that the inconsistency could be the result of a model failure. It would be difficult to come up with an explanation of some of the data in *Table 7.1* with any model. If the figures in *Table 7.1* are biased, the inferences that we have made from those data may need to be reconsidered. If the bias were one that generally affects figures on HIV prevalence by education, it would be extremely important for us to know about it. Unfortunately, we must leave the question about the origin of the inconsistency open for now. We hope better data in the future will help answer it. For now, we can only conclude that the data in *Table 7.1* may be biased in a way that overstates the extent of behavioral change among more-educated women.

The second important feature of *Table 7.4* is that prevalence is a lagging indicator of behavior. In other words, changes in prevalence reflect changes in behavior that happened in the past. To see the relationship between changes in behavior and changes in prevalence, let us look first at the "convergence" scenario. Under these conditions, the riskiness of sexual behavior for women with a secondary education or more converge to the riskiness of the behavior of women with a primary education or less over the period from 2001 to 2006. In 2006 and thereafter, the riskiness of behavior is the same in all three education groups. Among the least-educated women, prevalence rises in both age groups, even though the riskiness of their behavior has not changed. These rises are just part of the normal course of the HIV epidemic.

During the period of rapid behavioral change in the "convergence" scenario, from 2001 to 2006, the prevalence rate for women aged 20–24 with a secondary education decreases by 4 percentage points, while the prevalence for women aged 25–29 increases by 1 percentage point. Women with a tertiary education in the two age groups experience decreases in prevelence of 6 and 2 percentage points, respectively. Based on this information alone, it would be very hard to infer that 2001–2006 is a period of rapid behavioral change. Small percentage point changes could easily be overlooked or swamped by sampling error. Both examples clearly show the difficulty of making inferences about behavioral change from prevalence rates without the use of an appropriate model.

The "convergence" scenario was constructed such that all behavioral change stops after 2006. Nevertheless, most of the change in the prevalence rate is observed in the 2006–2011 period. Prevalence for women aged 20–24 with a secondary education falls from 54 percent in 2006 to 47 percent in 2011. For women aged 25–29, the decline in prevalence continues for even longer after behavioral change has ended. The prevalence rate for these women decreases from 71 percent in 2006 to 64 percent in 2011 and then to 60 percent in 2016. For women with a tertiary education in both age groups, the fall in prevalence is significantly more pronounced in the decade after behavioral change stops than it is during the 5-year period during which the behavioral change occurs.

The "crossover" and "differential" scenarios show much the same thing. In the "crossover" scenario, behavioral change happens over a 10-year period (2001–2011), while in the "differential" scenario it occurs only over a 5-year period (2001–2006). In both, behavioral change is reflected in the prevalence rates only with a lag. From around 5 years after the change begins, large effects are visible and continue for 10–15 years after the behavioral change has come to a halt.

The third important feature of *Table 7.4* is the limited effect of the use of medication on the prevalence rate data of women under the age of 34. The two medication scenarios produce prevalence rates that are hardly different from those of the "convergence" scenario on which they are based. To squeeze more information into *Table 7.4*, we omit women aged 20–24 when we consider the medication scenarios and include women aged 30–34 instead. First, compare the prevalence rates for women aged 25–29 in the "convergence" scenario with their counterparts in the two medication scenarios. The rates are within a few percentage points of one another. Medication programs increase HIV prevalence because they keep people with the disease alive longer and because the people on medication can still infect others. Still, *Table 7.4* shows that the increases in prevalence in the age groups considered are small.

When we compare the prevalence rates for women aged 30–34 in the "medication no educational differentials" ("medication1") and the "medication with educational differentials" ("medication2") scenarios, we again see small differences. Women with a tertiary education have higher prevalence under the "medication2" scenario because their use of medication is higher in that scenario. Women with a primary education have lower prevalence under the "medication2" scenario because their use of medication is lower in that scenario. Even though the differences in usage rates are significant (20 percentage points higher for women with a tertiary education, and 20 percentage points lower for women with a primary education), the difference in prevalence rates does not exceed 3 percentage points. Potentially, we would be able to see more of a difference for older women. In reality, this is unlikely to work. As all the available data come from pregnant women, biases associated with the nonrepresentativeness of women who bear children at age 35 and older would, most likely, render suspect any inferences about behavior and medication use from prevalence rate observations on those women.

Table 7.4 shows the following:

- The predicted pattern of HIV prevalence by education is not consistent with that observed for Zambia.
- Changes in prevalence rates do not imply contemporaneous changes in behavior, even in the absence of medication use.
- It is difficult to observe the effects of medication use in prevalence rate data, even when there are strong differences in use by education.

7.5   Previous Findings

Other work using the same model for Botswana has implications for our understanding of the connections between HIV/AIDS and education. We briefly consider four of these here:

- HIV/AIDS will not cause catastrophic economic damage in Botswana.
- A large antiretroviral medication program is affordable in Botswana.

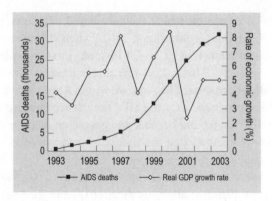

Figure 7.5. Rates of growth of real gross domestic product and annual AIDS deaths, Botswana 1993–2003. The rate of growth for 2003 is a Botswana Institute for Policy Analysis forecast and the rate of growth from 2002 is preliminary. Annual AIDS deaths are computed using the model described in the text. For more information, see Sanderson (2002b). *Sources of growth rates*: 1993, Botswana Institute for Development Policy Analysis (1998, p. 4); 1994–2003, Botswana Institute for Development Policy Analysis (2002b, p. 4).

- Such an antiretroviral medication program by itself cannot, in the long run, bring female life expectancy in Botswana above 40 years.
- Even with the expected massive AIDS deaths, continued urbanization and per capita income growth will require some combination of increased water transport infrastructure and further water-conservation measures to ensure that the capital city, Gaborone, will not have water-shortage problems by the year 2021.

The effect of HIV/AIDS on the economy of Botswana is discussed in IIASA (2001) and Sanderson (2002b).[10] Since its independence in 1966, Botswana has had spectacular economic growth. This growth continues to be fueled by mineral exports (primarily diamonds), but it would not have occurred without wise macroeconomic management strategies. Botswana's economic success provides a picture of what many mineral-rich African countries could have achieved. Nevertheless, the question on many people's minds today is not the past sources of Botswana's economic miracle, but whether its current extraordinarily high rate of HIV/AIDS prevalence will cause an economic catastrophe. The short answer to this question is "no."

---

[10] The discussion of Botswana's economy draws heavily on these two sources.

The recent history of the relationship between economic growth and AIDS deaths is shown in *Figure 7.5*. It shows what we call the "Botswana Paradox," the persistence of high rates of economic growth with high and increasing numbers of AIDS deaths from 1993 through 2002. The growth rates in *Figure 7.5* are high and show no tendency to fall even as the number of AIDS deaths was increasing dramatically from year to year. In 2002, almost 2 percent of the population of Botswana died of AIDS and the annual rate of economic growth was still around 5 percent. Since the rate of population growth in Botswana in 2002 was practically zero, the annual rate of per capita GDP growth was also around 5 percent, a very respectable rate indeed and one of the highest in Africa. To understand, first, how such rapid economic growth could exist while the number of AIDS deaths was sky-rocketing and, second, the likely future rate of economic growth in Botswana, it is crucial that we discuss the factors that drive that growth.

Botswana's economy is driven by mineral exports. Some of the revenues from these exports are appropriated by the government of Botswana and spent in a wide variety of areas, such as running governmental offices, drought relief, water infra-structure, housing, health care, and education. The revenue flows from diamond exports and the amount of government expenditure required to meet the twin objectives of economic growth and low inflation relative to its main trading partners generally do not match. In each year, the economy of Botswana has a certain capacity to absorb government spending productively. If the government of Botswana tried to push the economy beyond its capacity, the result would be inflation and very little additional output. If the government did not spend enough, the result would be growth slower than necessary and more unemployment. The genius of Botswana's macroeconomic policies has been to control government spending so as to keep the economy close to its continually growing productive capacity.

At any moment, the capacity of the Botswana economy to absorb spending depends mainly on three factors:

- The quantity of skilled labor.
- The size and distribution of the current capital stock.
- Export opportunities.

The availability of unskilled labor has not been a constraint on growth in the past because of high rates of unemployment and underemployment among the un-skilled. HIV/AIDS, of course, affects the quantity of skilled labor. The rapid eco-nomic growth in the late 1990s was driven by two of those three factors. First, de-spite the HIV/AIDS epidemic, the quantity of skilled labor grew rapidly because of previous investments in education. Second, export conditions were improving over the period 1993–2002 because of increasing diamond prices, increased diamond production, and the success of the government's diversification policies.[11]

To understand the future of the Botswana economy, we need to know how both the educational composition of the labor force and exports will evolve. Even with the epidemic, the number of working-age people with a secondary education or more will continue to rise rapidly. There will certainly be a shortage of more-educated workers relative to the likely number without the epidemic, but it is unlikely that there will be a shortage of them relative to the economy's requirement for continued growth.

The question concerning the future of exports is more difficult to answer. Diamond prices may still continue to rise, but little change is expected in diamond production in the near-term future, because there are no plans for new mines or for expanding existing ones. In any case, the labor force involved in mineral production is such a small fraction of Botswana's total labor force that a shortage of miners because of HIV/AIDS is unlikely. However, the effect of the HIV/AIDS epidemic on diversification of the economy toward nonmineral exports is unclear. Diversification continued throughout the 1990s. If behavioral changes lead more-educated people to have lower infection rates, it is possible that export diversification will continue apace.

Botswana is a fortunate and unique country. The driving forces behind its economic growth (strong mineral exports and increases in human capital, managed by wise and adaptive government policies) seem likely to survive the epidemic. There is no economic catastrophe on the horizon.

Botswana is fortunate and unique in another way as well: it can afford the national antiretroviral medication campaign it has begun. We came to this conclusion by combining the population-forecasting model in this chapter with a general equilibrium model of Botswana's economy. The costs of programs to combat HIV/AIDS will certainly be significant, but, at least for the next 15 years, it is unlikely that they will exceed the government's ability to bear them (IIASA 2001).[12] This is, importantly, because of the increases in productivity associated with higher education. In other countries, such as Namibia for example, affordability could depend crucially on the interactions between education and HIV.

Although our findings show that a national antiretroviral program is affordable in Botswana, they also show that, without behavioral change, even the most successful program will not raise life expectancy to over 40 years for women in Botswana (Sanderson 2002a). Clearly, medication alone is not the answer to the HIV/AIDS epidemic. For female life expectancy to rise above 40 years, behavioral

---

[11] For information on the diversification of the Botswana economy, see Botswana Institute for Development Policy Analysis (2002a, pp. 3–4).

[12] Currently, Botswana receives much of its antiretroviral medication free of charge through donations from Merck & Co., Inc., and others.

change is required. For female life expectancy to rise above 60 years, so much behavioral change is required that any medication program would be of relatively minor significance. If policy makers were to set a goal of raising life expectancy in Botswana to over 60 years, their prime concern would need to be how to help generate the required behavioral change. Here again, we return to the importance of understanding the connections with education.

Finally, education is an important determinant of locational choice. People with a secondary education or more are not likely to be satisfied with jobs herding livestock. Instead, they are more likely to locate in cities, where the skills that they learned in school can be put to more productive use. We applied this idea in forecasting the number of Batswana who would be living in urban areas and the number who would be living in the capital city of Gaborone. Using both the expected numbers of people living in Gaborone and expected income growth, we made estimates of the demand for water in Gaborone. These estimates were compared with detailed hydrological models of water supply to produce estimates of the future water balance for Gaborone (Hellmuth and Sanderson 2001; IIASA 2001). Future rainfall and temperature are uncertain, so we used a probabilistic approach to the study of water balance, which included our uncertainty about the nature of upcoming global weather patterns.

Our analysis of the probabilistic water balance figures for Gaborone showed that, even with the highest HIV/AIDS prevalence rate in the world, additional steps will need to be taken to insure against water shortages there. The government of Botswana is well aware of this. The North–South Water Carrier project was designed to be implemented in two stages. The first has already been completed. The construction of the second stage has, wisely, been delayed until future water demands can be foreseen more accurately. Whether the second stage will need to be built or whether conservation and the present water infrastructure will suffice to eliminate potential water shortages depends on the course of the HIV/AIDS epidemic, in general, and particularly on the interactions between education, behavioral change, and medication use.

The HIV/AIDS epidemic, even in severely affected countries such as Botswana, is not likely to bring urban population growth to an end. In Botswana, and elsewhere, the problems associated with bringing clean water and services to growing urban populations will still need to be addressed. In a companion study on Namibia, another country hard hit by the HIV/AIDS pandemic, our findings show that without strong conservation measures and an augmented water infrastructure, there is a substantial likelihood of future water shortages in Windhoek, the country's capital (IIASA 2001).

Education plays a role in virtually all aspects of the HIV/AIDS epidemic, from understanding how prevalence rates by education will evolve, to how the economy will be affected, to whether or not medication programs will be affordable, to the best mix of prevention and treatment programs, to rural–urban migration, and to the demand for urban infrastructure. We are in the position to make simulations of all these things and to compare our predictions with observations where they exist. Nevertheless, without information on education and HIV in Botswana, policies will have to be developed in the dark.

7.6   Conclusions

When the HIV/AIDS epidemic began to spread in sub-Saharan Africa, the more-educated people may have had higher prevalence rates than those with less education. That differential may have been shrinking, and it is plausible that it could have already reversed, with educated people changing their behavior more quickly and using available medication more readily and more efficiently. Many sub-Saharan African countries have anti-HIV programs that encourage behavioral change and make medication use more affordable and accessible. These programs influence people at different levels of education differently. We cannot possibly understand where programs are succeeding or failing without including education as a key variable. Nevertheless, the data to do this are still far too scarce and fragmentary. The calculations in this chapter, which clearly illustrate what a difference education makes to the dynamics of the epidemic, hopefully may contribute to providing the rationale for collecting such information in the future.

In the 1990s, the HIV/AIDS pandemic spread at a pace previously unimagined. The disease raced forward, while policy making lagged far behind. The Sentinel Surveillance system of data collection from small groups of pregnant women was inexpensive, easy to set up, and served the initial objective of ascertaining whether HIV/AIDS was spreading. We are now well past that phase. In Botswana and elsewhere, governments are mounting serious programs to lower HIV prevalence. This stage in the battle requires new tools and new forms of analysis, but inadequacies in previous data collections severely hamper our ability to develop these today. Under no circumstances should we let inadequate efforts today hamper our ability tomorrow.

It is important to understand that good intentions are not sufficient to design good anti-HIV programs. Some programs can even magnify the misery already caused by the epidemic (Sanderson 2002a). The need to take action quickly is not an excuse for taking action blindly, and with respect to education and HIV, we are surely flying blind in most countries.

Understanding usually takes time. In the case of HIV, data collection methods have to be designed, data have to be collected and analyzed, and ideas have to be tested and refined. Without a holistic understanding of what their effects are, anti-HIV programs can fail. Future generations in sub-Saharan Africa, then, will surely ask why policy makers made a horrible situation even worse. More detailed information about the dynamics of the epidemic by education—probably the most important population dimension after age and sex—and quantitative models to assist decision making can make a useful contribution at this critical stage.

Appendix 7.1:
Transition Rates between States

The prevalence–incidence relationship in 1995

In practice, it is possible to use information on the HIV prevalence rates of women by age at two dates to infer the intervening average age-specific incidence rates. For Botswana, we use 1993 and 1997 as those dates because reasonably comparable information is available for them. The data that we use come from Sentinel Surveillance Surveys, which derive information from a sample of women who sought prenatal care. These data are biased in a number of ways and have to be corrected before they can be used. If HIV prevalence rates early in Botswana's epidemic were not the same for all education groups, it is crucial that this be taken into account in correcting the observed prevalence rates. The Sentinel Surveillance data and how they were corrected are discussed below.

Age- and education-specific HIV incidence rates for women are derived from adjusted age- and education-specific prevalence rates using the formula

$$ir\left(a, e, 1995, susc\right) = 1 - \left\{ \frac{1 - \frac{pr(a+2,e,1997)}{susc(1995-a)}}{1 - \frac{pr(a-2,e,1993)}{susc(1995-a)}} \right\}^{0.25} \tag{7.1}$$

where $ir\left(a, e, 1995, susc\right)$ is the incidence rate among susceptible women of age a and education level e in 1995, $pr\left(a - 2, e, 1993\right)$ is the adjusted prevalence rate for women of age $a - 2$ and education e in 1993, $pr\left(a + 2, e, 1997\right)$ is the analogous rate for those women four years later, and $susc\left(1995 - a\right)$ is the proportion of the cohort born in year $1995 - a$ susceptible to acquiring HIV. For simplicity, Equation (7.1) assumes that all women are sexually active. When the proportion sexually active increases with age, as it does for teenagers, the formula is more complex.

Although baseline prevalence and incidence rates for women can be estimated from data, it is impossible to determine the appropriate relationship between prevalence and incidence rates. In sub-Saharan Africa, HIV/AIDS is transmitted predominantly between the sexes during unprotected intercourse. The prevalence rates relevant for determining the incidence rates of women of a given age and education are the prevalence rates of the men with whom they have unprotected intercourse.

One way to specify this relationship using the incidence rates in Equation (7.1) is

$$ir\left(a, e, 1995, susc\right) = \mu\left(a, e, 1995\right) \cdot$$

$$\left[pr\left(sex \ partners \ of \ women \ age \ a \ and \ education \ e, \qquad 1995\right)\right]^{\alpha} , \tag{7.2}$$

where $ir(a, e, 1995, susc)$ is the incidence rate among females of age a and education e in year 1995 who are susceptible to contracting HIV because of their risky sexual practices, $\mu(a, e, 1995)$ is a set of age- and education-specific constants that relate to women of age a and education e in 1995, $pr(sex\ partners\ of\ women\ age\ a\ and\ education\ e,\ 1995)$ is the prevalence rate of the men who are the sex partners of (susceptible) women of age a and education e in 1995, and α is a parameter that lies between 0 and 1 and reflects the heterogeneity in the riskiness of sexual behavior.

Two important features of Equation (7.2) need to be discussed here. First, because the $\mu(a, e, 1995)$ are age- and education-specific, they capture things that change across age and education groups in 1995. For example, if the frequency of sexual relations varied with age or more-educated women generally had more unsafe sexual contacts in 1995 than did less-educated women, these would be captured in the $\mu(a, e, 1995)$. We expect the μs to change over time with changes in behavior and with the implementation of antiretroviral medication programs. The second feature that must be mentioned here is the inclusion of the exponent α. When α is equal to 1.0, the incidence is proportional to the prevalence, holding age and education constant. When α is less than 1.0, but still greater than 0, the incidence rate among susceptibles increases less than proportionally. We determine the parameter α by fitting the forecasts beyond 1997 to observations.

Nothing on the right-hand side of Equation (7.2) is observable. Unfortunately, no nationwide African data on the HIV prevalence of men currently exist, and therefore the direct approach to specifying prevalence–incidence relationships through Equation (7.2) is foreclosed to us.

An indirect approach, staying close to the data that we have, utilizes the prevalence rates of women. Let us take 25-year-old women as an example. We can estimate the HIV incidence rate of these women from the existing data, but we cannot estimate the prevalence rate of the men with whom they have unprotected sexual relations. It seems plausible to assume that the men who have unprotected sexual relations with women who are 25 years old also have unprotected relations with somewhat older and younger women as well. Therefore, the prevalence rates of women similar in age to 25-year-old women can be taken as an indicator of the prevalence rates of the men with whom 25-year-old women have unsafe sex.

We can express this idea in equation form as

$$pr\ (f, a - 2\ to\ a + 2, e, 1995) = \lambda\ (a, e, 1995)$$

$$\cdot\ [pr\ (sex\ partners\ of\ women\ age\ a\ and\ education\ e,\ 1995)]\ ,\quad (7.3)$$

where $\lambda(a, e, 1995)$ is a set of age- and education-specific constants in 1995 and $pr\ (f, a - 2\ to\ a + 2, e, 1995)$ is the prevalence rate of females in the age group

$a - 2$ through $a + 2$, who have education level e in 1995. Nothing on the right-hand side of Equation (7.3) is observable either.

Combining Equations (7.2) and (7.3), we obtain

$$ir\,(a, e, 1995) = \left[\frac{\mu\,(a, e, 1995)}{\lambda\,(a, e, 1995)^{\alpha}} \right] \cdot pr\,(f, a - 2\ to\ a + 2, e, 1995)^{\alpha}\ . \quad (7.4)$$

Since the prevalence rates on the right-hand side of Equation (7.4) are observable from adjusted Sentinel Surveillance Survey data and the incidence rates on the left-hand side can be estimated using Equation (7.1), it is possible to compute the composite parameters $\kappa(a, e, 1995)$ from Equation (7.4), where

$$\kappa\,(a, e, 1995) = \left[\frac{\mu\,(a, e, 1995)}{\lambda\,(a, e, 1995)^{\alpha}} \right]\ . \quad (7.5)$$

In describing how we can estimate the $\kappa\,(a, e, 1995)$ terms, we have left out an important technical detail that concerns the interaction between those who exhibit risky behavior and those who do not. For the sake of exposition, imagine that 10 percent of all women do not engage in risky sexual practices. At one extreme, these women may have mutually monogamous relationships with an HIV-negative partner. In this case, their numbers are irrelevant for computing incidence rates. They and their partners do not interact with those who engage in risky sex. Therefore, the incidence rate for those who engage in risky sex depends only on the prevalence rate of those who engage in risky sex. At the other extreme, instead of viewing these women as having mutually monogamous relationships, they could have many different sex partners, always demanding that condoms are used. In this case, men who exhibit risky behavior sometimes encounter women who demand that a condom be used and sometimes do not. The incidence rate in this situation depends on the fraction of sex acts in which a condom is used. Over time, as a cohort ages, the proportion of women who always use condoms increases because of the high death rate among those for whom condom use is less regular.

We incorporate this by writing the equation for the prevalence rate in Equations (7.3) and (7.4) as

$$pr\,(f, a - 2\ to\ a + 2, e, 1995) =$$

$$\frac{HIV^{+}\,(f, a - 2\ to\ a + 2, e, unmed, 1995)}{Susc\,(f, a - 2\ to\ a + 2, e, 1995) + \beta \cdot Nonsusc\,(f, a - 2\ to\ a + 2, e, 1995)}\ , \quad (7.6)$$

where $HIV^{+}\,(f, a - 2\ to\ a + 2, e, unmed, 1995)$ is the number of HIV-positive females in the age range $a - 2$ to $a + 2$ and of education level e in 1995, $Susc\,(f, a - 2\ to\ a + 2, e, 1995)$ is the number of susceptible females in the age range $a - 2$ to $a + 2$ and of education level e in 1995 (including those who are

HIV-positive), and $Nonsusc\,(f, a-2\;to\;a+2, e, 1995)$ is the number of nonsusceptible females in the age range $a-2$ to $a+2$ and of education level e in 1995.

The parameter β reflects the interactions between susceptibles and nonsusceptibles. When β is equal to 1.0, nonsusceptibles are included in the denominator of Equation (7.6) in exactly the same way as susceptibles. This means that nonsusceptibles behave exactly like susceptibles, except that they always use condoms. When β is equal to 0.0, nonsusceptibles do not have intercourse with susceptibles, and therefore the number of nonsusceptibles has no influence on the incidence rate. The parameter β is, most likely, somewhere between the extremes. In the simulations presented here, we set β equal to 0.5 for all three education groups. It is possible that β could be different for different education groups, but we have no data that allow us to make even a rough guess as to how it might vary.

The numerator in Equation (7.6) refers to HIV-positive women in 1995 who were not on medication. The antiretroviral medications that we know today were not available in 1995, so no women in Botswana at that time were on medication. We included the term "unmedicated" in Equation (7.6) because when we make forecasts for the years after 1995, we will have to make a clear distinction between those on medication and those not on medication.

These equations provide us with the core of the structure of the prevalence–incidence spiral. We estimate 105 κs for 1995 (35 ages and three education groups). If there were no behavioral change and no medication use, the $\kappa\,(a, e, 1995)$ would be constant and we could use them for forecasting. For example, given the prevalence rate for women aged 20–24 by education at the beginning of 1993, Equation (7.4) can be used to forecast the incidence rate for 22-year-old women during 1993. This incidence rate, along with others (and additional information), is used to compute the prevalence rates at the beginning of 1994. The prevalence rates at the beginning of 1994 are the inputs into the calculation of the incidence rates during 1994, and so on.

Changes in prevalence–incidence relationships because of medication and behavioral change

Even when α, β, and the κs are constant, prevalence and incidence rates generally change over time, reflecting the internal dynamics of the HIV epidemic. Behavioral changes and medication use interact with these internal dynamics in complex ways. Let us begin our description of this with the addition of medication use. When antiretrovirals are used, Equation (7.6) has to be transformed into

$$pr\,(f, a-2\;to\;a+2, e, t) =$$

$$\frac{HIV^+\,(f, a-2\;to\;a+2, e, unmted,\;)+\gamma\cdot HIV^+\,(f, a-2\;to\;a+2, e, dnt\;\;)}{Susc\,(f,\;a-2\;to\;a+2, e, t)+\beta\cdot Nonsusc\,(f,\;a-2\;to\;a+2, e, t)}.\;(7.7)$$

Two changes distinguish Equation (7.7) from Equation (7.6). First, there is a new term in the numerator, $\gamma \cdot HIV^+ (f, a - 2\ to\ a + 2, e, m\varepsilon d,)$. The expression $HIV^+ (f, a - 2\ to\ a + 2, e\varsigma d\eta t\quad)$ is the number of women in the age group $a - 2$ to $a + 2$ who are on antiretroviral medication in year t and the parameter γ is the infectivity of people on medication relative to those who are not on medication. When γ is 1.0, people on medication are as capable of spreading HIV (per sexual act) as people not on medication. When γ is zero, people on medication cannot spread HIV.

It is certainly possible that γ depends on education. The relative infectivity of people on medication depends on the frequency of visits to physicians and on dosage compliance, both of which are likely to be correlated positively with education. There are no data on this, and the massive program of medication use in Botswana is just beginning. For simplicity, we assume that γ is independent of education. As a practical matter, this will have very little influence on what we say below.

As we saw earlier, there is evidence that the speed and possibly the ultimate extent of behavioral change differ by education. The model allows two sorts of education-specific behavioral changes, one along cohort lines and one along period lines. We represent cohort- and education-specific behavior change by varying the proportions of women, cross-classified by birth cohort and education, who do not engage in unsafe sexual practices. We represent period- and education-specific behavioral changes through proportional shifts in the κs estimated for 1995. Large-scale public education programs of the sort that the government of Botswana is just beginning are best modeled as influencing behavior in a period-specific way.

The κs reflect the riskiness of sexual behavior among the susceptibles. As a shorthand, we sometimes use phrases like "holding the riskiness of behavior constant." In terms of the mathematics of the model, this translates into keeping the κs constant. When we discuss decreases in the riskiness of sexual behavior, we mean decreases in the κs.

The framework that we have just sketched allows us to stay close to the data because the κs are estimated from observations. It also allows us to simulate the effects of differences in education on medication usage, and cohort- and period-specific behavioral changes.

Other transition rates

In *Figure 7.1*, we show that there are five kinds of transition rates in the model. We have just discussed the first of these, the incidence rates (the rates of transition from being uninfected to being infected). In this subsection, we discuss the other four:

the transition from being infected and asymptomatic to the onset of symptoms, the transition from the onset of symptoms to the initiation of medication use, the transition from being asymptomatic on medication to the recurrence of symptoms, and finally that from an unmedicated symptomatic state to death.

The transition rate from being infected, unmedicated, and asymptomatic to the onset of symptoms depends on the duration of infection. We generate the hazard rates by duration from an underlying normal distribution with a fixed mean and variance. In this chapter, the mean time from infection to symptoms in the unmedicated state is nine years with a standard deviation of two years. This is quite close to what it is in developed countries.

Once a person has passed through the asymptomatic and unmedicated state, there are two possibilities:

- initiate medication use, or
- become unmedicated and symptomatic.

The proportion that initiates medication use can differ with education and change over time. In this chapter, we have considered various possibilities for these proportions. Unfortunately, medication is not a cure for HIV/AIDS. It lengthens people's lives, but the disease can flare up at almost any time. There are no good data on the increase in life expectancy of people on medication, so we use the simplest specification possible. Some people begin medication and have to discontinue it after a short period because of the side effects. We do not consider these people as making the transition to medication use. Instead, they go into the unmedicated and symptomatic state. Those who use medication for a while are assumed to have a constant annual rate of attrition into the unmedicated and symptomatic state. This annual rate of attrition is just the inverse of the expected number of years in the medicated state. Here we assume that, on average, people spend 10 years in the medicated state. The 10-year period is just an average (e.g., some people will have their lives lengthened by only 2 years; others, by 20 years).

Once in the unmedicated symptomatic state, people have only a short time to live. They enter this state either when they become symptomatic and do not take medication or after they have taken medication and it has failed. We assume that, in this state, there is a fixed probability of dying during each year. In the simulations above, this probability is set at one-half. In other words, people with AIDS have a remaining life expectancy of two years.

The model also includes the transmission of HIV from mother to child and the use of medication to reduce the probability of that transmission, but we do not have the space to discuss this here.

Appendix 7.2:
The Prevalence Rate Data and Their Correction

The prevalence rate data used in this chapter and the most common form found in sub-Saharan Africa are from Sentinel Surveillance Surveys. In these surveys, women who attend prenatal care clinics have their blood tested anonymously for HIV. These data are substantially biased and cannot be used appropriately without adjustment. There are generally six main sources of bias:

- Women who seek prenatal care may not be a random sample of all pregnant women.
- Pregnant women are not a representative sample of all women of reproductive age.
- The Sentinel Surveillance sites are geographically unrepresentative.
- A correlation between HIV prevalence and fertility is induced by third factors, such as education.
- HIV itself has physiological effects on childbearing ability.
- A correlation between HIV prevalence and pregnancy in young women is caused by the timing of the onset of sexual activity.

Since over 85 percent of pregnant women in Botswana receive prenatal care, the magnitude of the first bias is likely to be low. As we do not have any other usable information on this score, we simply ignore this bias here. We solve the problem of age representativeness by using age-specific prevalence rates. The geographic bias in the data is mitigated by separating rural and urban Sentinel Surveillance sites and reweighting the observed age-specific prevalence rates using information on the location of the population from the 1991 census of Botswana.

It is crucial that we adjust the observed figures appropriately for the correlation between HIV prevalence and fertility that is induced by educational differences. It seems likely that at the beginning of the epidemic in Botswana, HIV prevalence rates were higher for more-educated women. We know, however, that these women had lower fertility than women with less education and, therefore, were a smaller proportion of prenatal clinic attendees than they were of the population. Since women with higher HIV prevalence rates had lower fertility, the HIV prevalence rates observed in the prenatal care clinics are biased downward. Education may not be the only factor to induce a bias in the observed rates. Other factors could matter too, but after correcting for education and rural–urban location, we think that the effects of other factors are likely to be small.

An important bias in the Sentinel Surveillance rates is generated by the HIV/AIDS infection itself. Fragmentary data suggest that HIV-positive women are less likely to bear children than otherwise similar HIV-negative women. This effect appears even in women who do not know their HIV status. It even seems to appear in women who are asymptomatic. It is easy to understand why symptomatic women are less likely to bear children. They know they are deathly ill, are fighting off opportunistic infections, and are certainly much less likely to be sexually active. The reduction in fertility of HIV-positive but asymptomatic women may be the result of HIV or it might be due to the strong positive relationship between being HIV-positive and the presence of other sexually transmitted diseases that reduce fertility.

The Sentinel Surveillance prevalence rates for women aged 15–19 have a significant upward bias because the sexually inactive women in that group can neither become pregnant nor contract HIV from an infected partner, and therefore do not show up in the Sentinel Surveillance data. The model used here adjusts for this bias. This is particularly important because the Sentinel Surveillance prevalence rate for those aged 15–19 is sometimes taken as an early indicator of the success of government programs.

Since, in Botswana, there are no national data from the 1990s on the relationship between HIV prevalence and education, we have to approximate them on the basis of plausible assumptions. This takes a number of steps. First, the observed prevalence rate of women of age a in 1995[13] is

$$OBR \quad (a, 1995) =$$

$$\frac{Births\,(a, positive, 1995)}{Births\,(a, positive, 1995) + Births\,(a, negative, 1995)}\,, \tag{7.8}$$

where $Births\,(a, positive, 1995)$ is the number of births to women of age a in 1995 who were HIV-positive, and $Births\,(a, negative, 1995)$ is the corresponding number of births to women who were HIV-negative.

We can write an equation for the number of births to HIV-positive women of age a in 1995 that distinguishes between births to HIV-positive women who are asymptomatic and those who are symptomatic:

$$Births\,(a, positive, 1995) =$$

$$Births\,(a, positive\ and\ asym, 1995) + Births\,(a, sym, 1995)\,. \tag{7.9}$$

Births to women of age a who are HIV-positive and asymptomatic can be expressed as

---

[13] We do not actually observe this rate, but it is computed from prevalence rates for 1993 and 1997.

$Births\,(a, positive\ and\ asym, 1995) =$

$$\sum_{e=1}^{3} HIV^{+}\,(a, e, asym, 1995) \cdot asfr\,(a, e, 1995) \cdot \delta\,(asym)\ , \qquad (7.10)$$

where $HIV^{+}\,(a, e, asym, 1995)$ is the number of HIV-positive and asymptomatic women of age a and education level e in 1995, $asfr\,(a, e, 1995)$ is the age- and education-specific fertility rate of HIV-negative women in 1995, and $\delta\,(asym)$ is a factor by which the fertility of HIV-positive and asymptomatic women is reduced relative to otherwise similar women who are HIV-negative.

Births to women of age a who have AIDS can be expressed analogously:

$Births\,(a, sym, 1995) =$

$$\sum_{e=1}^{3} HIV^{+}\,(a, e, sym, 1995) \cdot asfr\,(a, e, 1995) \cdot \delta\,(sym)\ , \qquad (7.11)$$

where $\delta\,(sym)$ is the factor by which the fertility of HIV-positive and symptomatic women is reduced relative to otherwise similar women who are HIV-negative.

Next, we have to express the unknown numbers of HIV-positive women by age and education in terms of numbers that we know and our assumptions. We do this by writing

$$HIV^{+}\,(a, e, 1995) = N\,(a, e, 1995) \cdot pr\,(a, 1, 1995) \cdot \rho\,(e, 1995)\ , \qquad (7.12)$$

where $HIV^{+}\,(a, e, 1995)$ is the number of HIV-positive women of age a and education level e in 1995, $N\,(a, e, 1995)$ is the total number of women of age a and education level e in 1995, $pr\,(a, 1, 1995)$ is the prevalence rate of women of age a and education level 1 in 1995, and $\rho\,(e, 1995)$ is ratio of HIV prevalence in education group e to that in group 1; clearly, $\rho\,(1, 1995)1=$.

What remains is to divide the HIV-positive women into those who are symptomatic and those who are not. Since the HIV epidemic did not begin to spread rapidly in Botswana until the end of the 1980s, relatively few women were symptomatic in 1995. For simplicity, we have assumed that all HIV-positive women in 1995 were asymptomatic.

Given assumptions about the ρs and combining Equations (7.8) through (7.12), we are left with one equation in one unknown, $pr\,(a, 1, 1995)$. All the other terms, such as the age- and education-specific fertility rates of HIV-negative women, are either observed or closely approximated from observed data. Solving the equation for $pr\,(a, 1, 1995)$ gives us the prevalence rate in 1995 for women with a primary education or less. Multiplying this rate by the appropriate ρ gives the prevalence rates for the other two education groups. These are the prevalence rates we use in computing the incidence–prevalence relationship discussed above.

References

Botswana Institute for Development Policy Analysis (1998). *BIDPA Briefing, 3rd Quarter*. Gaborone, Botswana: BIDPA. (Downloaded from www.bidpa.bw/)

Botswana Institute for Development Policy Analysis (2002a). *BIDPA Briefing, 2nd Quarter*. Gaborone, Botswana: BIDPA. (Downloaded from www.bidpa.bw/)

Botswana Institute for Development Policy Analysis (2002b). *BIDPA Briefing, 4th Quarter*. Gaborone, Botswana: BIDPA. (Downloaded from www.bidpa.bw/)

Cohen D (2002). *Human Capital and the HIV Epidemic in Sub-Saharan Africa*. Working Paper 2. Geneva: ILO Program on HIV/AIDS and the World of Work. (Downloaded on October 20th 2002 from www.ilo.org/public/english/protection/trav/aids/download/pdf/wp2_humancapital.pdf)

De Walque D (2002). How Does Educational Attainment Affect the Risk of Being Infected by HIV/AIDS? Evidence from Uganda and Zambia. Unpublished paper. Chicago: University of Chicago, Department of Economics.

Fylkesnes K, Musonda RM, Sichone M, Ndhlovu Z, Tembo F & Nonze M (2001). Declining HIV prevalence and risk behaviors in Zambia: Evidence from surveillance and population based surveys. *AIDS* **15**:907–916

Hellmuth M & Sanderson WC (2001). Southern Africa—water stressed by 2001? *APC-EU Courier* **189**:40–41.

IIASA (2001). *Botswana's Future, Mozambique's Future, Namibia's Future: Modeling Population and Sustainable Development Challenges in the Era of HIV/AIDS*. Population Project at the International Institute for Applied Systems Analysis. Web site: www.iiasa.ac.at/Research/POP/pde/index.html?sb=16.

Kilian AHD, Gregson S, Ndyanabangi B, Walusaga K, Kipp W, Sahlmüller G, Garnett GP, Asime-Okiror G, Kabagame G, Weis P & von Sonnenburg F (1999). Reductions in risk behavior provide the most consistent explanation for declining HIV-1 prevalence in Uganda. *AIDS* **13**:391–398.

Lutz W, Sanderson WC & Wils A (2002). Conclusions: Toward comprehensive P-E studies. In *Population and Environment. Methods of Analysis*, eds. Lutz W, Prskawetz A & Sanderson WC, pp. 225–250. A Supplement to *Population and Development Review*, **28**, 2002. New York, NY, USA: The Population Council.

Sanderson WC (2001a). The mixed blessing of antiretroviral treatment in Botswana. *AIDS Analysis Africa* **11**.

Sanderson WC (2001b). How many Batswana will be alive in 2021? *APC-EU Courier* **188**:42–43.

Sanderson WC (2002a). *The Demographic Impact of HIV Medication Programs: With Examples from Botswana*. Paper presented at the Population Association of America Meetings, 9 May 2002, Atlanta, Georgia, USA.

Sanderson WC (2002b). *Death, Diamonds, and the Botswana Paradox*. Paper presented at the Population Association of America Meetings, 9 May 2002, Atlanta, Georgia, USA.

Chapter 8

China's Future Urban and Rural Population by Level of Education

Gui-Ying Cao and Wolfgang Lutz

8.1 Introduction

China is the world's most populous country, with currently one out of five people in the world living within its borders. For this reason alone, the future of China's population is closely linked to the future of the world population. However, China's population trends are also remarkable for at least three major structural changes—called "revolutions" by the Chinese—that have been happening at a speed unsurpassed in any other country, despite the sheer size of the population involved:

- A very rapid fertility decline to below replacement level.
- Massive rural–urban migration.
- Significant improvements in educational enrolment.

All three mega-trends will continue to transform the Chinese society and economy significantly over the coming decades.

While there have been many studies on each of these major population changes and their possible longer-term impacts, no study so far has linked these three mega-trends to draw a more comprehensive picture of China's future population, human capital, and settlement structure. In this chapter, we present a unified analysis of these three aspects by means of multistate population projections by age, sex, urban or rural place of residence, and level of education. The interaction among these four demographic dimensions is of specific relevance and interest in China, more so than in many other countries. In traditional Chinese society, age and sex have both been very important sources of social stratification. With respect to place of residence, many people refer to urban and rural China as two different worlds. And differential education is important as a main determinant of income differentials.

A number of projections for China's future population have been produced by demographers at the United Nations (UN) and other international institutions, as well as in China. The projection presented here is different from other forecasts. One very important feature of this study is that it explicitly includes the educational status of the population and rural or urban place of residence in the process. It does not simply superimpose an assumed structure on exogenously given population forecasts, as, for example, the UN does in its projections of urban and rural populations (United Nations 2001) or the World Bank does in its projections of level of education (Ahuja and Filmer 1995). The multistate population projection method considers fertility, mortality, and migration separately for each educational group in urban and rural areas, and projects these eight distinct subpopulations by age and sex, with individuals allowed to move between groups throughout the projection. To our knowledge, this is the first time that the educational composition by age, sex, and place of residence has been used systematically for cohort-component projections in China.

The projections by urban or rural place of residence are important in their own right. Under the centrally planned economy, Chinese cities were closed off to farmers by the "invisible walls" of the household registration system (Chan 1997). Levels of socioeconomic development have differed greatly between rural and urban regions. The result of these "invisible walls" is that China has become a highly segmented society, divided by the geographic division of urban and rural sectors. Until recently, the urban household registration system, which determines where one can live and work, has prevented a tidal wave of rural migrants, who cannot be absorbed fully in the urban areas. But socioeconomic differences between rural and urban regions have increased during the recent period of economic reform, significantly increasing the incentive for migration in the future.

8.2   Salient Demographic Features in Contemporary China

China can be considered one of the developing countries most advanced in the process of demographic transition. Fertility rates declined from 4.2 births per woman in 1974 to below replacement level (down to 1.85), in 1995. There is not yet a generally accepted fertility estimate based on the 2000 census. The raw data so far show unbelievably low fertility rates of between 1.3 and 1.4 births per woman, but there clearly has been some undercounting. The as yet unresolved question is, By how much should these estimates be adjusted? The fertility transition in China has been largely attributed to the government's population policies and family planning programs. However, one can also assume that it has been driven by socioeconomic development, particularly by the recent rapid economic changes resulting from China's new economic reforms. In urban regions, these reforms have increased the benefits of having fewer children.

It is interesting to ask why fertility patterns and trends differ in urban and rural China despite the uniform implementation of population policies throughout the nation. These fertility differentials result from differences in socioeconomic conditions. It seems likely that these factors tend to favor government efforts to make information, supplies, and services accessible in urban areas (Cheng and Maxim 1992). In rural areas, the substitution of the household responsibility system of production for the commune system has increased productivity and household income, but has weakened the government's ability to regulate fertility.

Among other factors, education is an important determinant of fertility reduction. Studies have shown that education affects several aspects of fertility in China. First, educational development has had a substantial effect on the age at which women marry, because they stay in school longer and because education widens their employment opportunities in the labor market. Second, higher educational levels have raised the investment costs of children substantially, especially for parents who wish to ensure good career prospects for their children. Finally, education promotes a rational view of family formation and the acceptance of contraception to either space births or limit the number of children.

In the following, we briefly view changes in education in China over recent decades and address fertility, migration, aging, and the sex ratio by comparing rural and urban regions.

8.2.1   Development of education

As there have been such stunning recent improvements in education in China— the world's most populous country—it is worth taking a closer look at the process that led to this "education revolution." Education in China begins with kindergarten (ages 3–6) and continues with primary education (ages 6–12) and secondary education (ages 12–18), which includes junior and senior secondary schools, specialized secondary schools, vocational secondary schools, and technical training schools. Tertiary education, which includes universities and colleges as well as college for

Table 8.1. Population aged six and older, by educational level in 1964, 1982, 1990, and 1995.

Educational	1964		1982		1990		1995	
level	Millions	%	Millions	%	Millions	%	Millions	%
No schooling[a]	258.05	51.80	283.68	31.88	182.25	18.77	179.38	16.02
Primary	192.00	39.30	355.35	39.94	420.21	43.25	475.26	42.45
Secondary	41.46	8.32	244.73	27.50	353.27	36.36	439.97	39.29
Tertiary	2.88	0.58	6.04	0.68	15.76	1.62	25.06	2.24
Total	494.39		889.80		971.49		1,119.67	

[a]Includes the illiterate and semi-literate. No schooling in 1990 covers only population aged 15 and older.
Sources: Population Institute (1985); State Statistical Bureau (1986, 1993a, 1998); Yao and Hua (1995); Office of Population Survey (1997).

postgraduates, requires 4–5 years for a bachelor's degree, 7–8 years for a master's degree, and 10–11 years for a Ph.D.

In China, education is considered to be "a project of vital and lasting importance, calling for a good educational foundation" (*People's Daily*, 15 May 1987). For decades, the educational policy has been to "enable everyone who receives an education to develop morally, intellectually and physically" (Liu 1989). One of the most remarkable changes seen in China today is in the increasing percentages at all levels of education (*Table 8.1*). The percentage with no schooling has declined from 52 percent in 1964 to 16 percent in 1995. The most profound change is at the level of secondary education, where attendance has risen from only 8.32 percent in 1964 to 39.29 percent in 1995—almost five times as many students as in 1964.

The education system in China is under the authority and guidance of the Ministry of Education of the central government. At the provincial level, education is administered by the Education Bureau of the provincial government. Government expenditure on education has increased significantly over the past four decades. In 1953, the share of total government expenditure spent on education was 8.8 percent; in 1994 it had increased to 16.91 percent (State Statistical Bureau 1995). Associated with the economic reform of the mid-1980s, the central government advocated the financing of parts of universities by various institutions under the supervision of the Ministry of Education or the authority of education at the provincial level. The objective of this policy was to expand higher education to suit the needs of social and economic development. Government policies have focused in particular on two aspects of the education of the population:

- Eradicating illiteracy and promoting nine years of education for the population.
- Encouraging and improving the education of women.

8.2.2 Eradication of illiteracy and implementation of the nine-year education policy

In the 1950s, there was a widespread movement to eradicate illiteracy to better the listening and writing abilities of Chinese citizens. Around 70 percent of the total population was without formal schooling after China's civil war (1945–1949). In the 1960s, an obligatory nine-year education policy was implemented, calling for six years in primary school and three years in junior secondary school. This policy has been consistently realized in urban regions. However, in terms of financial assistance, the system did not develop in the manner originally planned in rural regions. In 1986, the State Council set up and issued a "law of obligatory nine-year education of citizens" to meet the Chinese "four modernizations" (industry, agriculture, science, and technology). Under this law, all persons are obliged to complete nine years of education, and the authorities at all levels must make this possible for everyone free of charge. Since then, concrete action to support nine years of education has been taken in all rural regions. As a result, China has reached near universal enrolment of children of primary school age and has rapidly increased the number of students in secondary schools. In 1997, 98.9 percent of children were enrolled in primary schools; in 1952, that figure was only 49.2 percent. In 1957, 44.2 percent of primary school graduates entered junior secondary school; this figure increased to 93.7 percent in 1997 (State Statistical Bureau 1998). Unfortunately, despite the rapid expansion in education, illiteracy in rural China still exists, especially among the elderly population.

8.2.3 Education of women

An outstanding feature of the changes in education in China is the increased participation of women. An important aspect of the state policies has always been their encouragement of female enrolment in schools at all levels. In China, a woman's level of education is one of the most important indicators of her social status. A woman's employment and domestic status depend heavily on her training and education. The Chinese government has made deliberate efforts to improve women's status by ensuring equal opportunities in education. As a consequence, the past four decades have witnessed a remarkable improvement in the education of females.

Figure 8.1 shows a significant increase in the proportion of females among all students at all levels of education. In 1997, 37 percent of all students in higher education were female; in middle schools, 46 percent were female; and in primary schools, 48 percent were female. Compared with 1952, this indicates a strong decline in the gender gap in education; however, some gender differences still exist at all levels of education, especially in rural China.

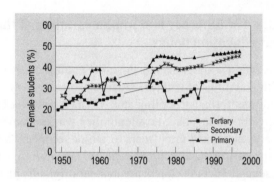

Figure 8.1. Development of female education: Percentage of female students. Data are not available for the years 1966–1972 and 1989. *Sources*: Chinese Ministry of Education (1984, 1998); China All Women's Federation (1991); State Statistical Bureau (1993b, 1996, 1998).

8.2.4 Regional disparity

Another important aspect of education in China is that it is unbalanced regionally; the disparities are particularly large between rural and urban areas. The educational distributions by age and rural or urban place of residence, calculated from the *National 1% Population Sample Survey 1995* (Office of Population Survey 1997), are shown in *Figures 8.2* and *8.3*. These two figures illustrate that the level of education is much higher for the urban than for the rural population. Obviously, a much larger proportion of the urban population has a secondary education in each age group. Also, the rural versus urban disparities by gender are pronounced. The rural population with low levels of education shows the highest gender differences. There are many more women than men without schooling at the higher adult ages.

8.2.5 Fertility differentials by rural or urban place of residence

The differences in total fertility rates (TFRs) between urban and rural populations over the past few decades are shown in *Figure 8.4*. The government's first family planning campaign took place in the mid-1950s, when the government began to manufacture contraceptives and relax restrictions on induced abortion. The urban fertility transition began as early as 1954, when the TFR was 5.72. It then fell to 5.67 in 1955, to 5.33 in 1956, and to 5.25 in 1958. The urban TFR was very low (2.98) in 1961—half the 1957 level—as a consequence of the years of agricultural crisis and starvation between 1959 and 1961. Urban fertility as a proportion of rural fertility dropped greatly in the 1960s, from 76 percent in 1962 to 53 percent in 1969. This disparity demonstrates the relatively early timing of the urban fertility

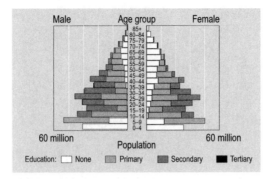

Figure 8.2. Population of rural China by age, sex, and level of education, 1995.
Source: Office of Population Survey (1997).

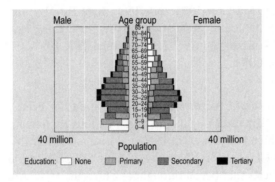

Figure 8.3. Population of urban China by age, sex, and level of education, 1995.
Source: Office of Population Survey (1997).

transition. In 1963 there was still unusually high fertility, possibly in reaction to the earlier years of depression. Since then, urban China has experienced unprecedented fertility declines. By the mid-1970s, the urban fertility rate had already reached replacement level. By this time, the government had given full attention to and taken concrete action on family planning by enacting policies that encouraged late marriages and fewer births. The rapid urban fertility decline during the 1970s coincided not only with the intensification of the family planning program, but also with the development of education and other socioeconomic modernization.

Fertility changes in China have been categorized either as "induced" or as "natural" (Wang 1991). The former reflects government intervention that hastened fertility decline, and the latter reflects a fertility transition caused by socioeconomic development, such as increased family income, improvement of education, and promotion of social welfare services. While the urban fertility decline can be

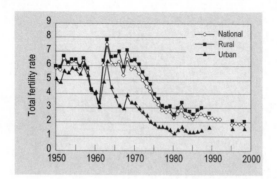

Figure 8.4. Differences in TFRs between urban and rural populations, 1950–2000. *Sources*: For 1950–1979, State Family Planning Commission (1982); for 1980–1988, State Family Planning Commission (1988); for 1989 and 1990, State Statistical Bureau (1993a); for 1991 and 1992, State Family Planning Commission (1992); for 1995, Office of Population Survey (1997); for 1998, State Statistical Bureau (1999) for urban and rural TFR; national TFR 1993, 1994, 1996–2000 estimated by Cao (2003).

interpreted as "natural," the rural fertility transition has been considered an "induced" decline. The rural population began its fertility transition from a level of 7.03 in 1968, which fell to 6.26 in 1969 and rose to 6.38 in 1970. After that year, the TFR in rural China declined rapidly with the full-scale implementation of family planning policies that began throughout China in 1971. Although the specific requirements of greater population control were not strictly adhered to during the 1970s, the rural TFR fell from 6.01 in 1971 to 3.05 in 1979. The TFR of rural China dropped to 2.48 in 1980, when the State Council put forward the strict family policy: only one child per couple. By 1995, the TFR of rural China had reached 2.0.

8.2.6 Fertility differentials by level of education

The association between a woman's education and her fertility is discussed extensively in Chapter 4 of this book. Here we focus only on the empirical data for rural and urban areas in China.

As can be seen in *Table 8.2*, in each age group there is an inverse relationship between fertility and level of education. In both urban and rural areas, a higher level of education is associated with a lower TFR. In China as a whole, the most dramatic change in fertility has occurred among women with a secondary or tertiary education. The TFR of women with no schooling is more than twice that of women with a tertiary education, and 1.5 times higher than that of women with a secondary

Table 8.2. Fertility differentials (total fertility rates) in China by education and urban/rural place of residence in 1990.

	Total	No schooling	Primary	Secondary	Tertiary
			Education		
China	2.29	2.96	2.52	1.99	1.32
Rural	2.58	3.00	2.59	2.43	1.59
Urban	1.59	2.55	2.08	1.48	1.31

Source: State Statistical Bureau (1991).

education. Thus, education appears to be an important factor influencing women's fertility, independent of the national family planning programs.

The Chinese experience has shown that education affects women's fertility by delaying marriage and thereby delaying a woman's entrance into her reproductive life. The age at first marriage is highly and positively correlated to education. According to the women's marriage survey in 1987 (Sha 1994, p. 72), the average age at first marriage was 25.89 years for women with a tertiary education, 23.05 years for women with a secondary education, 21.08 years for those with a primary education, and 20.14 years for women with no schooling. Women with a secondary or tertiary education are more likely to marry later and give birth to fewer children than their less-educated counterparts. Thus, educated women seem to use their human capital resources in the labor market while they reduce the time they allocate to familial roles, such as bearing and rearing children.

8.2.7 Fast-growing rural–urban migration

Since the mid-1980s, rural–urban migration has been an important factor in China's demographic change. A major consequence of the economic reforms in China has been a rise in population mobility. Rural–urban migration has become a dynamic force in the transition from a planned to a market-oriented economy.

Although there are numerous methodological problems in the classification of migration generally, the so-called floating rural laborers who move across provinces were estimated at around 56 million in the early 1990s (Jia and Meng 1996). Of these, 70–80 percent work in cities and other urban areas (Cai 1995). Thus, the number of rural migrant laborers in urban environments is estimated at approximately 45 million. Beijing, Shanghai, and Guangdong each host about 10 million migrants (Yang 1997). There are many socioeconomic reasons for this fast-growing rural–urban migration, most importantly the continuing population growth in rural areas, dramatic changes in the structure of agricultural production, and the rapidly growing urban economy.

Prior to 1978, the regional redistribution of the population resulted from the implementation of a traditional economic development strategy that made heavy industry a priority. This strategy created barriers for migration in two ways:

- Industrial growth by heavy industry created few employment opportunities to absorb surplus rural laborers.
- A planned labor force allocation made interregional and intersectoral migration impossible.

In addition, a household registration (*hukou*) system was introduced to prevent rural laborers from moving to cities. The *hukou* system, analogous to an internal passport system or a "green card" system, created different opportunities and constraints for holders of the urban and rural *hukou* status. Under the system, the rural population could not change their residential status and occupational identity as they liked. As a result, China's employment structure did not change in line with the changing composition of national economic output. While agricultural production dropped from 57.7 percent in 1952 to 32.8 percent in 1978, the agricultural labor force only decreased from 83.5 to 70.5 percent during that same period. Corresponding to this decrease in agricultural land was a rise in the level of urbanization: 17.9 percent in 1978 versus 12.5 percent in 1952. Since migration was strictly controlled, it was difficult for farmers to change their occupational identities and residential status. Hence, a large amount of surplus labor accumulated in the rural areas. Technological developments in agriculture, which made it less labor intensive, also contributed to the increase in rural unemployment and underemployment. According to estimates by the Population Institute of the Chinese Academy of Social Sciences, 32 percent of Chinese rural labor is surplus labor (Cai 1995). The differences between provinces are also substantial; the direction of migration appears to be from central and western China to the east, on top of the general rural–urban migration.

With the transition from a planned to a market-oriented economy, the household registration system in urban China has become a dual-track system, with a "planned" track and an "outside-of-planned" (or unofficial) track. In the planned track, rural–urban migration remains constrained by a highly controlled household registration system. Only *hukou* migration (i.e., migration with permanent residency rights) is considered to be planned migration. The scale of migration through the changing of permanent residence has not advanced enough to correct the distorted population distribution, so that unofficial migration has become a necessity. Migration without permanent residency rights is outside the state plans. Such migrants—the so-called floating population—are not supposed to stay in the area of destination permanently. However, the large unofficial migration actually plays a substantial role in the urban economy and the urbanization process. Urban industries demand low-wage labor from rural China in urban areas. Many construction companies hire their unskilled workers directly from rural areas. The booming towns and cities also offer numerous opportunities for rural laborers to start small private businesses within them.

8.3   Alternative Scenarios for China's Future

Chapters 2 and 3 of this book present probabilistic population projections for the China region up to 2100. This China region is broader than the mainland People's Republic of China in 1995 (i.e., without Hong Kong), which is the focus of this chapter. The China region in the global projections presented above also includes Cambodia, Laos, Mongolia, North Korea, Taiwan, Vietnam, and Hong Kong. Although China as defined in this chapter is home to almost 90 percent of the population of the China region, this difference in definition explains the difference in the aggregate population numbers presented in the different chapters of this book.

This chapter also presents very different kinds of population projections. Here, the aim is not to assess the aggregate level of uncertainty of the total population by age and sex. Instead, we delve much deeper into the structure of the population and produce projections that consider the differentiation by urban or rural place of residence and level of education, in addition to age and sex. Since we consider four educational categories and two residency categories (urban or rural), we have a total of eight subpopulations by age and sex projected independently (to provide for the possibility of moving among subpopulations), and we assume different age-specific fertility and migration schedules for each category.[1] This requires much more detailed empirical data for the starting conditions of the projections. Since these detailed data are not yet available from the 2000 census, we use data from the *National 1% Population Sample Survey 1995* (Office of Population Survey 1997) as the starting point. To estimate the fertility rates by level of education and urban or rural place of residence, we even had to use data from the 1990 national population census (State Statistical Bureau 1993a). In addition, information about migration, and especially estimates concerning the floating population, are derived from several special surveys.

A full account of the data sources used, the specific scenario assumptions made, and the detailed projection results is given in Cao (2003). Here, we only present selected findings for the year 2045, the end year of the projections, which start in 1995 and continue for 50 years.

---

[1]Mortality was assumed to be at the same level in all categories simply because no data on differentials were available.

Here, we make some comments about the assumed future fertility levels because of their overriding importance for the long-term population outlook, not only for China, but also for the world. Initial expectations in the 1980s were that Chinese fertility would continue to fall rapidly as a consequence of the government's highly successful anti-natalist policies. However, during the early 1990s there were some doubts as to whether these policies could actually be maintained under the conditions of rapid economic reform (Feeney 1996). These uncertainties, together with information about still-high desired family sizes in rural areas, led the population projections of the mid-1990s to assume that Chinese fertility would eventually increase to above 2.0 children (Lutz 1996; United Nations 1998). More recently, however, a number of important developments have suggested that long-term fertility in China will remain well below replacement level. The fertility decline now seems to have gained its own momentum and to be less dependent on strict government policies. Recent information indicates that fertility rates in some of the main urban areas are at incredibly low levels of around 1.0 or less. Also, survey information about desired family size shows strong declines among the younger generations. There are indications that, even in instances where the government has loosened its strict one-child family policy (e.g., when both prospective parents are single children themselves), such couples still overwhelmingly elect to have only one child. Finally, despite all economic liberalization, the government of China seems determined not to let fertility increase above the level of around 1.8 (personal communication with Jiang Zenghua, vice chairman of the People's Congress of China). All these new factors and arguments taken together allow us to assume that fertility in China will most likely remain below the replacement level for quite some time.

With the national population subdivided into eight categories, a large number of alternative scenarios can be defined for this interacting system, with a key question being the dependence or independence of the trends of the different subpopulations. As a pragmatic solution, we chose to define high (H), central (C), and low (L) scenarios for each subpopulation. These scenarios each reflect bundles of specific fertility, mortality, migration, and education scenarios, in which high education was combined with low fertility, low mortality, and low migration in the low scenario (L), and so on. This scenario was cross-classified with assumptions about the convergence of the fertility trends within educational groups. Hence, scenarios H2, C2, and L2 assume that women with different levels of education have similar levels of fertility by the end of the projection period, whereas scenarios H1, C1, and L1 assume that the relative magnitude of current educational fertility differentials is maintained. For rural–urban differentials no convergence is assumed, but two additional scenarios, C1m and H1m, are defined, which assume constant levels of rural–urban migration over the projection period. This was done because the

Table 8.3. China's total population and shares of urban and rural population under all eight scenarios, 2045.

Scenario	Assumptions	Urban (millions)	Rural (millions)	Total (millions)	Urban population (% of total)
Base-year population (1995)		344.22	860.36	1,204.57	28.58
Low scenario (L1)	No convergence	598.26	823.63	1,421.88	42.07
Central scenario (C1)	No convergence	701.65	778.47	1,480.12	47.40
High scenario (H1)	No convergence	946.96	620.87	1,567.83	60.40
Central scenario (C1m)	Constant migration	602.31	884.18	1,486.49	40.52
High scenario (H1m)	Constant migration	630.42	944.27	1,575.00	40.03
Low scenario (L2)	Convergence	597.45	849.86	1,447.31	41.28
Central scenario (C2)	Convergence	703.57	770.80	1,474.37	47.72
High scenario (H2)	Convergence	942.96	610.92	1,553.87	60.68

Source: Authors' calculations.

current estimate of rural–urban migration (around 1.3 million migrants per year) is significantly lower than the level assumed in the low scenario (an average of 5.1 million per year, compared with 10.5 million per year in the high scenario). These are only averages over the 50-year period, with the assumed trends being nonlinear. Again, all the specific numerical assumptions are presented and discussed in Cao (2003).

Table 8.3 gives the results for all eight scenarios in terms of the total, rural, and urban populations in 2045 and the proportions urban. The first line gives the situation for the base year (1995), when about 29 percent of China's 1.2 billion citizens lived in urban areas. Both China's total population and the proportion urban increase under all eight scenarios, but the scenarios show a considerable spread of alternative outcomes for the year 2045. The projected proportion urban for that year ranges from 40 to 60 percent of the total population. The 60 percent figure results from different versions of the high scenario, which are associated with a total population size of over 1.55 billion. This implies that under these scenarios the urban population of China in 2045 would be almost one billion, an increase by a factor of almost three from the current 344 million urban residents. The lowest rates of urbanization result from the constant migration scenarios, in which the urban population less than doubles and the total proportion urban is around 40 percent.

When these results of urbanization projections are compared with other projections, it must be kept in mind that the definition of what is an urban area has changed significantly over time. Here, we use the definition as given in the 1995

Table 8.4. Population (in millions) by level of education and urban or rural place of residence under the central scenario (C1), 2045.

	No education	Primary	Secondary	Tertiary	Total
Rural total	79	212	483	2	778
Males	33	85	256	1	376
Females	46	127	226	1	401
Urban total	45	94	490	71	701
Males	18	41	252	40	353
Females	27	52	237	31	348
China total	125	306	973	74	1,480
Males	52	127	508	41	729
Females	73	179	464	32	750

classification. Since then, it has changed in a way that classifies an additional 7 percent of the total population as urban.

The results for the rural population show a more diverse picture. Under six of the eight scenarios, the absolute size of the rural population declines from its current level of 860 million. The strongest declines result from the high scenarios, which also assume the highest migration. Under these scenarios, the number of people who live in rural areas will shrink by around 30 percent over the 50-year period. Only the two scenarios that assume constant rural–urban migration result in an increase of the total rural population by 3–10 percent. *Table 8.3* also shows that the assumption of convergence of educational fertility differentials has visible but minor impacts on total population size and proportions urban.

Table 8.4 gives the resultant educational distribution separately for rural and urban areas and for men and women. For space reasons, this is only done for the central scenario (C1). Among other things, *Table 8.4* clearly shows that major improvements in the average education of the population are expected not only in the urban areas, but also in the rural areas. While in the towns and cities of China some 80 percent of the population will have at least some secondary education, in the rural areas this figure will be about 60 percent under this scenario. *Table 8.4* also shows that the gender gap in education will remain higher in rural than in urban areas, although the difference is likely to diminish over time. Finally, the table shows that the population with a tertiary education is likely to live almost exclusively in urban areas.

Figure 8.5 gives the projected age pyramid by level of education for China's urban population in 2045 under scenario C1 (i.e., the central scenario assuming no convergence). In more detail than *Table 8.4*, it gives the age, sex, and education structure of the 701 million people who live in urban areas, corresponding to 47 percent of the total population of China under this scenario. This scenario implies that the young adult population between the ages of 20 and 40, both men and

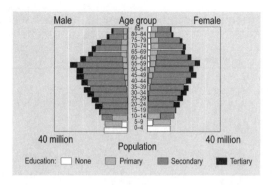

Figure 8.5. Population projection for urban China, 2045, central scenario. *Source*: Authors' calculations.

women, will universally have at least a secondary education. Urban inhabitants without any formal education can only be found in the 50 and older age groups and include significantly more women than men. This difference is particularly pronounced for women over the age of 60, a consequence of some gender bias in previous educational efforts. As we discuss in Chapter 4 of this book, however, this gender bias is much less pronounced in China than it is, for instance, in India.

The pyramid in *Figure 8.5* also shows that the urban population in 2045 will be significantly older than that in 1995 (see *Figure 8.3*). Actually, the largest age group in the entire urban population is likely to be the 55–59 age group. The youngest age groups are likely to be only half the size of that age group, which indicates a very significant degree of population aging. *Table 8.5* shows that under the central scenario, 30 percent of the urban population will be over age 60 in 2045. As we see from *Figure 8.5*, however, the cohorts over age 60 in 2045 are still relatively small, with the largest cohorts in the 40–60 age group. This implies that, beyond 2045, China will experience an acceleration of population aging, consistent with the probabilistic projections discussed in Chapter 3 of this volume.

Table 8.5 summarizes the age distributions for the urban, rural, and total populations under the L1, C1, and H1 scenarios (i.e., assuming no convergence). As expected, the proportion of children will be highest under the high scenario (H1) and lowest under the low scenario (L1). This holds for the urban and rural areas separately, although the difference is more significant for the rural areas. For the proportion over age 60, the pattern is the opposite. The low scenario for all areas results in more than 30 percent of the population over age 60, whereas under the high scenario this proportion is around 26 percent. The difference between urban and rural areas is most pronounced under the central scenario. Seen over the projection horizon, the proportion over age 60 is likely to increase by around a factor of three, for both the rural and urban areas. This is a very rapid and significant

Table 8.5. Age distribution under the low, central, and high scenarios, 2045.

		2045		
Age group	1995	Low scenario (L1)	Central scenario (C1)	High scenario (H1)
0–14				
Rural	28.72	17.28	19.74	25.86
Urban	21.76	10.34	11.21	13.74
Total	26.73	14.36	15.70	18.62
15–59				
Rural	61.29	52.08	52.43	48.16
Urban	67.64	58.43	58.65	59.67
Total	63.10	54.75	55.38	55.01
60+				
Rural	9.99	30.65	27.83	25.98
Urban	10.60	31.23	30.15	26.59
Total	10.17	30.89	28.93	26.37

Source: Authors' calculations.

population aging by any standard. The longer-range projection of Chapter 3 shows that this is not yet the end of the story: China is very likely to see further aging during the second half of the 21st century. The proportion over age 60 will likely reach around 40 percent, with the 80 percent prediction interval ranging from 27 to 53 percent for the whole China region.

8.4   Conclusions

The analysis in this chapter shows that the three remarkable structural changes in the Chinese population—the "revolutions" in education, urbanization, and family size—are all likely to continue into the future and even gain momentum. The analysis also shows that these three major transformations are linked directly to one another. This is why the simultaneous projection of the Chinese population by age, sex, education, and place of residence presented in this chapter not only is the first of its kind in a methodological sense, but is also highly important to understanding the dynamics of future population and human capital change in China.

China is clearly set to become one of the leading world powers in the 21st century. It will have not only a very large, but also a well-educated labor force. As discussed in Chapter 4, China will soon have more working-age men and women with a secondary or higher education than Europe and North America together. In addition, China is likely to see very rapid urbanization, with booming urban industry partly absorbing the great labor surplus in rural areas. And China will see very rapid population aging. While, over the coming few decades, China is still likely to benefit from the so-called demographic bonus—a combination of falling young-age dependency and still-low old-age dependency—the speed of aging will be daunting and require the development of social security systems that can replace the traditional exclusive support of the elderly by their children. With very low fertility and massive internal migration, an alternative to co-resident children clearly will have to be developed.

Not only will China be a superpower in terms of population and human capital, but the combination of rapid industrialization, growing per capita consumption, and the very large population will increasingly make China one of the world's leading contributors to global environmental change. This is the topic of Chapter 9.

References

Ahuja V & Filmer D (1995). Educational Attainment in Development Countries: New Estimates and Projections Disaggregated by Gender. Mimeo. Washington, DC, USA: The World Bank.

Cai F (1995). Determinants, trends and policies of population mobility in China. *Population Sciences of China* **6**:1–8.

Cao GY (2003). What Should We Say about the Level of Chinese Fertility from 1991 to 2000? Unpublished manuscript. Laxenburg, Austria: International Institute for Applied Systems Analysis.

Chan K (1997). *Studies on International Migration between City and Countryside in China*. Paper presented at the Symposium on Demography of China, October 1997. Beijing, China: China Population Association.

Cheng C & Maxim P (1992). Socioeconomic determinants of China's urban fertility. *Population and Environment* **14**:135.

China All Women's Federation (1991). *Statistics on Chinese Women, 1949–1989*. Beijing, China: China Statistical Press.

Chinese Ministry of Education (1984). *Data on Education, 1949–1981*. Beijing, China: China Encyclopedical Publishing House.

Chinese Ministry of Education (1998). *Education Statistical Yearbook of China 1998*. Beijing, China: China People's Education Statistical Publishing House.

Feeney G (1996). Fertility in China: Past, present, prospects. In *The Future Population of the World. What Can We Assume Today?*, Revised Edition, Ed. Lutz W, pp. 102–130. London, UK: Earthscan.

Jia S & Meng X (1996). The projection on China's labor force. *Population Sciences of China* **6**:26–30.

Liu J (1989). *Review on the Educational Policies*. Beijing, China: Institute of Population Studies, Chinese Academy of Social Sciences.

Lutz W (1996). *The Future Population of the World. What Can We Assume Today?*, Revised Edition. London, UK: Earthscan.

Office of Population Survey, State Statistical Bureau of China (1997). *National 1% Population Sample Survey 1995*. Beijing, China: China Statistical Press.

Population Institute, Chinese Academy of Social Sciences (1985). *China Population Yearbook 1985*. Beijing, China: Social Sciences Press.

Sha G (1994). *Studies on Population during the Economic Transition*. Beijing, China: Beijing University Press.

State Family Planning Commission (1982). *One-per-thousand Sample Survey on Fertility*. Beijing, China: State Family Planning Commission.

State Family Planning Commission (1988). *Two-per-thousand Sample Survey on Fertility and Contraceptives*. Beijing, China: State Family Planning Commission.

State Family Planning Commission (1992). *Population Sample Survey*. Beijing, China: State Family Planning Commission.

State Statistical Bureau (1986). *Bulletin of the 1964 Population Census*, Reprint. Beijing, China: China Statistical Press.

State Statistical Bureau (1991). *10 Percent Sampling Tabulation on the 1990 Population Census of the People's Republic of China, 1991*. Beijing, China: China Statistical Press.

State Statistical Bureau (1993a). *National Population Census 1990*. Beijing, China: China Statistical Press.

State Statistical Bureau (1993b). *China Statistical Yearbook 1993*. Beijing, China: China Statistical Press.

State Statistical Bureau (1995). *China Statistical Yearbook 1995*. Beijing, China: China Statistical Press.

State Statistical Bureau (1996) *China Statistical Yearbook 1996*. Beijing, China: China Statistical Press.

State Statistical Bureau (1998). *China Statistical Yearbook 1998*. Beijing, China: China Statistical Press.

State Statistical Bureau (1999). *China Population Statistics 1999*. Beijing, China: China Statistical Press.

United Nations (1998). *World Population Prospects. The 1996 Revision*. ST/ESA/SER.A/167. New York, NY, USA: United Nations, Department of Economic and Social Affairs, Population Division.

United Nations (2001). *World Urbanization Prospects. The 1999 Revision*. ST/ESA/SER.A/194. New York, NY, USA: United Nations, Department of Economic and Social Affairs, Population Division.

Wang Y (1991). *Rural Fertility in the Perspective of Family Economics*. Beijing, China: Institute of Population Studies, Chinese Academy of Social Sciences.

Yang Y (1997). *The Challenge of Unemployment*. Beijing, China: China Today Press.

Yao X & Yin H (1995). *Basic Data of China's Population*. Beijing, China: China Population Press.

Chapter 9

Population, Greenhouse Gas Emissions, and Climate Change

Brian C. O'Neill, F. Landis MacKellar, and Wolfgang Lutz

9.1 Introduction

The threat of human-induced climate change, popularly known as global warming, presents a difficult challenge to society over the coming decades. The production of so-called greenhouse gases (GHGs) as a result of human activity, mainly the burning of fossil fuels (e.g., coal, oil, and natural gas), is expected to lead to a generalized warming of the Earth's surface, rising sea levels, and changes in precipitation patterns. The potential impacts of these changes are many and varied—more frequent and intense heat waves, changes in the frequency of droughts and floods, increased coastal flooding, and more-damaging storm surges—all with attendant consequences for human health, agriculture, economic activity, biodiversity, and ecosystem functioning.

Since the impacts of climate change are expected to be global and potentially severe, and because energy production from fossil fuels is a fundamental component of the world economy, the stakes in the issue are high. At the same time, a number of aspects of climate change complicate the problem:

- First, while much is known about the factors that govern climate, considerable uncertainty remains in projections of the extent of climate change, of how severe the impacts will be, and of how costly it would be to reduce GHG emissions.

- Second, because the impacts of today's GHG emissions will be felt for decades into the future, it is not possible to wait and see how severe impacts will turn out to be before taking preventive action. Therefore, if emissions are reduced now, the costs will be borne in the near term while the (uncertain) benefits will be realized largely in the long term.

- Third, sources of GHG emissions are dispersed widely among nations: no single country could reduce future global climate change significantly just by reducing its own emissions. Even reductions in the more developed nations as a group, which have been responsible for the bulk of historical emissions, would not lead to a stabilization of atmospheric concentrations of GHGs. Any solution to the problem must eventually be global.

In this chapter, we briefly review the principal anthropogenic GHGs, the distribution of current sources, and the projections of future emissions trends. We then use population projections from the International Institute for Applied Systems Analysis (IIASA) to perform a simple sensitivity analysis intended to illustrate how the potential effect of different population paths on future emissions compares to the potential effect of factors that might alter per capita emissions rates. This analysis illustrates how changes in age structure and interactions between population growth rates and economic growth rates could affect our conclusions on climate change. We also summarize how changes in population growth rates might affect the ability of societies to adapt to climate change impacts, before concluding with thoughts on the implications of these results for links between climate change and population policy.

9.2   Climate Change and Greenhouse Gas Emissions

The most important anthropogenic GHGs are carbon dioxide (CO_2), methane (CH_4), nitrous oxide (N_2O), and halocarbons. *Table 9.1* summarizes some key characteristics of these gases. After water vapor, CO_2 is the second most important gas that produces the Earth's natural greenhouse effect. Direct measurements of atmospheric CO_2 over the past several decades, as well as measurements obtained from older air trapped in ice sheets, show that CO_2 concentrations have increased about 30 percent from their pre-industrial level, higher than at any time in the past 420,000 years (Petit *et al.* 1999). This increase has been driven by emissions from the burning of fossil fuels, as well as by changes in land use (principally deforestation) that release carbon to the atmosphere at a rate that accounts for about one-third

Table 9.1. Summary of main anthropogenic greenhouse gases.

Gas	Concentration (ppbv)[a]		Current growth (%/yr)	Lifetime[b] (yrs)	100-year global warming potential relative to CO_2
	Pre-industrial	1998			
CO_2	~278,000	365,000	0.5	~100 (50–75%)[c] $>10^4$ (25–50%)	1
CH_4	~700	1,745	0.4	12	23
N_2O	~270	314	0.3	114	296
CFC-12[d]	0	0.533	0.8	100	10,600

[a]Parts per billion by volume.
[b] Lifetime is defined as the average length of time a present emission will continue to affect atmospheric concentrations.
[c] From O'Neill *et al.* (1997). The response of the atmosphere to a CO_2 emission has a distinctly dual nature: at least half the effect of the emission is removed in about 100 years, while the remainder persists for tens of thousands of years or more. The exact fractions and timescales of persistence depend on the assumed future concentration scenario.
[d] CFC-12 is used here as a representative example of the chlorofluorocarbons, an important subclass of the halocarbons.
Sources: Ehhalt *et al.* (2001) and Ramaswamy *et al.* (2001), except as indicated in the notes.

of total CO_2 emissions (Houghton 2003). Carbon dioxide is removed from the atmosphere at a range of timescales. While half the effect of an emission is removed in a few decades, one-quarter to one-half the effect is essentially permanent on timescales relevant to climate change policy (O'Neill *et al.* 1997).

Methane also contributes to the Earth's natural greenhouse effect and is emitted from a range of natural sources, most notably as a product of anaerobic respiration in wetlands. However, current anthropogenic sources are estimated to account for more than half of total emissions and have led to more than a doubling of pre-industrial atmospheric CH_4 concentrations. Methane is released from a wide array of human activities, including raising livestock such as cattle and sheep (whose digestive systems use fermentation processes that produce CH_4), leakage from natural gas pipelines and coal mines, anaerobic respiration in rice paddies, and biomass burning, with a handful of other sources also contributing (Ehhalt *et al.* 2001). Methane has a relatively short atmospheric lifetime of about 12 years; its effect on climate is therefore shorter lived than that of CO_2.

Concentrations of N_2O have increased more than 15 percent through human activity. Sources of N_2O have not been well quantified, but the largest natural fluxes to the atmosphere are thought to be from soils (particularly in tropical forests), with a smaller but significant contribution from the oceans. Anthropogenic sources are estimated to be about two-thirds as large as natural sources and are dominated by fluxes from nitrogen-fertilized agricultural fields (Smil 1999), with additional contributions from a number of other sources including biomass burning, some industrial processes, and cattle and feed lots (Ehhalt *et al.* 2001). Nitrous oxide has a relatively long lifetime of about 120 years.

Halocarbons comprise a number of chlorine-, fluorine-, or bromine-containing gases with generally powerful heat-trapping properties. Halocarbons include chlorofluorocarbons (CFCs) and related compounds, such as hydrochlorofluorocarbons (HCFCs), hydrofluorocarbons (HFCs), and perfluorocarbons (PFCs), as well as carbon tetrachloride, sulfur hexafluoride (SF_6), and methyl chloroform. Historically, CFCs have been the most important halocarbons in terms of their warming effect. CFCs have no natural sources; they are synthetic compounds used as refrigerants, propellants, blowing agents in the manufacture of foams, and cleaning agents in the production of electronic components, and they have lifetimes of 50 years or more. They are the main culprits in stratospheric ozone (O_3) depletion. As O_3 is itself a GHG, this depletion offsets some of the warming effect of the CFCs. Emissions of CFCs have fallen as the industrialized nations, which are responsible for most of the global total, have complied with the Montreal Protocol on Substances that Deplete the Ozone Layer and its amendments to phase out production of these chemicals. However, while the HCFCs and HFCs often used as replacements are less efficient O_3 depleters, they are still effective GHGs.

As just mentioned, O_3 is also a GHG. Although about 90 percent of total O_3 is present in the stratosphere, tropospheric O_3 also has an important effect on climate. This "low-level" O_3 is produced through the oxidation of CH_4, as well as through reactions that involve a number of precursor gases (e.g., carbon monoxide, nitrogen oxides, and non-CH_4 hydrocarbons), which are themselves produced in part by human activities such as biomass burning and fossil fuel combustion. In addition, O_3 is transported into the troposphere from the stratosphere. Production and destruction processes vary widely through space and time, so O_3 concentrations vary with geographic location, altitude, season, and even time of day, which makes estimation of global trends difficult. Available measurements and modeling studies suggest that tropospheric O_3 concentrations in the Northern Hemisphere, where anthropogenic sources are largest, may have doubled since pre-industrial times. Globally averaged, the increase has been about 35 percent (Ehhalt *et al.* 2001), although there is high uncertainty in this estimate and the effects from O_3 are highly regional.

Since the GHGs have different lifetimes and heat-trapping properties, changes in their abundances affect the Earth's energy balance to different degrees. *Table 9.1* shows their 100-year global warming potentials (GWPs), an index that takes into account the different lifetimes of the gases by measuring the cumulative warming effect (radiative forcing) each would contribute over a 100-year period after equal-weight emissions. The values in *Table 9.1* show that, ton for ton, CO_2 emissions will contribute much less to radiative forcing over the next century than will emissions of other GHGs. This comparison should be viewed with some caution because GWPs are subject to a number of uncertainties and are sensitive to, among other things, the choice of time horizon and the future atmospheric concentrations of GHGs (O'Neill 2000; Smith and Wigley 2000). Despite the relatively high GWPs of the other gases, CO_2 is responsible for most of the warming effect that results from the current excess concentrations of all GHGs, since the atmospheric CO_2 level has undergone a much greater absolute increase than have the levels of other gases. For the same reason, its share of responsibility for GHG forcing is expected to grow in the future, although the aggregate warming effect of the other gases is expected to be significant as well.

Any climate change induced by the accumulation of anthropogenic GHGs occurs against a background of changes caused by a number of other factors. Some of these factors amplify greenhouse warming, while others may offset part of it. Some may, at different times, do both. For example, aerosols are small airborne particles that both absorb and reflect radiation and therefore can affect climate directly. They can also affect climate indirectly by altering cloud cover. Aerosols are emitted naturally and by human activity, either as particles or as gases that eventually form droplets. Natural sources include soil dust and spray from the oceans; the most important anthropogenic aerosols are sulfates formed from sulfur dioxide gas produced by the combustion of fossil fuels. Incomplete fuel combustion and burning of biomass also contribute significant aerosol fluxes in the form of soot and organic carbon (Penner *et al.* 2001). Different aerosols are thought to have different net effects on climate. Soot from the burning of fossil fuels is estimated to exert a positive forcing, while aerosols from the burning of biomass and from sulfur emissions are thought to have a cooling effect. Taken together, aerosols are thought to exert a cooling effect on climate and therefore may mask some of the effect of GHGs. Since they generally spend just a few days in the troposphere before returning to the surface in rainfall or through dry deposition, aerosols are not distributed uniformly in the atmosphere, but are concentrated near source regions (such as heavily industrialized areas). Their climate effect is therefore also regional, which makes it difficult to determine their global contribution to the enhanced greenhouse effect. It is estimated that anthropogenic aerosols may exert a direct cooling effect that is, on average, about 20 percent as large as the warming effect of GHGs released through human activity. However, indirect effects (e.g., on cloud reflectivity) could exert a cooling effect up to four times larger than the direct effects of aerosols, although the uncertainty in these effects is very large (Ramaswamy *et al.* 2001).

A number of natural factors affect climate as well, including strong volcanic eruptions, which inject large amounts of sulfurous gases into the stratosphere, where they are transformed into sulfate aerosols that can lead to a cooling of the climate for several years (Minnis *et al.* 1993). The sun's output varies slightly over an

11-year cycle associated with sunspots, and presumably over longer time periods
as well. While many researchers have proposed and investigated potential mechanisms that could amplify this small solar forcing into significant climate effects,
none are considered well established (Ramaswamy *et al.* 2001). In addition, even if
climate were not being influenced by any human activities whatsoever, it would still
vary from year to year, decade to decade, and even from one century to the next.
This natural variability may be caused by external influences, such as solar variability or volcanic eruptions, but it may also arise from complicated internal couplings
between different parts of the climate system. For example, links between atmospheric and oceanic circulation can produce variations in climate over a time scale
of years or decades. A well-known example is the so-called El Niño–Southern Os-
cillation (ENSO), a periodic change in the temperature of eastern Pacific surface
waters that occurs on average every 4.5 years, within a range of 2–10 years, as
a result of complex interactions with the atmosphere. Although natural variability could amplify or dampen human-driven climate change from year to year or
from one decade to the next, it is not likely to reverse the long-term trend toward a
warmer climate expected to occur as a result of rising concentrations of GHGs.

9.2.1   The distribution of current greenhouse gas emissions

Current and historical emissions of GHGs have been dominated by the production
of CO_2 from fossil fuel use, primarily in the more developed countries (MDCs).
However, when considering other sources of CO_2, as well as emissions of other
GHGs, emissions are distributed much more evenly between developed and developing regions.

Table 9.2 shows that, in 2000, MDCs emitted 5.2 billion tons (gigatons) of
carbon equivalent (GtCeq) GHGs, while less developed countries (LDCs) emitted
slightly more, at 5.5 GtCeq. LDCs are a larger source of CH_4 emissions and CO_2
emissions from land-use change than are MDCs, which more than compensates
for the MDC dominance of fossil fuel CO_2 emissions. Current emissions are not
necessarily the best indicator of contributions to warming effects, however, since
GHGs accumulate in the atmosphere over time and the climate system responds
with some delay to increases in GHG forcing. When measured in terms of contribution to temperature change, which integrates the effects of current and past
emissions, as well as the differences in warming effects across gases, estimates of
the MDC contribution range from about 60 to 75 percent (Den Elzen and Schaeffer
2002).

Table 9.2 highlights an additional difference between emissions patterns in the
two regions: MDCs are high emitters per capita and low emitters per unit gross
domestic product (GDP), while the situation is reversed in LDCs. In per capita
terms, the average MDC resident emits (so to speak) over three times more GHGs

Table 9.2. Estimated annual greenhouse gas emissions in gigatons carbon equivalent (GtCeq) by world region in 2000. Results are shown for two different regional breakdowns: four world regions and two world regions (MDCs/LDCs).[a]

Gas	OECD[b]	Eastern Europe & FSU[c]	Asia	Africa & Latin America	MDCs	LDCs
CO_2	3.20	0.91	2.03	1.83	4.11	3.86
Fossil fuels	3.20	0.91	1.78	1.01	4.11	2.79
Land use	0.00	0.00	0.26	0.82	0.00	1.07
N_2O	0.21	0.05	0.21	0.10	0.25	0.31
CH_4	0.46	0.24	0.79	0.53	0.71	1.32
HFCs/PFCs/SF_6	0.09	0.01	0.02	0.01	0.11	0.03
Total	3.96	1.21	3.04	2.48	5.18	5.52
Per capita	4.31	2.90	0.93	1.63	3.87	1.16
Per unit GDP	0.19	1.46	1.12	0.93	0.24	1.03

[a] Emissions of non-CO_2 gases are converted to units of GtCeq using 100-year global warming potentials from Ramaswamy *et al.* (2001). Units for per capita emissions are tCeq per person. Units for emissions per unit GDP are tCeq per US$1,000 GDP, in 1990 US$. The OECD region is defined by the group of member countries as of 1990.
[b] Organisation for Economic Co-operation and Development members in the Pacific region.
[c] European part of the former Soviet Union.
Source: Nakicenovic *et al.* (2000).

than the average LDC resident. Per capita emissions in MDCs are high because of the high level of economic production per capita. On the other hand, each unit of economic output produced in the MDCs contributes to global warming less than one-fourth as much as a unit of economic output produced in the LDCs.

Data for aggregated regions obscure variation within regions. For example, per capita emissions of CO_2 from energy use are twice as high in North America as in Europe, and twice as high in China and Latin America as in the rest of the developing world. Emissions related to deforestation are not spread evenly throughout the LDCs, but are concentrated heavily in a small number of countries (e.g., Brazil). Aggregated data also hide extremes. For example, per capita CO_2 emissions in the United States, one of the better-off and most energy-intensive MDCs, are 200 times higher than those in Bangladesh, one of the poorest LDCs. Within countries, there is further heterogeneity between rich and poor and between rural and urban regions (Murthy *et al.* 1997).

9.2.2   Future greenhouse gas emissions

Projecting future climate change begins with projecting GHG emissions, an exercise that must take into account a large number of factors, including population and economic growth, technological change, energy supply and prices, and land-use patterns. Future trends in these factors are highly uncertain, so the most common approach is to define a range of scenarios for each. When combined in different ways, these different underlying assumptions produce a range of GHG emissions scenarios that are not predictions of the future, but instead answer "what if?" questions about possible future emissions rates. Models of the GHG cycles are then used to translate the emissions projections into a range of future GHG concentrations. In turn, the concentration scenarios are used to drive climate models and produce a range of possible climate effects.

The most recent set of long-term emissions scenarios was produced by the Intergovernmental Panel on Climate Change (IPCC). The writing team for the *Special Report on Emissions Scenarios* (SRES) defined four "storylines" for future scenarios and quantified the basic driving forces for each storyline (see below). A number of modeling teams used the storylines and driving-force scenarios to produce scenarios of GHG emissions. Results revealed a wide range of possible futures, with CO_2 emissions in 2100 varying from 3 to 35 GtC over the full range of scenarios and models. The variation in all GHG emissions, when converted into radiative forcing of climate and used as input for climate models, produced changes in global average surface temperature by 2100 that ranged from 1.4 to 5.8°C. About half that range results from uncertainty in the future emissions path (i.e., assuming no policies to reduce climate change are put in place), and the other half resulted from uncertainty in the response of the climate system. Broadly speaking, demographic change, changes in economic output, and changes in the GHG intensity of the global economy are the forces that drive GHG emissions. Each of these is, in turn, influenced by a number of important indirect variables.

9.3   Population and Greenhouse Gas Emissions

Most analyses of the role of population in GHG emissions have taken the approach of applying the "I=PAT" (see discussion below) framework to historical or projected trends in emissions and driving forces, and decomposing emissions into contributions from various factors. However, this approach suffers from a number of serious flaws. Below, we briefly review I=PAT decompositions and conclude that these flaws make them of limited value. We then discuss alternative ways to investigate demographic influences on emissions and illustrate the sensitivity analysis approach, in which alternative emissions scenarios that differ by the assumptions for one or more variables are compared using a simple model that combines assumptions about population growth and age structure, economic growth, and technological change. We consider first the direct scale effect of population on GHG emissions. We then modify the model to explore the role of households, as distinct from individuals, in generating emissions and to examine indirect effects such as the possible link between the rate of population growth and the rate of growth of per capita GDP.

9.3.1 I=PAT decompositions

A method commonly used to evaluate the contributions of population growth or other demographic factors to energy use and CO_2 emissions is the decomposition of emissions rates into components caused by each of several "driving forces" of emissions. Decompositions have been performed on national and regional data on historical emissions, on scenarios of future emissions, and on cross-sectional data to decompose differences in emissions among countries or regions. All such decompositions begin with a multiplicative identity that describes emissions as the product of two or more driving forces. These identities are all variations of the well-known I=PAT equation as applied to CO_2 emissions. I=PAT describes the environmental impact (I) of human activities as the product of three factors: population size (P), affluence (A), and technology (T). It was developed in the early 1970s during the course of a debate between Barry Commoner and Paul Ehrlich and John Holdren. Commoner argued that environmental impacts in the United States were caused primarily by changes in production technology following World War II, while Ehrlich and Holdren argued that all three factors were important and emphasized in particular the role of population growth (O'Neill 2001).

9.3.2 Identity versus explanation

Since the early 1970s, I=PAT has been employed by many researchers in the analysis of a wide range of environmental issues in all regions of the world, including automobile pollution (Commoner 1991), fertilizer use (Harrison 1992), energy (Pearce 1991), air quality (Cramer 1998), and land use (Waggoner and Ausubel 2001), to name just a few. Formulating analyses in terms of an I=PAT-type identity has several benefits. Perhaps the most important is that it serves as a useful orienting perspective, simplifying the conceptualization of environmental impacts by dividing driving forces into a small number of broad categories. For example, CO_2 emissions are often expressed as the result, broadly speaking, of four general categories in what is known in the climate change literature as the Kaya identity (Kaya 1990):

$$C = P \times \frac{GDP}{P} \times \frac{E}{GDP} \times \frac{C}{E}, \qquad (9.1)$$

where C is carbon emissions per year, P is population size, GDP is GDP, and E is total energy use. This identity expresses CO_2 emissions as the product of population, per capita economic production (taken to be equal to per capita income), the amount of energy produced per unit of economic production (energy intensity), and the amount of carbon emitted per unit of energy produced (carbon intensity). Each category encapsulates a subset of influences. For example, energy intensity reflects the structure of an economy (a service-oriented economy will generally be less energy intensive than an economy in the early stages of industrialization) and the efficiency of its energy system. Carbon intensity reflects the fuel mix of the energy system, in particular the share of renewables and the reliance on carbon-intensive coal or less carbon-intensive natural gas.

The I=PAT formulation also illustrates an important consequence of the multiplicative relationship between driving forces: each variable amplifies changes in any other. As a result, a given change in technology may have only a small absolute effect on emissions in a society with a small, low-income population, while the same change would have a much greater effect in a populous, affluent society. Likewise, a given increment in population would have a much greater impact in affluent societies than in low-income countries, assuming similar levels of technology.

Despite these benefits, I=PAT has been criticized strongly for a number of perceived flaws. Although as an identity it is always true by definition, when it is used as an explanatory model it assumes implicitly that there are only three relevant variables (or four in the case of the Kaya identity), all related in a simple linear fashion. Critics assert that its lack of social science content, particularly the influence of policies and institutions on environmental outcomes, render it misleading at best. Some researchers have suggested that the P, A, and T variables be thought of as proximate (direct) causes of environmental impact, which are themselves influenced by a wide range of indirect, but more fundamental, ultimate causes that include income distribution, land-management practices, urban–rural settlement patterns, prices, political empowerment, trade relations, attitudes and preferences, and wars (Shaw 1989; Harrison 1994). These factors may be critical to environmental outcomes and differ widely across settings, which makes the equation ill-suited to analysis at the micro level and casts doubt on the results of larger-scale studies. Nonetheless, that data for the P, A, and T variables are generally available across a range of settings has invited widespread use of I=PAT for cross-site studies and studies at large spatial and temporal scales.

9.3.3 Decompositions

The I=PAT model was developed to quantify arguments that sought to apportion responsibility for environmental impacts among contributing factors, and has been widely used for this purpose ever since. The goal in such exercises is to rank the importance of the P, A, and T variables, usually to prioritize policy recommendations for reducing impacts. However, such exercises suffer from a long list of mathematical ambiguities inherent to decomposing index numbers (such as the I in

I=PAT), which makes the results difficult, if not impossible, to compare (MacKellar *et al.* 1998; O'Neill *et al.* 2001). These ambiguities also have allowed attacks on the methods of quantitative analysis to fuel wider debates without bringing them closer to resolution.

A fundamental problem is that there are a number of ways to perform the decomposition, and each method leads to a different result. In the initial Ehrlich–Holdren–Commoner exchanges, for example, the decomposition method used was a comparison of the ratios of final to initial values of each of the variables over a given time period. A problem with this approach is that the changes in the driving forces do not add up to the change in impact, which confounded attempts to divide up blame for I among P, A, and T. To circumvent this problem, first Commoner (1972) and later Holdren (1991) and many subsequent researchers converted the multiplicative I=PAT relation into an additive one based on average annual growth rates over a given time period. The contribution of each factor was expressed as the ratio of its own growth rate to the growth rate of I. This growth-rate decomposition methodology has been applied to data on GHG emissions by several researchers. Probably the most widely cited study is that of Bongaarts (1992), who concluded that 50 percent of the growth in global CO_2 emissions from fossil fuels between 1985 and 2025 resulted from population growth. Over the entire simulation period (1985–2100), population growth accounted for 35 percent of growth in CO_2 emissions. Other authors (Holdren 1991; Harrison 1992; MacKellar *et al.* 1995) used the same method on similar data sets and arrived at a range of conclusions on the contribution of population growth to growth in energy consumption or GHG emissions.

Yet another approach to I=PAT decompositions is to judge the relative importance of variables according to their effect on impact growth over the entire period. One method, which has been applied to CO_2 emissions (Bartiaux and van Ypersele 1993) and CH_4 emissions (Heilig 1994), is to freeze the variable of interest at its initial value and calculate how much the growth in total impact is reduced as a result. An alternative, which has been applied to energy demand (Howarth *et al.* 1991; Ang 1993) and CO_2 emissions (Moomaw and Tullis 1998), is to freeze all variables except the one of interest and calculate the resultant change in growth in impact.

Each of these methods produces different results. There is, in fact, no single correct method. Decomposing I=PAT belongs to a larger class of problems related to index numbers for which results are influenced by several factors (Fisher 1922; MacKellar *et al.* 1998; O'Neill *et al.* 2001). We review a few of the problems here, but this list is not exhaustive.[1]

---

[1] Additional issues are the choice of variables, approximation methods, and alternative normalizations. For a full discussion see MacKellar *et al.* (1998) and O'Neill *et al.* (2001).

Heterogeneity

The level of aggregation at which an analysis is performed can influence the results strongly. If population growth and per capita environmental impact are negatively correlated, as is the general case with GHG emissions, calculations at the global level generally assign a larger proportion of the blame to population growth than do more disaggregated analyses (Lutz 1993). The global view overlooks that population growth is generally fastest where per capita impact is lowest. On the other hand, if per capita impact is positively correlated with population growth, as, for example, in the case of land degradation caused by fuelwood harvesting, a large-scale analysis underestimates the role of population.

The Offset Problem

Decomposition exercises become particularly difficult to interpret when not all the variables move in the same direction. For example, if there are three variables on the right-hand side of the equation and one shrinks over the time period in question, the contribution of one of the growing variables is offset, and so the third variable apparently accounts for a very large proportion of total environmental impact. This problem often arises in decomposing CO_2 emissions trends, since carbon intensity of GDP (the product of energy intensity and carbon intensity of energy supply) is projected to fall in most regions of the world while both population and income are expected to rise. Many authors (Holdren 1991; Bongaarts 1992; MacKellar *et al.* 1995; Raskin 1995) sidestep the problem by collapsing carbon intensity and income into a single, more slowly growing "per capita emissions" term; however, this approach artificially inflates the importance of population and discards important information about the more rapid trends of consumption growth and declining resource use per unit output.

Interaction between Variables

Even the earliest users of the I=PAT equation explicitly recognized that it made the simplifying assumption that P, A, and T behaved independently. Arguments have since been made for the existence of bi-directional relationships among all the variables. A few studies have tested the I=PAT relationship as applied to CO_2 emissions against national-level data. Dietz and Rosa (1997), in a multiple regression analysis on 1989 data for 111 countries, found that the impact of population size on emissions was roughly linear, and if anything became disproportionately large for the most populous nations. Affluence also had a roughly proportional effect on emissions up to a transition point around US$10,000 per capita, beyond which its influence stabilized or even declined. DeCanio (1992) also estimated an I=PAT-type model, based on cross-sectional data from the late 1980s, to examine the sensitivity of emissions to alternative scenarios for per capita income. Regression analysis indicated an inverted U-shaped relationship between per capita emissions and per capita income, with the turning point at around US$17,000 per capita.

Implausible Scenario Comparison

All decomposition exercises aimed at producing policy-relevant results suffer from the shortcoming that they do not take into account how much change in a particular variable is plausible. Instead, they estimate the contribution of one variable to total impact by implicitly comparing a particular set of data to a hypothetical scenario in which that variable remains constant at its initial level. While this may shed light on the narrower (but still important) question of the source of absolute changes in environmental impact, decomposition results do not necessarily translate directly into priorities for intervention. From a policy point of view, it is much more relevant to ask how much a realistic scenario change for one variable, relative to a baseline path, would change the impact over a given period of time. Realistic alternative scenarios account for, among other things, momentum built into population age structures that make immediate population stabilization impossible, as well as momentum in technological systems and patterns of consumption.

9.3.4 Population and emissions scenarios

An alternative to decomposing historical or projected trends in emissions is to assess the role of population by analyzing alternative scenarios for future emissions. Sets of scenarios can be generated from alternative assumptions about exogenous variables, or alternative model parameters or structures. Comparing results can provide insight into the importance to emissions of particular demographic factors and their links to other variables. Scenario analysis avoids the mathematical ambiguity inherent to decomposition exercises, and the interpretation of results is, in this sense, more straightforward. Yet it is potentially subject to some of the same problems that plague decompositions—heterogeneity bias, the treatment of interactions between variables, and interpretations of the plausibility of alternative scenarios—so transparent assumptions regarding these aspects of the analysis are essential. In addition, scenario analysis can be carried out with different levels of complexity, and several aspects of the methodology must be taken into consideration in interpreting results.

For example, the starting point for investigations into this topic is usually what Keyfitz (1992) called the "direct scale effect of population"—that is, all else being equal, a larger (smaller) population will require more (less) energy and therefore lead to more (less) GHG emissions. This is obviously the simplest approach, and it is a logical starting point for more complex analyses. While simple, the approach can still take into account a number of fundamental issues, including heterogeneity (by sufficiently disaggregating the population of interest), inertia, and other dynamics of demographic, economic, and technological systems (by employing realistic scenarios for each of these factors).

A second methodological aspect is to consider other demographic factors in an internally consistent manner. If other demographic factors, in addition to size, matter to emissions (age structure or urban–rural distributions are good examples), the effects of all these factors should be taken into account in an internally consistent manner. For example, a low population growth path generally implies a more rapidly aging population. It may also be likely to be associated with more rapid urbanization. Knowledge of how different demographic factors are related to one another can be taken advantage of by considering their joint effects on emissions.

Third, there may be relationships between demographic variables, such as population size, growth rate, or age structure, and other proximate determinants of emissions, or driving forces, such as the growth rate and scale of economic output, energy intensity, or technical progress. This complicates the analysis of the role of demographics in emissions, because demographics contribute both directly and indirectly (through their effect on other factors) to emissions trends. However, to the extent these links are understood, they can contribute importantly to gauging more realistically the likely effect of an alternative population path on emissions—here, the "all else being equal" restriction is eased.

Finally, demographic factors may themselves be influenced by other variables. Some of these include other factors typically considered driving forces, such as economic growth (defining a dynamic system with bi-directional influences). However, one can also easily imagine a set of factors that simultaneously influence population and one or more additional driving forces. Globalization is one example. It may well be the case that increasing the interdependence of economies around the world would provide a boost to economic growth while also accelerating the diffusion of new technologies and speeding up fertility declines by facilitating the spread of modern ideas about lifestyles, the role of women, and desired family size. Another example might be population-related policies such as female basic education. While this type of socially desirable policy is not motivated by its demographic effects, it would likely lead to lower fertility; in addition, it probably would also affect economic growth by increasing the supply of human capital. In cases such as these, the question is no longer, What would be the effect of an alternative population path on emissions?, but rather, To what extent are particular population paths likely to be associated with particular paths for other driving forces, and hence emissions? The answer to the latter question depends on assumptions made about the range of other factors presumed to influence the driving forces, either directly or indirectly.

A comprehensive, quantitative analysis of demographics and emissions therefore requires the quantification of an extensive set of direct and indirect connections among demographic, socioeconomic, and technological variables, and a thorough analysis of the emissions outcomes that result from possible alternative futures. Such an exercise could lead to broad conclusions about the kinds of emissions paths most likely to be associated with different population scenarios. No such analysis has been carried out, and it cannot be attempted here in a single chapter. Instead, we first discuss the most comprehensive emissions scenario analysis yet produced, the SRES from the IPCC (Nakicenovic *et al.* 2000). While the SRES does not focus on demographic factors per se, it demonstrates the current state of the art in incorporating population variables in emissions scenarios and illustrates how such an analysis could be carried out to answer specific questions related to demographics. Next, we perform our own sensitivity analysis to illustrate the simpler aspects of population–emissions analyses aimed at examining the likely effect of alternative population paths, taking into account the direct scale effect of population, internally consistent considerations of aging and its effect on household size, and possible links between variables. We leave for future work any attempt to quantify a more extensive set of links that could account for broad socioeconomic factors driving simultaneous changes in the proximate determinants of emissions.

9.3.5   Population and emissions in the SRES

Faced with links between variables that are too uncertain to quantify, the SRES took a partially qualitative approach. A set of narrative "storylines" about the future were developed, each with a particular internal logic by which combinations of driving forces were associated with one another. The storylines were quantified by deciding on common paths for fundamental variables, such as population and economic growth rates. Independent modeling teams, using six models representative of integrated-assessment frameworks found in the scenario literature, then quantified the emissions likely to be associated with these fundamental variables within the context of the storylines. The result is a range of emissions scenarios for each individual storyline. The overall range of all scenarios from all storylines is representative of the range of emissions in the scenario literature. This approach is one way to reflect the uncertainty inherent in emissions projections: a set of alternative storylines reflects uncertainty in the fundamental demographic, socioeconomic, and technological driving forces, while the multi-model approach to quantifying each storyline accounts for uncertainty because of differing characteristics of models.

The SRES results generally support the conclusion that high (low) population growth tends to be associated with high (low) emissions growth (Nakicenovic *et al.*

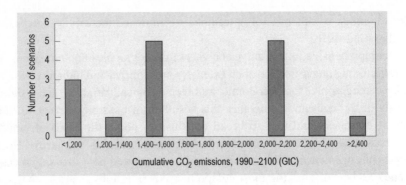

Figure 9.1. Distribution of cumulative global CO_2 emissions, 1990–2100, for SRES scenarios following the A1 storyline. *Source*: Nakicenovic *et al.* (2000).

2000, p. 36). However, there is an important qualification to this broad tendency. The SRES results show that similar population and GDP paths can produce widely varying emissions levels. For example, the family of scenarios that follow the A1 storyline (which assumes "convergence among regions, capacity building, and increased cultural and social interactions, with a substantial reduction in regional differences in per capita income" [Nakicenovic *et al.* 2000, p. 28]) all assumed low population growth and rapid economic growth, but produced cumulative CO_2 emissions over the 1990–2100 period that ranged from 1,050 to 2,500 GtC (see *Figure 9.1*). In addition, the SRES showed that similar emissions levels could result from different combinations of driving forces. Thus, a low population path cannot be assumed to be associated with low emissions, nor a high population with high emissions. A crucial question, however, is, How likely is it that a low population path would be associated with lower or higher emissions? The SRES does not attempt to answer this question.

Sensitivity analysis addresses a separate question: All else being equal, what is the likely effect of an alternative population path? Within a scenario development framework such as the SRES, one might imagine that such a question would be addressed by comparing scenarios from the same storyline, but with different population paths. This would be analogous to the kind of exercise carried out for the A1 storyline, in which similar assumptions about population and economic growth, and to a lesser extent final energy demand, were coupled with a range of assumptions about future energy systems, which clearly illustrated the great sensitivity of emissions to technological change. If a group of integrated assessment modeling teams were to evaluate scenarios that shared similar economic growth and technological change assumptions, but differed in population assumptions, conclusions could be drawn about the potential for demographic developments to influence emissions levels.

9.3.6   Population sensitivity analysis

Lacking such a comprehensive assessment, we perform our own set of simplified sensitivity analyses, based on the observation that most models incorporate population in an essentially linear fashion. This conclusion is supported by a review of the few studies that have carried out population sensitivity analyses within a single modeling framework (O'Neill *et al.* 2001), which concludes that models are sensitive to population assumptions and that lower population growth leads to lower emissions, at least within the framework of individual models. This conclusion is also supported by direct inspection of the structure of many models, which essentially scale emissions linearly with population size. Our sensitivity analysis illustrates the implications of this general structure.

To examine the extent to which alternative population paths could affect GHG emissions, we combine three different population projections with three different projections of per capita emissions. For both variables, the three projections are intended to be representative of a range of plausible future values over time. For the population paths, we use the scenarios from IIASA (Lutz 1996) that were employed in O'Neill *et al.* (2001). While the more recent probabilistic projections from IIASA foresee generally less population growth than these scenarios, what is important in this exercise is the relative difference between the three paths, and the variance in projected population has changed much less in the IIASA projections than in the absolute levels. For the per capita emissions paths, we use the central, high, and low projections from the IS92 scenarios developed by the IPCC. While the SRES offers more recent scenarios, the per capita emissions range of the earlier set of IS92 scenarios is similar to the full range of SRES scenarios (excluding the extremely fossil fuel-intensive A1C and A1G scenarios; see *Figure 9.2*). In addition, the IS92 scenarios were developed within a single model, the Atmospheric Stabilization Framework (ASF; Lashof and Tirpak 1990; Leggett *et al.* 1992). Since our analysis is intended to represent the relationships between demographics and other factors typically incorporated within single models, we use the IS92 scenarios. The treatment of population in the ASF model is very simple: in most sectors, population simply scales economic activity up or down, with no endogenous feedback of population on per capita income. In noneconomic sectors of the models, such as emissions from agriculture, the relationship between population size and emissions is also direct and linear. Therefore, while total emissions are a function of population size, per capita emissions are largely independent of population. Results are also available for these scenarios on a disaggregated basis (nine world regions rather than the four regions for which the SRES results are published).

We first examine a linear model by calculating the emissions that would result by assuming per capita emissions that follow a central path while population

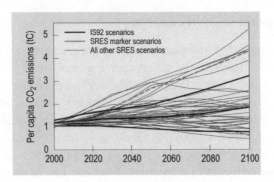

Figure 9.2. Global per capita CO_2 emissions in IS92 scenarios (black lines) and SRES scenarios (thick gray lines, marker scenarios; thin gray lines, all other scenarios). *Source*: Authors' calculations based on Nakicenovic *et al.* (2000) and Leggett *et al.* (1992).

follows one of the three alternative demographic scenarios. We compare these results with changes in emissions that would result from a central population path and three alternative per capita emissions scenarios. Next, we test the robustness of the results by relaxing the "all else being equal" assumption inherent in the linear model in two ways:

- First, we examine the influence of the different age structures of the different population paths. One implication of alternative age structures relevant to consumption and emissions is that older populations are likely to have smaller average household sizes. The smaller number of children relative to adults and the growing proportion of elderly (who are more likely in many societies to live alone or as a couple without children) are likely to lead to smaller households, with implications for energy use and emissions.
- Second, we also investigate the result of incorporating into the model an assumed relationship between the growth rates of population and per capita GDP. This relationship could be taken to represent the economic growth induced by a slower growth of population size, or by the investments in human capital that could be one cause of the slower growth in population.

9.3.7 A linear model

Figure 9.3 shows total GHG emissions for the world that result from combining the IPCC per capita emissions paths with the IIASA population scenarios using a linear model (i.e., per capita emissions are independent of population). Under the central

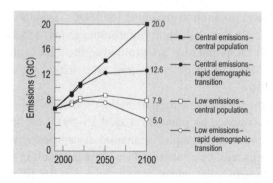

Figure 9.3. World greenhouse gas emissions from commercial energy, 1990–2100. *Source*: O'Neill *et al.* (2001).

emissions–central population scenario, GHG emissions are expected to rise from 6.6 GtC in 1990 to 14.1 GtC in 2050 and to 20.0 GtC in 2100. Regional results (not shown) indicate that the source of emissions will shift decisively to the South. In 1990, MDCs accounted for 75 percent of GHG emissions from commercial energy; according to the central emissions–central population scenario, MDCs will account for only 47 percent in 2050 and 39 percent in 2100. The main reason for this shift is that in the IPCC IS92 scenarios, while MDC per capita emissions remain well above LDC rates throughout the 21st century, the ratio of MDC to LDC per capita emissions falls from about 10 in 1990 to less than 4 in 2100.[2] This occurs primarily because in all the IPCC scenarios the ratio of MDC to LDC per capita income is assumed to fall from about 14 in 1990 to about 5 in 2100.

How does sensitivity of emissions to population and to per capita emissions compare? Based on the demographic and emissions scenarios employed here, in the near to medium term (up to 2050), the simulations show that total emissions are much more sensitive to plausible ranges of per capita emissions; under the central emissions scenario, the difference between emissions estimates that corresponds to the central and low population paths is slim. This results mainly from the momentum of population growth, which limits the rate of divergence of alternative population paths, and therefore of emissions as well. In contrast, under the central demographic scenario, the difference between emissions that result from the central and low per capita emissions scenarios is over 5 GtC. In the long term, however, alternative population paths can have a substantial effect on GHG emissions. Under the central emissions scenario, more rapid demographic transition reduces projected global emissions in 2100 by 37 percent. Results at the regional

---

[2] Accounting for sources of GHG emissions in addition to commercial energy, such as agriculture and deforestation, the ratio of MDC to LDC per capita emissions in the IS92a scenario remains stable at roughly 4:1 over the course of the 21st century.

level show that slower population growth in the MDCs accounts for nearly 40 per-cent of the global emissions reduction (in absolute terms) achieved in 2100, even though virtually all the population growth during the 21st century takes place in the LDCs. High MDC per capita emissions rates magnify the impact of MDC population reductions.

In the rapid demographic transition scenario, the elderly dependency ratio (pop-ulation over age 60 divided by population aged 15–59) is higher for both regions than it is in the central demographic scenario. It can be argued that this might reduce global savings and, by choking off investment, result in higher GHG emis-sions. A back-of-the-envelope calculation suggests that the difference between the two population scenarios is probably not great enough to support this view (O'Neill *et al.* 2001, Chapter 4). To translate population aging into environmental effects via the savings–investment link, it is necessary to hypothesize that more rapid aging slows the rate of technological progress, or shifts the structure of demand toward more carbon-intensive sectors, or leads to fiscal gridlock in the MDCs. Moreover, while the evidence is mixed, some research suggests that the lower LDC youth de-pendency ratio (population aged 0–14 divided by population aged 15–59) in the rapid demographic transition scenario substantially raises the supply of savings in these countries (Higgins and Williamson 1997).

9.3.8   Aging and households

The use of a model based on population size assumes that the environmental impact being modeled arises at the level of the individual, not that of the household or the community, for example. Yet, to take energy consumption as an example, there are substantial economies of scale at the household level. A significant proportion of residential energy consumption should be assigned to "household overhead"; that is, it is tied to the hearth, not to the number of household members. The possible rel-evance of alternative demographic denominators points toward a partitioned model in which emissions are driven partly by numbers of people and partly by numbers of households. O'Neill *et al.* (2001, Appendix II) review studies on household-level economies of scale in energy consumption. These lead us to employ a partitioned model approach in which half the emissions are assigned to individuals and half to households. We construct a projection of numbers of households by region by combining the population projections with age-specific household headship rates held constant at their 1990 levels. The essential feature of the projections is that population aging during the 21st century will reinforce a historical trend toward smaller average household size, since there will be a smaller proportion of younger individuals (who tend to live with their parents) and a larger proportion of elderly people (who tend to live alone). Thus, the number of households in both MDCs and LDCs is expected to grow faster than the population itself. This result is based on the assumption of constant age-specific headship rates; that is, the fraction of each age group that can be considered to be heading households does not change with time. If, instead, one assumes a continuation of historical trends toward living alone in given age groups, the number of households increases even more rapidly than is assumed here.

To create a scenario for emissions per household, we assume that per household emissions grow at the same rate as per capita emissions. This assumption reflects the general features of the effect of changes in household size on emissions. As household size falls, per capita emissions are expected to rise as economies of scale in energy use are lost. In our scenarios, the rise in per capita emissions caused by the consideration of households is equal to the rate of decline in household size (i.e., if household size declines 1 percent/year, per capita emissions rise 1 percent/year faster than they otherwise would). This particular assumption is arbitrary, but its magnitude is reasonable when compared with the results of more detailed studies available for a limited number of case studies of developed countries (Vringer and Blok 1995; O'Neill and Chen 2002).

Figure 9.4 compares the results of the partitioned model with those of the standard linear model under the central emissions scenario. The partitioned model projects substantially higher GHG emissions than does the standard model. Global emissions in the partitioned model under the central population scenario rise to 16 GtC in 2050 and 25 GtC in 2100, 25 percent higher than in the standard model. This difference is driven by the growth rate of households, which is higher than the growth rate of population in both MDCs and LDCs. However, the simulations show that, in the near term, the difference between emissions estimates that correspond to the central and rapid demographic transition scenarios is small regardless of whether the projections are made with the standard or partitioned model. However, the long-term sensitivity to population displayed by the standard model is nearly as strong in the partitioned model. In both MDCs and LDCs, more rapid demographic transition reduces the projected emissions in 2100 by about one-third, little different from the 37 percent reduction projected by the standard model. In other words, considering age-structure effects that increase the number of households does not alter the conclusion that alternative demographic futures can substantially influence GHG emissions in the long run. At the same time, however, the marked difference in absolute emissions levels between the standard linear model and the partitioned model illustrates the need to account for age-structure effects in emissions projections.

9.3.9   Relationships between variables

Criticisms of linear models generally assert that the problem has been oversimplified (e.g., Shaw 1993). If the implied *ceteris paribus* assumptions were replaced

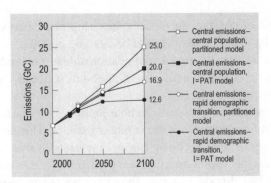

Figure 9.4. World greenhouse gas emissions from commercial energy, 1990–2100, I=PAT versus a partitioned model. *Source*: O'Neill *et al.* (2001).

with more realistic relationships between variables, the reasoning goes, the results would change. Failure to take account of possible relationships between variables is perhaps the linear I=PAT model's weakest point; it is certainly the model's most often criticized limitation. However, to gauge the effect of nonlinearities, the obvious starting point is to determine the implications of unadorned linear relations. The problem is not so much starting with linear relations as not progressing to more complicated links.

Several important *ceteris paribus* assumptions built into the I=PAT model assume away any substantial links between these broad variables. Potentially important links that are ignored include a possibly bi-directional relationship between P and A. The relationship between fertility, mortality, and per capita income is far from well understood; indeed, the relationships may be so dependent on conditional variables as to be nearly incomprehensible. However, the least likely theory is that there is no relationship at all. Mutual influences between A and T are likely as well. The core result of the neoclassic economic growth model is that, in the long-run equilibrium, the rate of per capita economic growth will be given by the rate of technological progress, where the latter is defined as the rate of increase in economic output, the level of all inputs remaining the same. In the opposite direction, researchers have observed very strong associations between economic growth and the pollution intensity of the economy (Chenery and Syrquin 1975; Maddison 1989; Pandit and Cassetti 1989). For example, environmental impact per unit GDP has been found either to decline monotonically with the level of development or to follow an inverted U-shaped path; that is, it first rises, then falls (World Bank 1992). This path reflects not only changes in economic structure, but also the fact that rising income stimulates demand for environmental quality. The combination of changing economic structure and rising demand for environmental quality defines an "environmental transition" (Ruttan 1991; Antle and Heidebrink

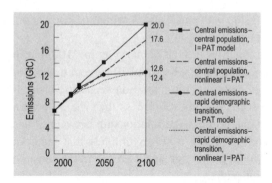

Figure 9.5. World greenhouse gas emissions from commercial energy, 1990–2100, standard versus nonlinear I=PAT. *Source*: O'Neill *et al.* (2001).

1995) in which economic growth is associated with environmental deterioration when a country is poor, but with environmental improvement after a critical point in national economic development has been reached.

However, while lists of possible interactions are easy to generate, formalizing and validating them within a quantitative model is another matter (Schneider 1997). To test the importance of indirect effects, we modified the I=PAT model to incorporate potential relationships between the rates of growth of the variables on the right-hand side of the equation. As we are concerned here primarily with the effect of alternative demographic futures, we limit our analysis to the potential relationships between the growth rates of P and A. *Figure 9.5* compares the results of the standard I=PAT model with the results of a model that assumes that each percentage point deceleration in the rate of population growth increases the rate of per capita economic growth by 0.25 percentage points, a relationship based on neoclassic economic growth models commonly employed in climate change assessments (Nordhaus 1994). In all cases, the baseline is the central emissions scenario. However, in the nonlinear model, per capita income is altered from the path assumed by the central emissions scenario as a result of the assumed relationship between P and A, which results in slower-growing total emissions whenever the population increases and faster-growing emissions whenever the population declines.

Both models project similar levels of GHG emissions: in 2100 the central population scenarios produce emissions levels that differ by just over 10 percent (20.0 GtC in the standard model versus 17.6 GtC in the nonlinear model), while the rapid demographic transition scenarios produce emissions levels that differ only marginally (12.6 GtC versus 12.4 GtC). The assumed relationship between P and A has almost no effect on long-term emissions under the rapid demographic transition scenario because population actually declines in that scenario over the second half of the 21st century, which reverses any divergence in emissions produced by the assumed relationship between P and A while the population grew over the first half of the 21st century.

The projected reduction in GHG emissions in 2100 that results from slowed population growth remains at a substantial 30 percent in the nonlinear model (12.4 GtC under the rapid demographic transition scenario versus 17.6 GtC under the central population scenario), not much less than the 37 percent projected by the standard I=PAT model. Unless the relationship between P and A is far stronger than current research suggests, it seems unlikely that incorporating this particular indirect effect would make a great difference in the sensitivity of emissions to alternative population paths.

Based on this set of sensitivity analyses, we conclude that alternative population paths can have a substantial effect on future GHG emissions. In particular, lower population growth is likely to lead to lower emissions. One should keep in mind that this is different from a guarantee that low population growth will be associated with a world with low emissions, or high population growth with high emissions. As demonstrated by the SRES scenarios, the range of possibilities remains wide even with a particular population scenario. However, for a world with a given set of economic growth and technological system characteristics, current modeling frameworks indicate that slower population growth is likely to lead to reduced emissions.

9.3.10   Population and adaptation

Historic GHG emissions have committed the world to some climate change even if aggressive mitigation policies are put into place immediately. Societies therefore have an incentive to plan for adaptation to climate change impacts no matter how much emissions are reduced. How might demographic factors affect the ability of societies to cope with climate change? O'Neill *et al.* (2001) focus on one aspect of this question by asking whether slower population growth would enhance the ability of institutions, especially in developing countries, to adapt to the likely impacts of climate change. In 20, 50, and certainly in 100 years, some countries that are currently poor will no longer be so. However, others will, and large subpopulations may remain poor even in countries that attain average living standards much higher than they have today. In considering the impacts of climate change, it is important to impose a hypothetical unfavorable climate not on the world of today, but on the world as it may be decades in the future. Nonetheless, both the geographic distribution of expected climate change impacts and a concern for equity suggest a focus on low-income settings.

The expected impacts of climate change could threaten agriculture, health, and environmental security, especially in LDCs. This does not mean that climate change is expected to make living conditions worse than they are today; rather, conditions are expected to be worse than they would have been in the absence of climate change. While living conditions in today's LDCs are bound to improve greatly over the time frame considered here, that improvement would be facilitated if there were no climate change. Against the negative impacts of climate change must be set institutional and social responses through the market, government agencies, the legal system, household structure, etc. A case can be made that lower fertility at the household level and slower population growth at the regional and national levels would ease the challenges faced by these institutions.

Consider the case of agriculture. By placing growing demands on the world food system, population growth raises the stakes in global climate change. Given population trends, food availability will have to increase three- or fourfold by the middle of the 21st century to achieve the goals of improved diet and enhanced food security. This implies that the 2 percent long-term rate of increase in world food supplies since the mid-1930s—an astonishingly rapid rate of increase by historic standards—will have to be maintained in the coming decades. While climate change may be neutral at the global level, it is likely to make attaining the necessary agricultural growth more difficult in the poor regions that need it most. Maintaining global agricultural production under conditions of climate change may require an increase in the relative price of food, which hurts the poor.

Population has impacts at the household and macro scales. At the household level, high fertility might impair the capacity for innovation and constructive agricultural intensification. Even if it does not, research indicates that household-based innovation alone is insufficient to cope with rapid population growth. At the national (and global) level, the question is whether rapid population growth encourages or impedes the development of effective institutions—such as markets, research laboratories, extension services, transportation networks, and the like—to enhance agricultural growth. This is closely related to the broader question of whether population growth hinders general economic development and progress. As the distribution of food and agricultural resources is an important component of the overall distribution of wealth and income in LDCs, there is also the important question of whether slower population growth would make it easier for policy makers to make difficult allocational decisions.

On balance, the research described above suggests that slower demographic growth would ease the pressure on the world food system and make it more resilient to the stresses expected from climate change. On the other hand, the situation is far too complex and contingent on local circumstances and institutions to support any claim that reducing the rate of population growth is a key strategy in this area. There are too many other avenues of improvement to be pursued, including the reduction of gross inefficiencies in food production, storage, distribution, and consumption.

In the case of health, the evidence suggests that reducing high fertility would have some beneficial effects on health at the household level. Some policies that tend to lower fertility, such as maternal and child health programs or programs to promote the education of girls, may also have beneficial impacts on health independent of their impacts on fertility. Healthier societies with stronger health institutions are more likely to be resilient to the impacts of climate change.

However, simply slowing the rate of population growth is unlikely, in and of itself, to be a very effective policy for improving health for a number of reasons:

- First, it cannot substitute for a more equitable distribution of available health resources.
- Second, there is a danger that the population aging that follows from slower population growth will require additional resources without improving the overall health of the population; indeed, it may sharpen the conflict between expenditure for curative care, which benefits mostly aged patients and the middle and upper classes, and the demand for preventive care, which benefits mostly young persons and poor households. By the middle of the 21st century, the proportion of the LDC population that is elderly (aged 60 and older) will have grown sharply. Policies that have the impact of lowering fertility in LDCs will significantly raise the elderly share, with accompanying stress on health care institutions (World Bank 1994).
- Third, a wide range of more direct measures to improve resilience to the health impacts of climate change is available. For example, in the case of malaria these include surveillance, improved treatment, open-water management, and applications of pesticides (although the acceleration of the life cycles of parasites allows quicker development of resistant strains). Better and larger-scale public health monitoring systems are also needed (Haines *et al.* 1993). Interventions need not be designed to reduce the incidence of disease directly, but rather to reduce its impact on the community. For example, where malaria eradication is infeasible, interventions designed to improve the nutritional status of an undernourished population may be more appropriate than vector-control interventions. As in the case of agriculture, the importance of local capacity and institutions must be stressed.

In the case of environmental security, the concept of "environmental refugees" has attracted wide interest. While its definition may be too broad, it reflects the general conclusion of research in the area: rising environmental pressures encourage out-migration (Lonergan 1998), and if a virtuous out-migration response is stifled, then rapid environmental deterioration and a resultant distress migration are possible. A similar observation applies to violent conflicts over natural resources:

scarcity invariably gives rise to conflicts between stakeholders; if these are not resolved by institutions, including the market, then violent conflict becomes a distinct possibility. Stresses associated with global change will probably intensify the pressures that already drive internal, regional, and intercontinental migration, and policy makers and societies will be forced to come to terms, one way or another, with these rising pressures. Both virtuous and vicious adjustment paths are available, and it would be wrong to jump to the conclusion that global climate change presages a century of massive refugee movements and violent conflicts. However, lower fertility and slower population growth would contribute to relieving the proximate causes of distress migration (e.g., soil degradation) and ease the institutional adjustments alluded to above.

In all three areas, then, slower population growth is likely to be beneficial to societies faced with adapting to climate change impacts. However, in none of the three areas considered are policies that affect fertility likely to be key strategies, since more direct means of improving resilience are available. Among these are better management of agricultural resource systems, more equitable distribution of available health resources, and elimination of rigidities that trap impoverished populations in environmentally unstable environments.

9.4   Conclusions and Policy Implications

The two principal conclusions of this chapter—that alternative population scenarios would substantially influence GHG emissions in the long run and affect the ability of societies to adapt to climate change impacts—suggest that it is worth considering links between population and climate change policy. The consideration, in broad terms, of the policy relevance of population to environmental matters is not new, but no international agreements have translated the recognition of these linkages into specific recommendations. On the environment side, Agenda 21, signed at the Earth Summit in 1992 and intended as a blueprint for sustainable development, recommends only that nations take demographic factors into account in the policy-making process. On the population side, the Programme of Action agreed to at the International Conference on Population and Development in Cairo in 1994 also discusses population–environment links, but does little more than repeat the language of Agenda 21. One logical forum for analysis of relationships between population and climate change is the IPCC, which is charged with assessing the science of climate change and its potential impacts, as well as formulating response strategies. Yet it has paid little attention to population. There are likely a number of reasons for this omission, not least the tension between North and South over the relative contribution of population and consumption to environmental problems (Bongaarts *et al.* 1997).

The analysis of population and GHG emissions suggests that under conditions of rapid demographic transition (lower fertility and lower mortality, which result in slower population growth and an older population age structure), GHG emissions would be reduced relative to emissions in a baseline demographic scenario. While moderate in the short run, the difference between the two emissions paths is significant in the long run. The basic conclusion that more rapid demographic transition translates into lower emissions is found to be robust in a number of simple sensitivity tests. More direct means of reducing emissions (such as improving energy efficiency) are available, and these arguably have less pervasive social and economic effects than policies designed to slow population growth. On the other hand, there is a case that the adjustment burden on these more direct policy interventions will be lighter in a world characterized by slow population growth. The analysis of the role of population in adaptation to environmental stress, based in large part on vicious-circle models, concluded that lower fertility would improve the ability of developing countries to adapt to the expected impacts of climate change. Symmetrically, more direct policy interventions are available to strengthen institutions such as markets, government agencies, the family, etc. However, the adjustment burden on such institutions will probably be lighter in an environment of low fertility and moderate population growth.

Many population-related policies—such as voluntary family planning and reproductive health programs, and investments in education and primary health care—improve individual welfare among the least well-off members of the present generation. Since these also have climate change benefits, they easily qualify as no-regrets policies of the sort identified for priority action by the IPCC. The existence of a climate-related external cost to the fertility decisions of individuals lends support to such programs, not only because they assist couples in having the number of children they want, but also because they tend to lower desired fertility.

These conclusions do not necessarily imply that population policies are the most effective or equitable policies with which to address climate change. Throughout our discussion, we stress that there are more direct ways to reduce GHG emissions and enhance the functioning of institutions. However, a portfolio approach suggests that policies related to population should be part of a broad range of policies to mitigate and adapt to climate change, and to global environmental change in general, especially given that many of these are win–win strategies.

References

Ang BW (1993). Sector disaggregation, structural effect and industrial energy use: An approach to analyze the interrelationships. *Energy* **18**:1033–1044.

Antle JM & Heidebrink G (1995). Environment and development: Theory and international evidence. *Economic Development and Cultural Change* **43**:603–623.

Bartiaux F & van Ypersele J-P (1993). The role of population growth in global warming. In *Proceedings of the International Population Conference Montreal 1993*, Vol. 4, pp. 33–54. Liege, Belgium: International Union for the Scientific Study of Population.

Bongaarts J (1992). Population growth and global warming. *Population and Development Review* **18**:299–319.

Bongaarts J, O'Neill BC & Gaffin SR (1997). Climate change policy: Population left out in the cold. *Environment* **39**:40–41.

Chenery H & Syrquin M (1975). *Patterns of Development, 1950–1970*. Oxford, UK: Oxford University Press.

Commoner B (1972). Response. *Bulletin of the Atomic Scientists* **17**:42–56.

Commoner B (1991). Rapid population growth and environmental stress. In *Consequences of Rapid Population Growth in Developing Countries*. Proceedings of the United Nations/Institute d'études démographiques Expert Group Meeting, New York, 23–26 August 1988, pp. 161–190. New York, NY, USA: Taylor and Francis.

Cramer JC (1998). Population growth and air quality in California. *Demography* **35**:45–56.

DeCanio SJ (1992). International cooperation to avert global warming: Economic growth, carbon pricing, and energy efficiency. *Journal of Environment and Development* **1**:41–62.

Den Elzen M & Schaeffer M (2002). Responsibility for past and future global warming: Uncertainties in attributing anthropogenic climate change. *Climatic Change* **54**:29–73.

Dietz T & Rosa EA (1997). Effects of population and affluence on CO_2 emissions. *Proceedings of the National Academy of Sciences* **94**:175–179.

Ehhalt D, Prather M, Dentener F, Derwent R, Dlugokencky E, Holland E, Isaksen I, Katima J, Kirchhoff V, Matson P, Midgley P, Wang M, Berntsen T, Bey I, Brasseur G, Buja L, Collins WJ, Daniel J, DeMore WB, Derek N, Dickerson R, Etheridge D, Feichter J, Fraser P, Friedl R, Fuglestvedt J, Gauss M, Grenfell L, Grübler A, Harris N, Hauglustaine D, Horowitz L, Jackman C, Jacob D, Jaeglé L, Jain A, Kanakidou M, Karlsdottir S, Ko M, Kurylo M, Lawrence M, Logan JA, Manning M, Mauzerall D, McConnell J, Mickley L, Montzka S, Müller JF, Olivier J, Pickering K, Pitari G, Roelofs GJ, Rogers H, Rognerud B, Smith S, Solomon S, Staehelin J, Steele P, Stevenson D, Sundet J, Thompson A, van Weele M, von Kuhlmann R, Wang Y, Weisenstein D, Wigley T, Wild O, Wuebbles D & Yantosca R (2001). Atmospheric chemistry and greenhouse gases. In *Climate Change 2001: The Scientific Basis*, Eds. Houghton JT, Ding Y, Griggs DJ, Noguer M, van der Linden PJ, Da X, Maskell K & Johnson CA, pp. 239–287. Cambridge, UK: Cambridge University Press.

Fisher I 1922 (1967 reprint). *The Making of Index Numbers*. New York, NY, USA: Augustus M Kelley Publishers.

Haines A, Epstein PR & McMichael AJ (1993). Global health watch: Monitoring the impacts of environmental change. *Lancet* **342**:1464–1469.

Harrison P (1992). *The Third Revolution: Environment, Population and a Sustainable World*. London, UK: ID Tauris and Company in association with Penguin Books.

Harrison P (1994). Towards a post-Malthusian human ecology. *Human Ecology Review* **1**:265–276.

Heilig GK (1994). The greenhouse gas methane (CH_4): Sources and sinks, the impact of population growth, possible interventions. *Population and Environment* **16**:109–137.

Higgins M & Williamson JG (1997). Age structure dynamics in Asia and dependence on foreign capital. *Population and Development Review* **23**:261–293.

Holdren J (1991). Population and the energy problem. *Population and Environment* **12**:231–255.

Houghton RA (2003). Revised estimates of the annual net flux of carbon to the atmosphere from changes in land use and land management 1850–2000. *Tellus* **55B**:378–390.

Howarth RB, Schipper L, Duerr PA & Strom S (1991). Manufacturing energy use in 8 OECD countries: Decomposing the impacts of changes in output, industry structure and energy intensity. *Energy Economics* **13**:135–142.

Kaya Y (1990). *Impact of Carbon Dioxide Emissions Control on GNP Growth: Interpretation of Proposed Scenarios*. Paper presented to the IPCC Energy and Industry Subgroup, Response Strategies Working Group, Paris, France.

Keyfitz N (1992). Seven ways of making the less developed countries' population problem disappear—In theory. *European Journal of Population* **8**:149–167.

Lashof DA & Tirpak D (1990). *Policy Options for Stabilizing Global Climate*. Washington, DC, USA: Hemisphere Publishing Corp.

Leggett J, Pepper WJ & Swart RJ (1992). Emissions scenarios for the IPCC: An update. In *Climate Change 1992: The Supplementary Report to the IPCC Scientific Assessment*, eds. Houghton JT, Callander BA & Varney SK, pp. 68–95. Cambridge, UK: Cambridge University Press.

Lonergan S (1998). The role of environmental degradation in population displacement. *Environmental Change and Security Project Report*, Issue 4 (Spring), pp. 5–15. Washington, DC, USA: The Woodrow Wilson Center.

Lutz W (1993). Population and environment—What do we need more urgently: Better data, better models, or better questions? In *Environment and Population Change*, eds. Zaba B & Clarke J, pp. 47–62. Liege, Belgium: Derouaux Ordina Editions for the International Union for the Scientific Study of Population.

Lutz W (1996). *The Future Population of the World: What Can We Assume Today?*, Revised Edition. London, UK: Earthscan.

MacKellar FL, Lutz W, Prinz C & Goujon A (1995). Population, households, and CO_2 emissions. *Population and Development Review* **21**:849–865.

MacKellar FL, Lutz W, McMichael AJ & Suhrke A (1998). Population and climate change. *Human Choice and Climate Change, Vol. 1: The Societal Framework*, eds. Rayner S & Malone EL, pp. 89–193. Columbus, OH, USA: Battelle Press.

Maddison JM (1989). *The World Economy in the 20th Century*. Paris, France: Organisation for Economic Co-operation and Development.

Minnis P, Harrison EF, Stowe LL, Gibson GG, Denn FM, Doelling DR & Smith WL (1993). Radiative climate forcing by the Mt. Pinatubo eruption. *Science* **259**:1411–1415.

Moomaw WR & Tullis DM (1998). Population, affluence, or technology: An empirical look at national carbon dioxide production. In *People and Their Planet*, eds. Baudot B & Moomaw W, pp. 58–70. New York, NY, USA: MacMillan.

Murthy WS, Panda M & Parikh J (1997). Economic growth, energy demand, and carbon dioxide emissions in India: 1990–2020. *Environment and Development Economics* **2**:173–193.

Nakicenovic N, Alcamo J, Davis G, de Vries B, Fenhann J, Gaffin S, Gregory K, Grübler A, Jung TY, Kram T, Lebre La Rovere E, Michaelis L, Mori S, Morita T, Pepper W, Pitcher H, Price L, Riahi K, Roehrl A, Rogner H-H, Sankovski A, Schlesinger M, Shukla P, Smith S, Swart R, van Rooijen S, Victor N & Dadi Z (2000). *Special Report on Emissions Scenarios*. Cambridge, UK: Cambridge University Press for the Intergovernmental Panel on Climate Change.

Nordhaus WD (1994). *Managing the Global Commons*. Cambridge, MA, USA: MIT Press.

O'Neill BC (2000). The jury is still out on GWPs. *Climatic Change* **44**:427–443.

O'Neill BC (2001). I=PAT. *Encyclopedia of Global Change*, Vol. 1, ed. Goudie A, pp. 702–706. Oxford, UK: Oxford University Press.

O'Neill BC & Chen BS (2002). Demographic determinants of household energy use in the United States. In *Population and Environment. Methods of Analysis*, eds. Lutz W, Prskawetz A & Sanderson WC, pp. 53–58. A Supplement to *Population and Development Review*, **28**, 2002. New York, NY, USA: The Population Council.

O'Neill BC, Oppenheimer M & Gaffin SR (1997). Measuring time in the greenhouse. *Climatic Change* **37**:491–503.

O'Neill BC, MacKellar FL & Lutz W (2001). *Population and Climate Change*. Cambridge, UK: Cambridge University Press.

Pandit K & Cassetti E (1989). The shifting patterns of sectoral labor allocation during development: Developed versus developing countries. *Annals of the Association of American Geographers* **79**:329–344.

Pearce DW (1991). *Blueprint 2: Greening the World Economy*. London, UK: Earthscan.

Penner JE, Andreae M, Annegarn H, Barrie L, Feichter J, Hegg D, Jayaraman A, Leaitch R, Murphy D, Nganga J, Pitari G, Ackerman A, Adams P, Austin P, Boers R, Boucher O, Chin M, Chuang C, Collins B, Cooke W, DeMott P, Feng Y, Fischer H, Fung I, Ghan S, Ginoux P, Gong S-L, Guenther A, Herzog M, Higurashi A, Kaufman Y, Kettle A, Kiehl J, Koch D, Lammel G, Land C, Lohmann U, Madronich S, Mancini E, Mishchenko D, Nakajima T, Quinn P, Rasch P, Roberts DL, Savoie D, Schwartz S, Seinfeld J, Soden B, Tanré D, Taylor K, Tegen L, Tie X, Vali G, Van Dingenen R, van Weele M & Zhang Y (2001). Aerosols, their direct and indirect effects. In *Climate Change 2001: The Scientific Basis*, eds. Houghton JT, Ding Y, Griggs DJ, Noguer M, van der Linden PJ, Da X, Maskell K & Johnson CA, pp. 289–348. Cambridge, UK: Cambridge University Press.

Petit JR, Jouzel J, Raynaud D, Barkov NI, Barnola JM, Basile I, Bender M, Chappellaz J, Davis M, Delaygue G, Delmotte M, Kotlyakov VM, Legrand M, Lipenkov VY, Lorius C, Pepin L, Ritz C, Saltzman E & Stievenard M (1999). Climate and atmospheric history of the past 420,000 years from the Vostok ice core, Antarctica. *Nature* **399**:429–436.

Ramaswamy V, Boucher O, Haigh J, Hauglustaine D, Haywood J, Myhre G, Nakajima T, Shi GY, Solomon S, Betts R, Charlson R, Chuang C, Daniel JS, Del Genio A, van Dorland R, Feichter J, Fuglestvedt J, Forster PM de F, Ghan SJ, Jones A, Kiehl JT, Koch D, Land C, Lean J, Lohmann U, Minschwaner K, Penner JE, Roberts DL, Rodhe H, Roelofs GJ, Rotstayn LD, Schneider TL, Schumann U, Schwartz SE, Schwarzkopf MD, Shine KP, Smith S, Stevenson DS, Stordal F, Tegen I & Zhang Y (2001). Radiative forcing of climate change. In *Climate Change 2001: The Scientific Basis*, eds. Houghton JT, Ding Y, Griggs DJ, Noguer M, van der Linden PJ, Da X, Maskell K & Johnson CA, pp. 349-416. Cambridge, UK: Cambridge University Press.

Raskin PD (1995). Methods for estimating the population contribution to environmental change. *Ecological Economics* **15**:225–233.

Ruttan VW (1991). Sustainable growth in agricultural production: Poetry, policy and science. In *Agricultural Sustainability, Growth, and Poverty Alleviation: Issues and Policies*, eds. Vosti S, Reardon T & von Urff W, pp. 13–28. Washington, DC, USA: International Food Policy Research Institute.

Schneider SH (1997). Integrated assessment modeling of global climate change: Transparent rational tool for policy making or opaque screen hiding value-laden assumptions? *Environmental Modeling and Assessment* **2**:229–248.

Shaw RP (1989). Rapid population growth and environmental degradation: Ultimate versus proximate factors. *Environmental Conservation* **16**:199–208.

Shaw RP (1993). Review of Harrison 1992. *Population and Development Review* **19**:189–192.

Smil V (1999). Nitrogen in crop production: An account of global flows. *Global Biogeochemical Cycles* **13**:647–662.

Smith S & Wigley TML (2000). Global warming potentials: 1. Climatic implications of emissions reductions. *Climatic Change* **44**:445–457.

Vringer K & Blok K (1995). The direct and indirect energy requirements of households in the Netherlands. *Energy Policy* **23**:893–902.

Waggoner PE & Ausubel JH (2001). How much will feeding more and wealthier people encroach on forests? *Population and Development Review* **27**:239–257.

World Bank (1992). *World Development Report 1992: Development and Environment*. Washington, DC, USA: The World Bank.

World Bank (1994). *Averting the Old Age Crisis*. Washington, DC, USA: The World Bank.

Chapter 10

Conceptualizing Population in Sustainable Development: From "Population Stabilization" to "Population Balance"

Wolfgang Lutz, Warren C. Sanderson, and Brian C. O'Neill

How we think about population in sustainable development matters. It matters to how we organize our observations, and it matters, most importantly, to the formulation and implementation of appropriate policies. Unfortunately, the rationales for those policies are now in considerable disarray. There is no unified framework within which to think about population in sustainable development; only partial approaches are used to deal with specific situations.

This confusion is exacerbated by the current situation of mixed demographic regimes. Some countries still have high fertility and are experiencing rapid population growth. This growth will continue for a long time, even if fertility declines in the near future, because of the momentum generated by past high fertility. Some countries—mostly in Africa—still have high fertility but, because of the HIV/AIDS pandemic, will see little or no population growth. Still another sizeable group of countries, including some in almost every income range, already has fertility below replacement, the level needed to avoid population shrinkage in the long run. To make matters even more complex, the populations of some of the low fertility countries are still growing because of their young age distributions (the momentum effect). In other countries, longer periods of low fertility have already altered the age distribution to such an extent that, without immigration, there will be fewer and fewer women of reproductive age for a while, even in the unlikely case that fertility immediately recovers to two children per woman. This is a case of negative population momentum. Lutz *et al.* (2003) recently showed that the European Union switched to negative momentum around the year 2000. This means a new force has been added to those that already cause population aging and shrinkage.

In addition, the old view that poor countries have growing populations and rich countries have stable or shrinking populations no longer holds. Over the coming decades, China, still a poor country by any standard, is expected to experience a lower population growth rate and considerably faster population aging than the United States. None of the conceptual frameworks that we currently have allows us to see the underlying unity in this diversity. How can we make sense of these seemingly confusing trends? We need a conceptual basis that allows us to put these observations into a broader perspective and to derive an appropriate policy framework.

We attempt to provide some insight into the situation in two ways. First, we review the basic rationales for population policy in the second half of the 20th century and examine the current situation in light of these. Second, we introduce the concept of "population balance." Population balance unifies many of the separate dimensions within a common conceptual framework that includes human capital as an integral part. It allows us to see that the concerns about too rapid a population growth and those about the consequences of too rapid a population aging are not completely separate issues, but really two different aspects of population imbalance. Population balance is introduced here in two complimentary ways: in qualitative terms and through the discussion of a highly simplified quantitative model.

10.1 Changing Population Policy Rationales[1]

Historically, population policies related to fertility have received the most attention in international conferences and policy fora. In principle, public policies can affect all three components of population change: fertility, mortality, and migration. However, mortality-related policies are less contentious, since decreases in mortality are considered a universal goal. Nobody argues that mortality reductions should be slowed because they contribute both to continued population growth and to rapid population aging. Generally, migration policies are considered to be internal affairs

---

[1]This section draws heavily on O'Neill *et al.* (2001).

and are rarely subject to international policy discussions, with the exception of humanitarian issues associated with refugees and asylum seekers. Even international labor migration, which has recently received much public attention, has not been the subject of much international policy making. A long-planned United Nations (UN) conference on migration continues to be postponed because most countries find it too controversial a topic for anything to be gained from an international meeting.

We therefore focus on fertility in this brief review of the major rationales for population policy over the past several decades. Until recently, these rationales were based mainly on presumed links between fertility and aggregate-level impacts of demographic trends on economic development and the environment. In the 1990s, the focus shifted to a rationale based on individual welfare. The Cairo Programme of Action, the statement that emerged from the 1994 International Conference on Population and Development, reflected the new consensus on this approach. We summarize these rationales and mention ways they may again become relevant, given the emerging focus on aging and divergent demographic conditions around the world.

10.1.1 The geopolitical rationale

The history of international population policy is linked inextricably with the history of the international family planning movement, which emerged in the 1920s as a complex amalgam of eugenicists, public health advocates, and social reformers (Adams 1990; Hodgson 1991). Scientific advances in genetics and large-scale human rights abuses in Germany under National Socialism thoroughly discredited both eugenics and policies derived from it. As a result, the international population movement was in disarray after World War II (Kühl 1997).

In reconstructing itself, the early postwar international family planning movement relied heavily on two justifications for public support of voluntary family planning. One justification was the health and well-being of women, children, and young families. The second justification, seldom stated openly, but always in the background, was geopolitical in nature. During the 1950s, new census data revealed staggering rates of demographic increase in India and other less developed countries (LDCs). With the Cold War as background, policy makers in the West feared that rapidly expanding Third World populations would be fertile breeding grounds for political instability. Early international assistance for family planning from the US government was justified internally in these political terms (Donaldson 1990).

Concerns over national economic and political standing have also sometimes served as the basis for pronatalist policies, such as generous parental leave, child allowances, public provision of day care, etc. (Teitelbaum and Winter 1985). In the

1960s and early 1970s, for example, a number of East European countries, alarmed by the prospect of population decline, restricted abortions and put in place financial incentives for childbearing. With many more developed countries (MDCs) facing labor-force shrinkage and even possible overall population decline, pronatalism may begin to rise in coming decades.

10.1.2   The macroeconomic rationale

At the Bucharest population conference in 1974 (see *Box 10.1*), MDCs argued that higher fertility in LDCs was an impediment to macroeconomic growth. By 1984, when the next international population conference was held in Mexico City, virtually all countries with the exception of the United States had adopted this view.

There is a long-standing argument about whether there is an inverse relationship between the rate of population growth and the rate of economic growth. Empirical research on time series up to the 1980s did not provide compelling support for this proposition (United States National Research Council 1986). More recent studies indicate that in Africa during the 1990s, economic growth and population growth were inversely related, and that in some Asian countries transitory age-structure changes that resulted from fertility declines contributed positively to economic growth (Bloom and Williamson 1998; Bloom *et al.* 2000; Kelley and Schmidt 2001). In any case, the perceived positive economic consequences of fertility reductions have been one rationale for both national population policies and international population assistance.

The macroeconomic consequences of population aging, while uncertain, are of increasing concern to MDCs, which must cope with overcommitted pension and health systems. While no country has justified pronatalist policies explicitly in terms of population aging, this rationale may be at the back of policy makers' minds. Impacts of population aging on LDCs are an emerging policy concern.

10.1.3   The social welfare rationale: Externalities to childbearing

The consequences of fertility that affect society as a whole, including future generations, but that do not influence parents in any other way are externalities. These externalities can be a problem because the value of an additional child to its family is different from its value to society as a whole, which leads parents to have too many or too few children compared with what would be best from a broader perspective. In the case of a negative net externality (net social benefits of a birth are less than net private benefits), the magnitude of the externality is equal to the per child tax that a government should theoretically levy on parents to maximize social welfare. In the case of a positive net externality (net social benefits of a birth are greater than net private benefits), the magnitude of the externality represents the

Box 10.1. Evolution of international population policy documents in the context of sustainable development.

The World Population Conference held in Bucharest in 1974 brought population issues to the forefront of international concern. At the time, the relationship between population growth and economic growth was the overriding issue. Nevertheless, considerable debate about the impact of population growth on the environment took place as well, with concern centered on the depletion of nonrenewable resources and food scarcity (United Nations 1997). The Bucharest Plan of Action eventually adopted, however, made no prominent reference to the issue, noting only that national population goals and policies should consider natural resources and food supply along with the more established considerations of economic and social factors.

At the International Conference on Population held in Mexico City in 1984, delegates met to discuss progress on and obstacles to implementation of the Bucharest Plan of Action. While links between population and economic development continued to dominate the agenda, environmental issues were given more prominence, with concern shifting somewhat from local to global impacts. The conference declaration recommended that, in countries where imbalance existed between population growth and the environment, governments should "adopt and implement specific policies, including population policies, that will contribute to redressing such imbalance."

The International Conference on Population and Development in Cairo in 1994 produced a new Programme of Action. Its emphasis was on individual rights, particularly the rights of women. Environmental considerations were perhaps more prominent than in previous population documents, but essentially relied on language that appeared in Agenda 21 (the document resulting from the 1992 Earth Summit held in Rio de Janeiro), which called, in broad terms, for the integration of population policies into sustainable development programs.

In preparation for the World Summit on Sustainable Development, held in Johannesburg in 2002, the Global Science Panel on Population and Environment (see below), sponsored by the International Institute for Applied Systems Analysis (IIASA), the International Union for the Scientific Study of Population (IUSSP), and the United Nations University (UNU), produced a statement on "Population in Sustainable Development" (Lutz and Shah 2002; Lutz *et al.* 2002b) that built a bridge between the Cairo focus on individual rights and the concerns about environmental change. Key to this bridge is the concept of differential vulnerability, which recognizes that environmental problems affect the weaker members of society to a greater extent than they affect stronger members. The statement noted that education was one of the most important tools for reducing the vulnerability of the poor.

payment that a government should theoretically make to parents. More generally, a range of incentives and disincentives to childbearing can be employed to cope with the externality problem. Generous West European family policies, while publicly framed in terms of social welfare, not demography, may be interpreted in part as a way to cope with the positive net externality to childbearing in societies characterized by subreplacement fertility. Negative externalities to childbearing in LDCs could be reduced or eliminated through population policies, including those that act indirectly to reduce fertility, such as improved maternal and child health.

More controversial are direct antinatalist incentives, which have been employed in a small number of LDCs (Chomitz and Birdsall 1991). Taxation according to the number of children is likely to hurt the poor more than the wealthy, and family-size penalties can unfairly penalize children of higher birth order. Incentives for sterilization, which have been utilized in Bangladesh, India, and Sri Lanka, raise the issue of entrapment. Poor women may accept payment for sterilization, but later regret the decision. More generally, incentives may be viewed as unethical because they inject financial considerations into an area that involves fundamental human rights.

10.1.4   The ecological rationale: Scale and ecological concerns

The scale of human activity depends, in part, on population size. McNicoll (1995) and many ecological economists point to the lack of sensitivity to scale as a potential deficiency in neoclassical economic approaches to issues that involve demographic and economic futures. Demeny (1986) makes a similar point and argues that the inability to deal with long-term population change is a serious failing of the neoclassical framework.

Scale is closely related to the concept of carrying capacity. The relationship between scale and carrying capacity may be one reason for the adoption of goals and targets for total population size. China, for example, has adopted targets for total population size as one basis for its population policies, which involve birth quotas, disincentives for large families, and incentives for small families. However, some have accused the Chinese approach (more specifically, the one-child policy) of being in violation of human rights.

There is no agreed formula to determine a sustainable population size. From the ecological point of view, the range of global carrying-capacity estimates has widened, rather than narrowed, over time (Cohen 1995). A small economic literature on optimal population size has made welfare comparisons between populations of different sizes, but has not come to any clear conclusions (Dasgupta 1986, 1998).[2] On the positive side, rapid population growth can give rise to economies of scale and what are called Boserup–Simon effects (Boserup 1981; Simon 1981) in the form of accelerated technological progress. The empirical evidence in this area

---

[2]The impediment is relevant to optimization models for the evaluation of climate change policy, because these models will face this problem if they are to incorporate population as an endogenous variable (Wexler 1996).

has not been strong, and, in any case, the time horizon of policy makers is too short for such effects to serve as a basis for policy.

10.1.5 The individual welfare rationale

Over the past decade the view that policies affecting population should above all stress the welfare of individuals, as opposed to demographic trends and their macro-consequences, has gained primacy. In this view, ensuring access to health care and education, fostering the empowerment of women and guaranteeing reproductive rights are ends in themselves, not means to achieve particular demographic goals (Bok 1994). Overemphasis on "number," according to this school of thought, has led to coercive practices and insufficient attention to contraceptive safety, with consequences that fall largely on women. Voluntary family planning programs, for example, are now seen as a way to guarantee the rights of individuals and couples to have the number of children they desire, not as a way to reduce fertility. They are viewed as just one part of what should be a broad provision of reproductive health services that also includes

- pre- and postnatal health care;
- treatment of infertility and other reproductive health problems, including sexually transmitted diseases; and
- education and counseling on all aspects of pregnancy, childbirth, infant and women's health, and parenting.

Population policies are also justified in this view if their aim is to improve the well-being of children. In some circumstances, high fertility can set off a self-reinforcing series of responses at the household level that impairs the health and education of children. If parents are not informed fully about the costs of high fertility to children (a form of intergenerational externality), or if the parents' need for the economic contributions made by children is stronger than their altruism toward their offspring, intervention may be justified to alleviate the conditions that lead to high fertility (Birdsall and Griffin 1993).

The individual welfare rationale heavily influenced the Cairo Programme of Action (McIntosh and Finkle 1995). In it, voluntary choice in matters of childbearing was enshrined as a basic right and a wide range of initiatives that addressed reproductive health was called for. Gender issues, such as improving the status of women through education and economic opportunities, and securing reproductive rights, were given prominence.

Some have lamented the lack of urgency within the Cairo document concerning the rapid population growth in LDCs and its consequences (Westoff 1995). The dominance of women's issues came at the expense of the traditional focus on the demographic rationale for population policies, and it has been argued that this shift risks the loss of support for international population programs (Harvey 1996). Environmentalists pointed out the lack of attention to the environment in the Cairo Programme of Action (Earth Negotiations Bulletin 1994); the page or two of text relating to the environment contains little of substance beyond generic calls for integration of environmental, economic, and demographic concerns.

Yet the Programme of Action does set a number of quantifiable goals for the target year 2015: the elimination of unmet needs for contraception; reductions in infant, child, and maternal mortality; increased life expectancy; and universal completion of primary education. In keeping with its focus on the welfare of women as opposed to demographic consequences, there is no discussion of what impact the attainment of the targets might have on global population size, except to say that it would result in a global population below the UN medium projection at the time of the Conference. The Programme of Action also calls for increased spending to achieve these goals. It is estimated that a total of US$17 billion annually by 2000, rising to over US$20 billion by 2015, would be required to fund the basic reproductive health programs outlined in the Cairo document. One-third of that amount was to come from international donors and the rest from developing countries themselves. Based on current trends, however, only a small fraction of this amount is likely to be provided.

The achievement of the aims of the Cairo document would probably lead to a reduction in fertility and a slowing of population growth, so common ground exists between those most concerned with individual rights and those most concerned with the consequences of population growth. The statement on "Population in Sustainable Development" produced by the Global Science Panel on Population and Environment explicitly links the two goals. The Panel, which consists of a group of leading scientists and members of the policy community from both the population and environment fields, was convened by three international organizations: IIASA, IUSSP, and UNU. Its task was to summarize the state of the art of population policy and give guidance to decision makers about priorities that would be appropriate under the different demographic regimes (Lutz and Shah 2002; Lutz *et al.* 2002b). The Panel came to a consensus on the importance of population to development and the environment, and in particular that policies should be targeted to those populations most vulnerable to environmental and socioeconomic stress. In addition, the Panel concluded that education and reproductive health care, including voluntary family planning, would benefit both people and the environment, and therefore should receive the highest policy priority.

The approach represented by the Global Science Panel statement confirms the relevance of the individual welfare approach to population policy, but it recognizes that aggregate-level impacts between demography, development, and environment are also important. The future could see additional linkages made across various policy rationales, and perhaps previous concerns may be given new prominence but for different reasons. Geopolitical concerns driven by population shrinkage and, particularly, a decline in the working-age population in some industrialized countries may again become prominent. Macroeconomic concerns over the effects of aging are already apparent and eventually may lead policy makers to look at demographic measures as possible policy options. Yet at the same time, scale-driven ecological concerns are likely to hold sway in several major regions in which the population is likely to grow well into the 21st century. The mix of concerns, and of policy rationales, has not yet led to a unified approach. In the next section, we provide some initial steps in that direction.

10.2 Population Balance

The concept of population balance proposed here refers to the well-being of groups of individuals that belong to the same generation (cohort). This focus on the well-being of cohorts allows the unification of concerns about population growth, population shrinkage, aging, education, health, economic growth, and the environment, as well as intergenerational equity, which is the driving force behind the notion of sustainable development. Population balance shows us why both population growth and population aging that are too rapid can have serious negative consequences on human society and ultimately on individual welfare. Growth that is too rapid may put pressure on the educational system (as has been shown in many developing countries), while aging that is too rapid may bring dangerous stress for the old-age security system (the European Commission speaks of population aging as a sustainability issue). However, moderate growth or aging may not necessarily have negative implications, especially if environmental constraints are not yet relevant and productivity per person (which is closely related to education) increases over time. Population balance teaches us that consideration should be given to both population growth and aging; to both demographic and socioeconomic characteristics of individuals; and to demographic, socioeconomic, and environmental conditions of societies. Hence, population balance is one way to conceptualize the demographic component of sustainable development.

The concept of population balance originated from the merging of two research traditions at IIASA that are both of a rather formal and quantitative nature. The first was the work on multistate population projections, which was expanded to include variables such as education (see Chapter 4 of this volume). The second was a series of comprehensive in-depth population–development–environment case studies that were designed to help understand the determinants and consequences of population trends in specific situations (such as on the island of Mauritius and in five other places; see Lutz *et al.* [2002a] for a summary).

A highly stylized model distilled from these studies is discussed in the next section in an attempt to give a clear formal description of the essence of the concept of population balance. It is a simple simulation model in which production and consumption depend on age and education (with education being a cost in the short run, but with the educated labor force being more productive in the long run), and in which scale also matters with respect to environmental pollution. This simple model shows that both very high and very low fertility lead to lower long-term levels of cohort welfare, while there is a middle area, a rather flat optimum, with higher levels.

Is "population balance" the right phrase for such a concept broadened to describe the changing relationships of more population dimensions than just size? In a dictionary (see, e.g., the *Oxford Concise Dictionary*), many definitions of the word "balance" are given for different contexts. In the field of physics, balance has a rather static connotation and refers to a stability of equal weights; in finance, it means the difference between assets and debts. In the fields of art and music, one finds more inspiring definitions. In music, balance refers to the "relative volume of different sources of sound" (the balance button on your stereo); in art it even means "the harmony of proportion." Since demography is all about proportions, this might be translated directly to mean the relationship of different proportions of age groups or other subpopulations, such as generations or educational groups. Thus, the challenge is to find the mix (harmony) of these proportions that is most conducive to individual welfare and intergenerational equity over the long run. This mix may look quite different in various cultural, economic, and environmental settings.

As a metaphor, the notion of "balanced nutrition" also inspired this concept. One can live in good health with different kinds of diets as long as the diet does not become too extreme in any direction. Also, what may be considered an optimal diet depends on the climate, the culture, and personal lifestyle. Analogously, population balance may mean somewhat different things in densely populated and resource-poor regions than in rich and sparsely populated regions. It may mean different things in societies with rapidly increasing educational levels and productivity than in those with stagnant or deteriorating educational systems; and it may be seen differently at the local, national, and global levels. The empirical analyses and projections presented in the chapters of this book give many illustrations of this point through the discussions of regional and location-specific population prospects, changes in human capital formation, and interactions with the natural environment.

10.3   A Highly Simplified, Quantitative Population Balance Model

Population balance is a concept that considers the well-being of people over their entire life course. Operationalizing this concept in a formal model can be a daunting task because of the large number of factors that influence well-being. In this section, we present a highly simplified population balance model and discuss three of its implications. There is always a tension between formulating large models that encompass more aspects of reality but are difficult to analyze and creating small models that leave out more but are easier to understand. Here, we go to the extreme of producing a highly oversimplified model (see *Box 10.2*), because even it has important lessons to teach us.

It is crucial that we do not confuse the broader population balance framework with the elements of the specific model that we use here. Each particular equation has advantages and disadvantages, and we should not condemn the entire framework if we would prefer to write one or another equation somewhat differently. To make the distinction between the framework and the particular model as clear as possible, we begin with a verbal discussion of the framework's main features.

The most important aspect of the population balance methodology is our interest in the long-term well-being of people. When we speak about the well-being of people, we mean people's experience over their lifetimes. In demographic parlance, well-being is a cohort measure. We view human well-being as a composite of three factors:

- Consumption.
- Survival rates.
- Environmental quality.

We assume, other things being equal, that people prefer more consumption, a longer life, and a cleaner environment. We divide the human life cycle into three phases:

- Youth.
- Working ages.
- Retirement.

In all phases of the life cycle, people consume. In the youth phase, people have no income, so their consumption and education costs are financed out of the incomes of the other two groups. We assume that education increases economic productivity in the working-age phase. In the working ages, people receive income,

Box 10.2. Equations of a highly simplified population balance model.

1. Equations

Welfare Indicator $(c) =$

$$\sum_{ed=0}^{1} \sum_{a=0}^{99} \frac{N\,(a, a+c, ed)}{Births\,(c)} \cdot Consumption\,(a, a+c)^{\alpha} \cdot EnvQuality\,(a+c) \quad (10.1)$$

$$Output\,(t) = \bar{Y} \cdot \left[\sum_{a=20}^{64} N(a, t, 0) + (1+r) \cdot \sum_{a=20}^{64} N(a, t, 1) \right] \quad (10.2)$$

$$Output\,per\,capita\,(t) = \bar{Y} \cdot [s_2\,(t) \cdot (1 + r \cdot efract\,(t))] \quad (10.3)$$

Consumption $(a^*, t) =$

$$\frac{Output\,per\,capita\,(t) - s_e\,(t) \cdot ed\cos t\,(t) \cdot efract\,(t)}{s_1\,(t) \cdot \rho_1 + s_2\,(t) + s_3\,(t) \cdot \rho_3} \quad (10.4)$$

$$20 \leq a^* \leq 64 \quad (10.5)$$

$$Consumption\,(a^{**}, t) = \rho_1 \cdot Consumption\,(a^*, t) \quad (10.6)$$

$$0 \leq a^{**} \leq 19 \quad (10.7)$$

$$Consumption\,(a^{***}, t) = \rho_3 \cdot Consumption\,(a^*, t) \quad (10.8)$$

$$65 \leq a^{***} \leq 100 \quad (10.9)$$

$$Pollution\,(t) = \phi \cdot Output\,(t) \quad (10.10)$$

$$EnvQuality\,(t) = \frac{\beta + \gamma \cdot Pollution\,(t)}{\beta + Pollution\,(t)} \quad (10.11)$$

2. Definitions

Cohorts: A cohort is a group of people born in year c followed over their lifetime. This implies that $c + a = t$, where c is the year of birth of the cohort, a is the current age of people in that cohort, and t is the current year.

Age groups: There are three life-cycle stages: youth (ages 0–19), working ages (ages 20–64), and retirement (ages 65 years and older). Children are educated from ages 6 through 19. There are no school dropouts.

Box 10.2. Continued.

Education:

- There are two education groups, those with no education ($ed = 0$) and those who have attended school ($ed = 1$).
- $N(a, t, ed)$ is the number of people of age a, in year t, who have education level ed.
- $\bar{Y}$ is the annual output produced by a person with no education.
- $(1 + r)\bar{Y}$ is the annual output produced by a person with some education.
- ρ_1 and ρ_3 are the ratios of consumption in youth and retirement, respectively, to consumption in the working ages.
- $s_1(t), s_2(t), s_3(t)$, and $s_e(t)$ are the fractions of the total population who are in life-cycle states 1, 2, and 3, and the fraction who are being educated, respectively.
- There is only one sex in the model.

3. Parameters

Mortality rates are taken from the Coale and Demeny (1983, p. 53) model West female life table, level 23 (life expectancy at birth equals 75 years):

$$\alpha = 0.9, \quad r = 0.5, \quad \bar{Y} = 1, \quad ed\cos t = 0.8, \quad \rho_1 = 0.2, \quad \rho_3 = 0.9,$$
$$\beta = 10, \quad \gamma = 0.5, \quad \phi \text{ is calculated so that } Pollution\,(0) = 1.$$

---

consume, save, invest, and, of course, work. In retirement, people receive income and consume.

The consumption of people in the working ages depends upon a large number of factors, including their incomes as workers and owners of capital, their private savings, government programs that transfer resources to the young and the retired, and private transfers between and within families. Since the young have no income, their consumption depends on private and public transfers to them. Retirees consume out of income from capital, out of their savings, and also from public and private transfers. Generally speaking, consumption at each age depends in a complex way on income flows, government transfer programs, and private transfer payments.

Survival rates and environmental quality are also important components of well-being. In general, these change as a person ages, and they need to be taken into account in each year of life, just as consumption does. Well-being has many facets, and it is not difficult to think of several ways to further increase the dimensions considered. For example, we could add disability status to the determinants of well-being so that we would weight years in which a person was disabled differently from years in which he or she was not. Rather than elaborate the framework any further, we now take these ideas and translate them into simple specific functional forms.

A set of definitions and parameter values for the highly simplified model is given in *Box 10.2*. We do not present an equation-by-equation description of the model, but several areas do require comment. The model is set within the context of a closed economy with no financial assets or physical capital. All investment is in human capital. In the basic story told here, the most important feature of this investment is that it must be made prior to the working ages. In a broad sense, investment in human capital is much like investment in physical capital, because there needs to be a reduction in consumption first to finance the investment, which is followed then by a return that is spread over time.

The complex set of factors that relates incomes to consumption levels is grossly simplified by assuming that, through savings, government programs, and private transfers, the consumption levels in the three life-cycle stages are held in fixed proportions. A more satisfactory specification would involve many equations and would distract us from the business at hand.

Survival rates do not appear explicitly in the model. Instead, they are implicit in the $N(a, a+c, ed)$ terms—the numbers of people who survive to each age—that appear in the welfare indicator. The environmental quality function represents in a very simple way the effects of transitory pollution. Persistent pollution is also important to consider, but it would needlessly complicate the model.[3]

We use our simplified model only with stable populations. In the long run, a stable population is generated whenever age-specific fertility and mortality rates are fixed. In such a situation, the population grows or shrinks at a constant rate and the proportions of the population at each age are fixed. We could use the model to deal with cases of demographic transitions instead of stable populations, but a full description and analysis of such situations would take many more pages than are available.

When we ran the model in *Box 10.2* with the parameters given there, we obtained the results plotted in *Figure 10.1*. Total fertility rates (TFRs) from 0.1 to 6.0 appear on the horizontal axis; the higher the TFR, the higher the rate of population growth. With the mortality rates used here, a TFR of 2.04 is consistent with no population growth. When TFRs are below 2.04, the population shrinks; when they are above 2.04, the population grows. Values of the welfare indicator computed over the entire life cycle appear on the vertical axis.

Three important findings can be seen in *Figure 10.1*. First, the welfare indicators have an inverted U-shape. When TFRs are relatively high, the population grows rapidly and the age structure is weighted heavily toward the young. When

---

[3]For a simple model with persistent pollution, see Sanderson (1994, 1995).

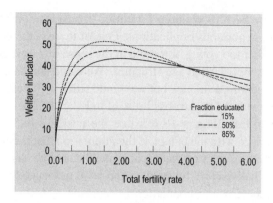

Figure 10.1. Welfare indictor for stable populations by fraction educated and total fertility rate, baseline parameters.

TFRs are well below the replacement level of 2.04 children per woman, the population shrinks and the age structure is weighted heavily toward the old. *Figure 10.1* shows that either extreme is bad for well-being. Some intermediate levels at which the age structure is neither too young nor too old are optimal. The curves have a relatively flat maximum, which means that, especially in the case of low education, it does not seem to make much difference where fertility is within the range from 1.3 to 3.0. However, beyond this range the welfare indicator falls rapidly, particularly on the low fertility side.

Leaving scale factors aside, *Figure 10.1* shows that the concerns about rapid population growth and population aging are really two sides of the same coin. The people who are concerned about rapid population growth and those concerned about population aging are really concerned about the same general phenomenon, an unbalanced age structure. Interest in age-structure effects dates back to the Coale and Hoover (1958) model of the effects of demographic change on economic growth, in which the increased dependency rate caused by rapid population growth was an important feature. With that exception, analysis of age-structure effects played a decidedly minor role in discussions about the effects of demographic change on economic growth until quite recently, when it become the center of attention in explaining the East Asian economic growth miracle (Bloom and Williamson 1998; Bloom *et al.* 2000) and economic growth patterns more generally (Kelley and Schmidt 2001). *Figure 10.1* is consistent with the recent re-emphasis on the importance of age-structure differences.

The human life cycle has natural phases, an early one during which children are educated and consume before they can produce, a productive middle portion, and a phase at the end of the life cycle in which little or nothing is produced. This life cycle is not the artifact of any model. There is no academic discussion about whether people are born as children or adults. Consideration of the human life cycle, by itself, has enormous implications. One of these is the possibility that the age structure is either too young or too old in the sense that welfare is lower than it would be with a more balanced age structure. We could add an enormous amount of complexity to our simple model, but we would still be left with the basic facts of the life cycle and, with them, the possibility of unbalanced age structures.

Another lesson from *Figure 10.1* is that the peaks of the inverted U-shaped welfare curves change with the extent of the population that is educated. The peak in the curve with 85 percent of the population educated occurs at a fertility level that is more than half a child lower than the level associated with peak welfare when only 15 percent of the population is educated. This teaches us that there is an interaction between age structure and education. The mix of lower fertility and higher education may be better for welfare than the combination of higher fertility and lower education. *Figure 10.1* also shows that with higher education, the maximum becomes less flat.

In models that include people's basic life-cycle phases, welfare is highest where there is a balance in the age structure of consumption and production. This balance changes with education. More-educated people are more productive during their working years, but the education costs money that must be spent when the people are young. Hence, with higher education the optimal mix of people of working age and those of school age changes in favor of the workers.

The interaction between the peak of the inverted U-shaped welfare curves and the level of education provides a distinct challenge to the idea that we ought to think of population stabilization as the universal goal for all countries, regardless of their levels of education. No single goal is appropriate for all countries at all times. Some countries could be at the peak of their curves with a growing population, while others could be at their peak with a shrinking population. The only goal that is reasonable for all countries is population balance. In other words, countries should not set zero population growth as their goal, but should instead aim at the rate of growth that is suitable under their particular conditions. These goals will, in general, differ from country to country. *Figure 10.1* shows that, from the point of view of the welfare of people, there is nothing special about zero population growth.

These considerations of population balance have been developed with a view to the real-world challenges of the 21st century. In the very long run, constant fertility below replacement will lead to extinction, in the same way that higher fertility will lead to an inevitable explosion. However, we should not think in terms of eternally constant trends. Real populations will always show fluctuations in their vital rates as well as adjustment to changing conditions. In this sense, the next challenge for population-balance calculations would be to apply them to a number of empirically observed current population structures instead of the stable conditions that underlie *Figure 10.1*.

A final lesson from *Figure 10.1* is derived from the observation that at higher TFRs, the welfare curves cross. At lower TFRs, education increases welfare, but at high enough TFRs, the reverse is true. This pattern is consistent with the broad facts of the demographic transition with which this book began. Earlier in history, before the beginning of the demographic transition, when fertility was high and the age structures were very young, we also see low levels of education. As the demographic transition proceeded, educational levels rose as fertility fell. Now that we come to the end of the volume, we have found possible reasons for these connections.

Our simple model cannot tell the whole story of the interaction between education and fertility. When the education of women rises, fertility tends to fall. Falling fertility makes education more valuable in terms of increasing welfare and so tends to increase education, which then has a further decreasing effect on fertility. For countries still in the process of demographic transition, this real-world virtuous cycle is not captured in our simple model.

The model that we present is by intention extremely simple. Nevertheless, it has important lessons to teach us as we think about demographic issues. We have learned the following:

- Concerns about population growth and population aging are not separate, but are really two aspects of unbalanced age distributions.
- From a welfare point of view, there is nothing special about zero population growth, and countries should set long-term goals appropriate to their particular circumstances.
- Fertility somewhat below replacement does not necessarily mean lower long-range welfare, if it is associated with better education.

10.4   Conclusions

In this book we argue that in the 21st century, population concerns are likely to move away from a focus on high fertility and population growth to concerns about population age structure, regional distribution, and the "quality" dimension (i.e., skills and human resources in a broader sense).

The transition from an older demographic regime characterized mainly by countries that are still in the process of demographic transition and experiencing population growth to another regime characterized by aging and shrinkage is happening gradually, with different parts of the world being at different stages of this secular development. We currently live in a world of mixed demographic regimes and also in a world in which the traditional division into poor countries with populations growing rapidly and rich countries with populations growing slowly is becoming obsolete—just think of China (poor but whose population soon will begin to shrink) and the United States (rich and with continuing population growth). This also has significant implications for the impact of human population trends on global environmental pollution; both population and environmental policies have to be rethought and their interdependence studied. A first step in this direction was recently taken by the Global Science Panel on Population and Environment (Lutz and Shah 2002; Lutz *et al.* 2002b), which identified two policies of empowerment that should have priority under both the old and the new regimes: improving reproductive health and education, especially the education of women.

The new and more complex population realities require new and more complex policies. Population balance provides a framework for thinking about and designing these policies. Only with such a broader policy approach will we be able to address the future challenges posed by population in the context of sustainable development.

References

Adams RM (1990). *The Wellborn Science: Eugenics in Germany, France, Brazil, and Russia.* New York, NY, USA: Oxford University Press.

Birdsall N & Griffin C (1993). *Population Growth, Externalities, and Poverty.* Policy Research Working Paper: Population, Health, and Nutrition, No. WPS 1158. Washington, DC, USA: The World Bank.

Bloom DE & Williamson JG (1998). Demographic transitions and economic miracles in emerging Asia. *The World Bank Economic Review* **12**:419–455.

Bloom DE, Canning D & Maleney P (2000). Population dynamics and economic growth in Asia. In *Population and Change in East Asia*, eds. Chu CY & Lee R, pp. 257–290. A supplement to *Population and Development Review* **26**. New York, NY, USA: The Population Council.

Bok S (1994). Population and ethics: Expanding the moral space. In *Population Policies Reconsidered: Health, Empowerment, and Rights*, eds. Sen G, Germain A & Chen LC, pp. 15–26. Boston, MA, USA: Harvard University Press.

Boserup E (1981). *Population and Technological Change: A Study of Long-Run Trends.* Chicago, IL, USA: University of Chicago Press.

Chomitz KM & Birdsall N (1991). Incentives for small families: Concepts and issues. In *Proceedings of the World Bank Annual Conference on Development Economics 1990*, eds. Fischer S, de Tray D & Shah S, pp. 309–349. Washington, DC, USA: The World Bank.

Coale AJ & Demeny P (1983). *Regional Model Life Tables and Stable Populations*, Second Edition. New York, NY, USA: Academic Press.

Coale AJ & Hoover J (1958). *Population Growth in Low Income Countries.* Princeton, NJ, USA: Princeton University Press.

Cohen J (1995). *How Many People Can the Earth Support?* New York, NY, USA: WW Norton.

Dasgupta PS (1986). The ethical foundations of population policy. In *Population Growth and Economic Development: Issues and Evidence,* eds. Johnson DG & Lee RD, pp. 631–659. Madison, WI, USA: University of Wisconsin Press.

Dasgupta PS (1998). Population, consumption, and resources: Ethical issues. *Ecological Economics* **24**:139–152.

Demeny P (1986). Population and the invisible hand. *Demography* **23**:473–487.

Donaldson PJ (1990). *Nature against Us: The United States and the World Population Crisis, 1965–1980.* Chapel Hill, NC, USA: University of North Carolina Press.

Earth Negotiations Bulletin (1994). *A Summary of the International Conference on Population and Development,* Volume 6, Number 39. New York, NY, USA: International Institute for Sustainable Development.

Harvey PD (1996). Let's not get carried away with "reproductive health." *Studies in Family Planning* **27**:283–284.

Hodgson D (1991). The ideological origins of the Population Association of America. *Population and Development Review* **17**:1–34.

Kelley AC & Schmidt RM (2001). Economic and demographic change: A synthesis of models, findings and perspectives. In *Population Matters—Demographic Change, Economic Growth and Poverty in the Developing World,* eds. Birdsall N, Kelley AC & Sinding S, pp. 67–105. New York, NY, USA: Oxford University Press.

Kühl S (1997). *The Internationalization of Racism: The Rise and Fall of the International Movement for Eugenics and Racial Purity in the 20th Century.* Frankfurt am Main, Germany: Campus-Verlag.

Lutz W & Shah M (2002). Population should be on the Johannesburg agenda. *Nature* **418**:17.

Lutz W, Sanderon W & Wils A (2002a). Conclusions: Toward comprehensive P-E studies. In *Population and Environment: Methods of Analysis,* eds Lutz W, Prskawetz A & Sanderson W, pp. 225–250. New York, NY, USA: The Population Council.

Lutz W, Shah M, Bilsborrow RE, Bongaarts J, Dasgupta P, Entwisle B, Fischer G, Garcia B, Hogan DJ, Jernelöv A, Jiang Z, Kates RW, Lall S, MacKellar FL, Makinwa-Adebusoye PK, McMichael AJ, Mishra V, Myers N, Nakicenovic N, Nilsson S, O'Neill BC, Peng X, PresserHB, Sadik N, Sanderson WC, Sen G, Torrey B, van de Kaa D, van Ginkel HJA, Yeoh B & Zurayk H (2002b). The Global Science Panel on Population in Sustainable Development. *Population and Development Review* **28**:367–369.

Lutz W, O'Neill BC & Scherbov S (2003). Europe's population at a turning point. *Science* **299**:1991–1992.

McIntosh CA & Finkle JL (1995). The Cairo Conference on Population and Development. *Population and Development Review* **21**:223–260.

McNicoll G (1995). On population growth and revisionism: Further questions. *Population and Development Review* **21**:307–340.

O'Neill BC, MacKellar FL & Lutz W (2001). *Population and Climate Change*. Cambridge, UK: Cambridge University Press.

Sanderson WC (1994). Simulation models of demographic, economic, and environmental interactions. In *Population, Development, Environment: Understanding Their Interactions in Mauritius*, ed. Lutz W, pp. 33–71. Berlin, Germany: Springer-Verlag.

Sanderson WC (1995). Predictability, complexity, and catastrophe in a collapsible model of population, development, and environmental interactions. *Mathematical Population Studies* **5**:259–279.

Simon J (1981). *The Ultimate Resource*. Princeton, NJ, USA: Princeton University Press.

Teitelbaum M & Winter J (1985). *The Fear of Population Decline*. Orlando, FL, USA: Academic Press.

United Nations (1997). *World Population Prospects: The 1996 Revision*. New York, NY, USA: United Nations.

United States National Research Council (1986). *Population Growth and Economic Development: Policy Questions*. Washington, DC, USA: National Academy Press.

Westoff C (1995). International population policy. *Society* **32**:11–15.

Wexler L (1996). Improving Population Assumptions in Greenhouse Gas Emissions Models. Working Paper WP-96-99. Laxenburg, Austria: International Institute for Applied Systems Analysis.

Index

About the Editors

Wolfgang Lutz is leader of the Population Project at the International Institute for Applied Systems Analysis (IIASA) and director of the Vienna Institute of Demography of the Austrian Academy of Sciences. He has published widely in the fields of population forecasting and population–environment analysis and is editor of *The Future Population of the World* (1996), co-author of *Population and Climate Change* (2001), and coordinator of the UNU/IUSSP/IIASA Global Science Panel on Population and Environment.

Warren C. Sanderson is a professor in the Departments of Economics and History at the State University of New York at Stony Brook and is co-chair of the Department of Economics there. He has published widely in the field of economic demography and is co-editor of *Population and Environment* (Population Council 2002).

Sergei Scherbov is a senior scientist at the Vienna Institute of Demography of the Austrian Academy of Sciences and a senior research scholar at IIASA. He has published numerous articles in the fields of demographic analysis and population forecasting.